Pulmonary Manifestations of Rheumatic Disease

Guest Editor

KRISTIN B. HIGHLAND, MD, MSCR

CLINICS IN CHEST MEDICINE

www.chestmed.theclinics.com

September 2010 • Volume 31 • Number 3

SAUNDERS an imprint of ELSEVIER, Inc.

W.B. SAUNDERS COMPANY
A Division of Elsevier Inc.

1600 John F. Kennedy Boulevard • Suite 1800 • Philadelphia, Pennsylvania 19103

http://www.theclinics.com

CLINICS IN CHEST MEDICINE Volume 31, Number 3
September 2010 ISSN 0272-5231, ISBN-13: 978-1-4377-2434-9

Editor: Sarah E. Barth
Developmental Editor: Jessica Demetriou

Clinics in Chest Medicine (ISSN 0272-5231) is published quarterly by Elsevier Inc., 360 Park Avenue South, New York, NY 10010-1710. Months of issue are March, June, September, and December. Periodicals postage paid at New York, NY and additional mailing offices. Subscription prices are $274.00 per year (domestic individuals), $432.00 per year (domestic institutions), $133.00 per year (domestic students/residents), $300.00 per year (Canadian individuals), $530.00 per year (Canadian institutions), $373.00 per year (international individuals), $530.00 per year (international institutions), and $186.00 per year (international and Canadian students/residents). International air speed delivery is included in all Clinics subscription prices. All prices are subject to change without notice. **POSTMASTER:** Send address changes to Clinics in Chest Medicine, Elsevier Health Sciences Division, Subscription Customer Service, 3251 Riverport Lane, Maryland Heights, MO 63043. **Customer Service: Telephone: 1-800-654-2452** (U.S. and Canada); **1-314-447-8871** (outside U.S. and Canada). **Fax: 1-314-447-8029. E-mail: journalscustomerservice-usa@elsevier.com** (for print support); **journalsonlinesupport-usa@elsevier.com** (for online support).

Reprints. For copies of 100 or more of articles in this publication, please contact the Commercial Reprints Department, Elsevier Inc., 360 Park Avenue South, New York, NY 10010-1710. Tel.: 212-633-3812; Fax: 212-462-1935; E-mail: reprints@elsevier.com.

Clinics in Chest Medicine is covered in *MEDLINE/PubMed (Index Medicus), Current Contents/Clinical Medicine, EMBASE/ Excerpta Medica, Science Citation Index,* and *ISI/BIOMED.*

Printed and bound by CPI Group (UK) Ltd, Croydon, CR0 4YY

Transferred to Digital Print 2011

Contributors

GUEST EDITOR

KRISTIN B. HIGHLAND, MD, MSCR
Associate Professor of Medicine, Divisions of
Pulmonary, Critical Care, Allergy and Sleep
Medicine and Rheumatology and Immunology,
Medical University of South Carolina,
Charleston, South Carolina

AUTHORS

VIVEK N. AHYA, MD
Medical Director, Lung Transplantation
Program, Assistant Professor of Medicine,
Division of Pulmonary, Allergy, and Critical
Care Medicine, University of Pennsylvania
School of Medicine, Philadelphia,
Pennsylvania

DANIELLE ANTIN-OZERKIS, MD
Assistant Professor of Medicine, Director, Yale
Interstitial Lung Disease Program, Internal
Medicine–Pulmonary and Critical Care
Division, Yale University School of Medicine,
New Haven, Connecticut

ROBERT BAUGHMAN, MD, FACP, FCCP
Professor of Medicine, Interstitial Lung Disease
and Sarcoidosis Clinic, University of Cincinnati
Medical Center, Cincinnati, Ohio

MARCY B. BOLSTER, MD
Medical Director, MUSC Center for
Osteoporosis and Bone Health, Professor of
Medicine, Division of Rheumatology and
Immunology, Medical University of South
Carolina, Charleston, South Carolina

ELZBIETA CHYCZEWSKA, MD
Professor, Department of Lung Diseases and
Tuberculosis, Medical University of Bialystok,
Bialystok, Poland

CATHERINE DECKER, PharmD, AE-C
Senior Clinical Pharmacist and Instructor,
Department of Pharmacy, University of
Wisconsin Hospital and Clinics, University of
Wisconsin School of Pharmacy, Adult
Pulmonary Clinic, Madison, Wisconsin

ARMIN ERNST, MD
Chief, Division of Interventional Pulmonary,
Beth Israel Deaconess Medical Center;
Associate Professor of Medicine and Surgery,
Harvard Medical School, Boston,
Massachusetts

JANINE EVANS, MD
Associate Professor of Medicine, Internal
Medicine–Rheumatology Division, Yale
University School of Medicine, New Haven,
Connecticut

H. JAMES FORD, MD
Assistant Professor of Medicine, Division of
Pulmonary and Critical Care Medicine,
University of North Carolina at Chapel Hill,
Chapel Hill, North Carolina

STEPHEN K. FRANKEL, MD
Chief, Division of Critical Care and Hospital
Medicine, National Jewish Health, Denver;
Associate Professor of Medicine, National
Jewish Health, University of Colorado Denver
School of Medicine, Aurora, Colorado

FAYE N. HANT, DO, MSCR
Assistant Professor of Medicine, Division of
Rheumatology and Immunology, Medical
University of South Carolina, Charleston,
South Carolina

LAURA B. HERPEL, MD
Assistant Professor of Medicine, Division of
Pulmonary, Critical Care, Allergy and Sleep
Medicine, Medical University of South
Carolina, Charleston, South Carolina

KRISTIN B. HIGHLAND, MD, MSCR
Associate Professor of Medicine, Divisions of
Pulmonary, Critical Care, Allergy and Sleep
Medicine and Rheumatology and Immunology,
Medical University of South Carolina,
Charleston, South Carolina

ROBERT J. HOMER, MD, PhD
Professor of Pathology and Internal Medicine
(Pulmonary), Yale University School of
Medicine, New Haven, Connecticut

DAVID JAYNE, MBBchir, MD
Director, Vasculitis and Lupus Clinic, Consultant
Nephrologist, Addenbrooke's Hospital,
University of Cambridge, Cambridge, UK

MEENA KALLURI, MD
Assistant Professor of Medicine, Division of
Pulmonary Medicine, University of Alberta,
Edmonton, Canada

DIANE L. KAMEN, MD, MSCR
Assistant Professor of Medicine, Division of
Rheumatology and Immunology, Medical
University of South Carolina, Charleston,
South Carolina

NAVEEN KANATHUR, MD
Department of Medicine, National Jewish
Health, Denver, Colorado

MARIA KOKOSI, MD
Senior Fellow, 3rd Pulmonary Department,
Sismanoglio General Hospital, Marousi,
Athens, Greece

KRZYSZTOF KOWAL, MD
Associate Professor, Department of
Allergology and Internal Medicine, Medical
University of Bialystok, Bialystok, Poland

OTYLIA KOWAL-BIELECKA, MD
Associate Professor, Department of
Rheumatology and Internal Medicine, Medical
University of Bialystok, Bialystok, Poland

JAMES C. LEE, MD
Assistant Professor of Medicine, Lung
Transplantation Program, Division of
Pulmonary, Allergy, and Critical Care Medicine,
University of Pennsylvania School of Medicine,
Philadelphia, Pennsylvania

TEOFILO LEE-CHIONG, MD
Department of Medicine, National Jewish
Health, Denver, Colorado

RICHARD A. MATTHAY, MD
Professor of Medicine, Internal
Medicine–Pulmonary and Critical Care
Division, Yale University School
of Medicine, New Haven, Connecticut

KEITH C. MEYER, MD, MS, FACP, FCCP
Professor of Medicine, Medical Director of
Lung Transplantation, Section of Allergy,
Pulmonary and Critical Care Medicine,
University of Wisconsin School of Medicine
and Public Health, Madison, Wisconsin

CHESTER V. ODDIS, MD
Professor of Medicine, Division of
Rheumatology and Clinical Immunology,
University of Pittsburgh, Pennsylvania

SAMAAN RAFEQ, MD
Division of Interventional Pulmonary, Beth
Israel Deaconess Medical Center, Boston,
Massachusetts

ELLEN C. RIEMER, MD, JD
Assistant Professor of Pathology and Director
of Pulmonary Pathology, Department of
Pathology and Laboratory Medicine, Medical
University of South Carolina, Charleston,
South Carolina

ROBERT A.S. ROUBEY, MD
Associate Professor of Medicine, Division of Rheumatology, Allergy and Immunology, and Thurston Arthritis Research Center, University of North Carolina at Chapel Hill, Chapel Hill, North Carolina

AMI RUBINOWITZ, MD
Associate Professor of Diagnostic Radiology, Department of Diagnostic Imaging, Yale University School of Medicine, New Haven, Connecticut

SALLY E. SELF, MD
Professor of Pathology and Laboratory Medicine, Department of Pathology and Laboratory Medicine, Medical University of South Carolina, Charleston, South Carolina

RICHARD M. SILVER, MD
Distinguished University Professor, Division Director, Division of Rheumatology and Immunology, Medical University of South Carolina, Charleston, South Carolina

CHARLIE STRANGE, MD
Professor of Medicine, Division of Pulmonary and Critical Care Medicine, Medical University of South Carolina, Charleston, South Carolina

DAVID TRENTHAM, MD
Division of Rheumatology, Beth Israel Deaconess Medical Center, Boston, Massachusetts

Contents

The proper use and interpretation of serologic testing for diagnosing autoimmune diseases presents a challenge to clinicians for several reasons. Most laboratory tests for autoimmune disease are significantly less than 100% sensitive or specific. In addition, different techniques for the same antibody test may give different results, such as indirect immunofluorescence and multiplex bead assay for antinuclear antibody. Autoantibody testing should only be performed in the context of the clinical workup of patients who have a reasonable likelihood of having the disease for which the testing is relevant. Otherwise, the predictive value of a positive test is too low. Particularly with antinuclear antibody and antineutrophil cytoplasmic antibody testing, clinicians must know the methodology through which the tests are being performed, and should develop a relationship with the laboratory pathologist so that inconsistent or surprising results can be investigated.

Pulmonary involvement is common in patients with connective tissue diseases (CTDs), and significantly contributes to morbidity and mortality in this patient population. There are different forms of lung pathology in CTDs, which include primary involvement such as interstitial lung disease or pulmonary hemorrhage, and pulmonary complications resulting from other CTD-related organ involvement including aspiration pneumonia due to muscle weakness or esophageal fibrosis. Moreover, iatrogenic lung disease, such as medication-induced hypersensitivity pneumonitis or opportunistic infections due to immunosuppression, may develop. Appropriate treatment of pulmonary complications in patients with CTDs requires careful diagnostic workup because different forms of lung involvement may overlap, causing similar clinical manifestations and similar radiological or functional impairment. Moreover, in view of the broad variability of clinical course of CTD-related interstitial lung disease, identification of biomarkers helpful in predicting prognosis becomes of key importance. In addition to radiological assessment and functional testing that provide information regarding localization and severity of lung disease, bronchoalveolar lavage (BAL) appears helpful in revealing the nature of lung pathology and intensity of lung inflammation through sampling of cells and fluid from the lower respiratory tract. The aim of this article is to critically review available data concerning the evaluation of BAL cytology in different forms of lung disease associated with CTDs.

Pulmonary manifestations are common in connective tissue diseases, and are associated with significant morbidity and mortality in this patient population. Systemic sclerosis (SSc) and mixed connective tissue disease (MCTD) are clinical entities for which the detection of lung involvement is essential to improve patient care and outcomes. This article discusses the pathogenesis, clinical presentation, and evaluation of the patient with pulmonary disease related to SSc and MCTD, with an emphasis on interstitial lung disease and pulmonary hypertension.

Pulmonary disease is a major source of morbidity and mortality in rheumatoid arthritis, manifesting most commonly as interstitial lung disease, airways disease, rheumatoid nodules, and pleural effusions. The diagnostic assessment of respiratory abnormalities is complicated by underlying risk for infection, the use of drugs with known pulmonary toxicity, and the frequency of lung disease related to rheumatoid arthritis itself. Evaluation and management of rheumatoid arthritis-associated pulmonary disease frequently necessitates a multidisciplinary approach.

Systemic lupus erythematosus (SLE) is a potentially severe, frequently disabling autoimmune disease with multiorgan involvement and a typically waxing and waning course. SLE is often considered the prototypical autoimmune disease. Although SLE has the potential to affect any organ, the lungs are commonly involved later in the course of the disease in the setting of other organ involvement. Pulmonary disease may complicate SLE and is an important cause of morbidity and mortality. The most common pulmonary manifestation attributable to SLE is pleuritis, but other pleural involvement can be seen, as well as parenchymal disease, pulmonary vascular disease, diaphragmatic dysfunction, and upper airway dysfunction. Finding the true prevalence of lung involvement with SLE is complicated by the high rates of pulmonary infections. This article reviews the diverse clinical symptoms and immunologic pulmonary manifestations of SLE.

Sjögren syndrome is a slowly progressing autoimmune disease. Pulmonary manifestations are frequent in primary Sjögren syndrome but often not clinically significant; the most common are xerotrachea, interstitial lung diseases, and small airway obstruction. Pulmonary manifestations in Sjögren syndrome have a slow progression and favorable prognosis, with the exception of primary pulmonary lymphoma and pulmonary hypertension.

Pulmonary involvement in myositis includes interstitial lung disease (ILD), respiratory muscle weakness, aspiration, infections, and drug-induced disease. ILD may precede myositis, and results in increased morbidity and mortality rates. Initial evaluation should include pulmonary function tests and high-resolution computed tomography. Nonspecific interstitial pneumonia (NSIP) is the most common histologic pattern on lung biopsy. Treatment usually consists of a combination of steroids and other immunosuppressive agents, and the response depends on the clinical presentation and underlying histology.

Osteoporosis is a common systemic disease whose presentation crosses many specialties in medicine. Low bone mass, (osteopenia) and osteoporosis increases a patient's risk of suffering from a fracture, and fragility fractures are known to have a significant effect on morbidity and mortality, with up to a 1-year 20% mortality risk. Early detection of osteoporosis is essential to reduce a patient's risk of fracture. Several diseases are associated with an increased risk of osteoporosis because of the medications used to treat these diseases, including but not limited to the prescribing of glucocorticoids. It is important to recognize which patients warrant therapy for bone health and to implement medical management as appropriate.

Systemic autoimmune diseases may be progressive and lead to organ system dysfunction and premature death. Current treatment paradigms are usually predominantly based on the administration of immunosuppressive and/or immunomodulatory drug therapy. Such therapy can stabilize systemic manifestations of connective tissue disease (CTD) and may put the disease into remission, and many of these agents are commonly used to treat CTD-associated interstitial lung disease (ILD). Although these agents have largely revolutionized the treatment of the systemic autoimmune diseases, adverse reactions, which can be serious and life threatening, to the various immunosuppressive agents used in the treatment of CTD can occur. Treating physicians must be aware of mechanisms of action of various immunosuppressive agents and be able to recognize the potential adverse reactions that may occur with therapy as well as potentially harmful effects on fetal development. Appropriate monitoring may prevent or limit toxicity from these agents, and knowledge of drug-drug interactions is essential when these agents are prescribed.

In the last 45 years, lung transplantation has evolved from its status as a rare extreme form of surgical therapy for the treatment of advanced lung diseases to an accepted therapeutic option for select patients. Although pulmonary fibrosis and pulmonary vascular diseases are important indications for lung transplantation, only a small percentage of transplants are performed in patients with collagen vascular diseases. The reasons for this low number are multifactorial. This article reviews issues relevant to all lung transplant candidates and recipients as well as those specific to patients with autoimmune diseases.

Clinics in Chest Medicine

THE CLINICS ARE NOW AVAILABLE ONLINE!

Access your subscription at:
www.theclinics.com

Preface

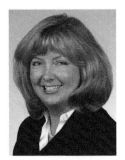

Kristin B. Highland, MD, MSCR
Guest Editor

At the Medical University of South Carolina, the pulmonary and rheumatology divisions share clinic space (and a conference table). As a result, our rheumatology fellows are well versed in interpreting pulmonary function testing and our pulmonary fellows routinely inject everyone's knees before their 6-minute walk! Kidding aside, a close collaboration between these 2 disciplines is paramount in taking care of the complex patient with rheumatic lung disease.

It has been 13 years since *Clinics in Chest Medicine* devoted an issue to the pulmonary complications of the connective tissue diseases. During this last decade, methods used to detect auto-antibodies have become increasingly sensitive, leaving the physician to wonder if she is dealing with an autoimmune disease confined to the lungs (autoimmune lung disease) versus a "false positive." Bronchoscopy for the diagnosis of alveolitis has fallen in and out of favor, but still remains an important research tool and is useful for exclusion of infection and/or alveolar hemorrhage. This decade has brought about new insights into the pathogenesis of the rheumatic diseases and their phenotypic expression. It has been an amazing time for the development of medications for the treatment of rheumatoid arthritis and the inflammatory arthropathies. At last, there was a positive randomized-placebo-controlled trial in scleroderma, a disease that has been notorious for being refractory to all therapy. We now also have more tools in our arsenal to treat the other connective tissue diseases and the vasculitides. Consequently, there is a heightened awareness of the potential pulmonary and nonpulmonary toxicity of these medications. There is also a greater

concern for the long-term complications of chronic glucocorticoid therapy. New interventional rigid and flexible bronchoscopic techniques have also resulted in advances in the treatment of difficult inflammatory airway lesions that are common in patients with relapsing polychondritis and some of the other rheumatic diseases. When all else fails, more and more rheumatic lung disease patients are being considered for lung transplantation.

This issue has an impressive lineup of both pulmonologists and rheumatologists with expertise in rheumatic lung disease. Furthermore, in this issue many of the articles are written in close collaboration between these 2 disciplines, allowing capture of both perspectives.

In addition to thanking the brilliant physicians that have contributed to this article and Sarah Barth who is a very patient and kind publisher, I would like to thank my colleagues that frequently sit around that conference table. In particular, my pulmonary (Charlie Strange) and rheumatology (Richard Silver) mentors, both of whom have fostered me during my career as a pulmo-rheumatologist. Or is it a rheumo-pulmonologist?

Kristin B. Highland, MD, MSCR
Divisions of Pulmonary, Critical Care
Allergy and Sleep Medicine and Rheumatology
and Immunology
Medical University of South Carolina
96 Johnathan Lucas Street, Suite 812 CSB
Charleston, SC 29425, USA

E-mail address:
highlakb@musc.edu

chestmed.theclinics.com

Autoantibody Testing for Autoimmune Disease

Sally E. Self, MD

KEYWORDS

• Autoantibody • Autoimmune • Serology • Rheumatic

GENERAL REMARKS

The proper use and interpretation of serologic testing for diagnosing autoimmune diseases presents a challenge to clinicians for several reasons. Most laboratory tests for autoimmune disease are significantly less than 100% sensitive or specific. In addition, different techniques for the same antibody test may give different results, such as indirect immunofluorescence and multiplex bead assay for antinuclear antibody (ANA). This problem was recently highlighted in a recent *New England Journal of Medicine* case record in which a diagnosis of systemic lupus erythematosus was confounded by a false-negative ANA using one method.[1]

Another challenge is considerable interlaboratory variability in quantitative indirect fluorescence titers. Although attempts have been made at standardization, indirect immunofluorescence, used in testing for ANAs and antineutrophil cytoplasmic antibodies (ANCAs), remains subjective, and titers will vary enormously among laboratories. It is not uncommon for College of American Pathologists proficiency surveys show ANA titers varying from 1:32 to greater than 1:5120 on the same specimen.

The biology of autoantibodies is an added problem. Low titers of autoantibodies are not uncommon in healthy individuals. The incidence and titer of autoantibodies in healthy individuals increase with age.[2] Overlap also occurs in disease specificity among different autoantibodies. Autoantibody testing should be performed selectively and only when historical and clinical findings support the diagnosis of an autoimmune disease.

Therefore, this article discusses autoantibody testing in the context of the specific autoimmune disease.

SYSTEMIC LUPUS ERYTHEMATOSUS

Testing for ANAs is the screening test for patients in whom systemic lupus erythematosus is suspected. It has a sensitivity of greater than 95%.[3] ANA testing can be performed using three major methods: indirect immunofluorescence, enzyme immunoassay (EIA), and multiplex bead flow cytometry. Indirect immunofluorescence on Hep-2 cells is the standard methodology and has the advantages of including all the nuclear antigens in the substrate and providing a pattern. The specificity will vary according to the screening titer used, with a reported false-positive rate of 32% when a 1:40 titer is used.[2] Higher screening titers result in a higher specificity at the cost of sensitivity.

Ideally, the screening titer should be determined by each laboratory based on the patient population and desired performance characteristics. However, this is not always practical. Indirect immunofluorescence is subjective and labor-intensive. The titers reported vary considerably among laboratories because of the subjectivity. EIAs and multiplex bead assays are more objective, much less labor-intensive, and more suitable for large-volume testing. For these reasons, many of the large referral laboratories have embraced these technologies.

The major disadvantage of these techniques is that they may not be able to detect all of the

Department of Pathology and Laboratory Medicine, Medical University of South Carolina, 165 Ashley Avenue, Suite 309, Charleston, SC 29425, USA
E-mail address: selfs@musc.edu

Clin Chest Med 31 (2010) 415–422
doi:10.1016/j.ccm.2010.04.001

antigens detectable with indirect immunofluorescence. Although the American College of Rheumatologists issued a position statement in February 2009 stating that ANA detected with indirect immunofluorescence is the gold standard, lively debate over this issue exists among laboratory directors.[4] Clinicians must be aware of which test is being performed when they order an ANA; what the weaknesses are of that technique; and when it is worthwhile to order an alternate technology.

The patterns seen when an ANA is performed using indirect immunofluorescence can provide information about the antigens involved.[5] The homogeneous pattern is associated with antibodies against double-stranded DNA (dsDNA) and histones, and is the most specific pattern for lupus and drug-induced lupus. The speckled pattern is the most common pattern, but the least specific. Many different antigens will result in a speckled pattern, including SS-A/Ro, SS-B/La, U1 ribonucleoprotein (RNP), and Sm. The nucleolar pattern is most often seen in association with scleroderma, whereas the centromere pattern is seen in the limited cutaneous or CREST (calcinosis, Raynaud's syndrome, esophageal immobility, sclerodactyly, and telangiectasia) variant of scleroderma (**Fig. 1**). The ANA patterns may be poorly reproducible, and more than one pattern

may exist in a sample. Therefore, testing for antibody to specific lupus-associated antigens is generally indicated after a positive ANA, and is performed simultaneously with some of the more automated assays, such as the multiplex bead assays.

More than 50 different autoantibody specificities have been reported in sera from patients with systemic lupus erythematosus, and on average a patient with lupus will have three different autoantibodies.[6] Anti-native or anti-dsDNA and anti-Sm (Smith) are usually measured with enzyme immunoassays or multiplex bead assays. Both anti-dsDNA and anti-Sm are fairly specific for systemic lupus erythematosus, but only occur in 70% and 25% to 50% of cases, respectively. Both are associated with lupus renal disease. The titer of anti-dsDNA tends to correlate with activity of disease.[6] Antibodies to histone are correlated with drug-induced lupus.

Other autoantibodies seen in lupus include, among others, those directed against single-stranded DNA, nuclear RNP, SSA/Ro, SSA/La, Ku, Ki, proliferating cell nuclear antigen (PCNA), ribosomal RNP, and Hsp90 (heat shock protein). The Sm and nRNP antigens are closely associated. Although the Sm antigen can be isolated, the nRNP antigen will usually have contaminating Sm antigen. Some assays then report anti-Sm/RNP

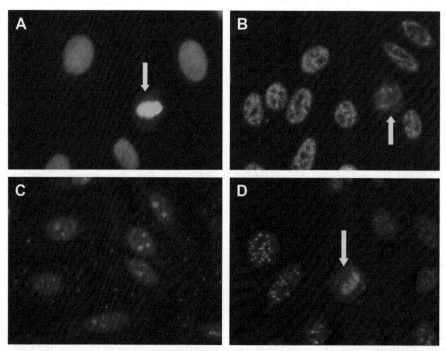

Fig. 1. ANA patterns detected using indirect immunofluorescence. (*A*) Homogeneous pattern. Note that the metaphase plate (*arrow*) is positive. (*B*) Speckled pattern. The metaphase plate in the speckled pattern is negative (*arrow*). (*C*) Nucleolar pattern. (*D*) An example of the centromere pattern. The centromeres line up along the metaphase plate (*arrow*).

for this reason. Anti-Ku antibodies are seen in 23% of patients with idiopathic pulmonary arterial hypertension (primary pulmonary hypertension).[7] Anti-Ki is seen in approximately 10% of patients with lupus and is also associated with pulmonary hypertension.[6] A summary of autoantibody specificities in lupus is presented in **Table 1**.

The traditional way to test for these antibodies is to perform an ANA screen using indirect immunofluorescence, and then if positive, to follow-up with testing for antibodies to dsDNA and extractable nuclear antigens. The extractable nuclear antigen panel usually includes tests for antibodies to Sm, Sm/RNP, SSA(Ro), SSB(La), and Scl-70. Elevated titers of antibody to dsDNA have been associated with increased disease activity, as have decreased concentration of serum complement C'3 and C'4.[6]

Antiphospholipid antibodies (APAs) are seen in approximately one-third of patients with lupus and can be tested for in several ways.[8] The antibodies to cardiolipin result in a false-positive test for syphilis when using cardiolipin-based assays (eg, rapid plasma reagin and venereal disease research laboratory tests). The lupus anticoagulant (which in vivo functions as a procoagulant) is measured through the prolongation of the partial thromboplastin time, which can be overcome by adding excess phospholipid.

The dilute Russell viper venom test can also be used to test for a lupus anticoagulant. Enzyme immunoassays for APA are also available. Included in these are tests for antibodies to phospholipid-binding proteins, which may be the real target for APAs. The most notable of these is β_2-glycoprotein 1.

Table 1
Selected autoantibodies in SLE

Antigen	Nature	Prevalence in SLE	Associations
Hep-2 cell nuclei	ANA	>95%	Numerous autoimmune diseases
dsDNA	Native, double-stranded DNA	40%–60%	High specificity for lupus, titers correlate with disease activity
Histones		50%–70%	Drug-induced lupus
Sm	Small nuclear RNAs complexed with protein	20%–30%	High specificity for lupus
Nuclear RNP (U1RNP)	Small nuclear RNAs complexed with protein	30%–40%	MCTD
SS-A(Ro)	Protein associated with RNA	30%–50%	Sjögren syndrome, subacute cutaneous lupus, neonatal lupus with heart block, SLE with interstitial pneumonia
SS-B(La)	Protein bound to small RNA	10%–15%	Sjögren syndrome
Ku	DNA binding proteins	10%–39%	MCTD, scleroderma, primary pulmonary hypertension
Ki	Nuclear protein	8%–31%	Arthritis, pericarditis, and pulmonary hypertension in patients with SLE
PCNA/cyclin	Cell cycle protein	3%	
Hsp90	Heat shock protein	50%	Polymyositis
P ribosomal protein, rRNP	Ribosomal phosphoprotein	10%	Neuropsychiatric SLE
ssDNA	Single-stranded DNA	70%	
β_2-glycoprotein 1	Anionic proteins, cardiolipin	25%	Lupus anticoagulant, arterial and venous thromboses, neurologic disease

Abbreviations: MCTD, mixed connective tissue disease; SLE, systemic lupus erythematosus; ssDNA, single-stranded DNA.

SYSTEMIC SCLEROSIS OR SCLERODERMA

Autoantibodies are seen in approximately 95% of patients with scleroderma and more than 30 specificities have been described. Most of these can be detected with a screening ANA using indirect immunofluorescence. The antigen specificity may be detected with enzyme immunoassay or multiplexed bead assay. The antigen specificities have been shown in some studies to correlate with pulmonary involvement, either interstitial fibrosis, pulmonary hypertension, or both.[9,10]

The nucleolar pattern according to immunofluorescence is relatively specific for systemic sclerosis, but is not seen in all cases. Target antigens giving the nucleolar pattern include anti-PM-Scl, antifibrillarin/anti-U3-ribonucleoprotein (anti-U3-RNP), anti-Th/To, and the anti-RNA-polymerases (variously called anti-RNAP or Pol 1-3). Of the latter, the Pol 3 antibody is more often seen in scleroderma. The centromere pattern can also be seen through indirect immunofluorescence. The antigen is CENP-B, which is associated with the CREST syndrome. CREST designation may not be as useful clinically as once thought, and currently systemic sclerosis is divided between limited cutaneous systemic sclerosis and diffuse cutaneous systemic sclerosis. Anticentromere antibodies are seen in more than 50% of limited cutaneous systemic sclerosis, and seldom in diffuse cutaneous systemic sclerosis. Anti-Scl-70, an antibody against topoisomerase 1, gives a speckled pattern on ANA indirect immunofluorescence.

Recently, anti–platelet derived growth factor receptor antibodies were described in systemic sclerosis.[11] Although intriguing from a pathogenic viewpoint, the testing for these antibodies was based on a functional assay and not generally available. The clinical significance of the presence of these antibodies to organ involvement and prognosis has not been determined.

A large series by Steen[10] related the antigen specificity to the development of lung disease, either pulmonary hypertension, interstitial fibrosis, or both. Patients who had anticentromere antibodies had a low incidence of pulmonary fibrosis but were likely to develop pulmonary hypertension late in their illness, with more than half of those who die from scleroderma-related illness dying of pulmonary hypertension. Patients with anti-Th/To develop pulmonary hypertension and interstitial fibrosis. Patients with antibodies to U3-RNP tend to be black and have severe lung disease with both pulmonary hypertension and interstitial fibrosis. Patients with antibody to topoisomerase (Scl-70) tend to have interstitial fibrosis without pulmonary hypertension. Patients with anti-Pol 3 have a low incidence of pulmonary fibrosis. An association does not seem to be present between titer of any to the autoantibodies and disease severity, nor does there seem to be any use for monitoring the autoantibodies over time. **Table 2** summarizes the autoantibodies seen in scleroderma. Several autoantibodies are associated with polymyositis/scleroderma overlap syndrome, including anti-PM-Scl, anti-U1-RNP, and anti-Ku.

POLYMYOSITIS/DERMATOMYOSITIS

Approximately one-third of patients with polymyositis and dermatomyositis will have interstitial lung disease.[12] Of patients with polymyositis or dermatomyositis, between 60% and 90% will have a positive ANA. The patterns vary according to the antigen specificity. Anti-PM-Scl will give a nucleolar pattern, whereas antibodies to Jo-1, PL-12, and Ku will give a speckled pattern.

The myositis-specific antibodies occur in 25% to 40% of patients with myositis. They can be divided into three groups: anti-tRNA synthetases (anti-Jo-1, anti-PL-7, anti-PL-12, and anti-OJ), anti-signal recognition particle (anti-SRP), and anti-Mi-2, a cytoplasmic antigen. Myositis-associated antibodies include anti-PM-Scl, anti-U1RNP, anti-U2RNP, and anti-Ku. Anti-SSA, anti-SSB, and anti-Sm antibodies may also be present. Antibodies to Jo-1 and SS-A(Ro) are significantly associated with interstitial lung disease.[12] **Table 3** summarizes the polymyositis/dermatomyositis-associated antibodies.

RHEUMATOID ARTHRITIS

The mainstays of the serologic testing for rheumatoid arthritis are rheumatoid factor and antibodies to cyclic citrullinated peptide (anti-CCP). As with other serologic tests for autoimmune disease, neither is entirely sensitive or specific.

Rheumatoid factor is an antibody (usually an IgM isotype, although IgG and IgA rheumatoid factor do occur) to the Fc portion of the IgG antibody. It can be measured using several techniques: latex agglutination, enzyme immunoassay, or nephelometry. Rheumatoid factor may be positive in several other conditions, including chronic bacterial infections, viral infection (eg, hepatitis C), hematologic diseases, and chronic inflammatory diseases of uncertain origin. The incidence of rheumatoid factor in healthy individuals increases with age.[13]

Anti-CCP is measured using enzyme immunoassay. Antibody testing for CCP was developed

Table 2
Selected autoantibodies in systemic sclerosis (scleroderma)

Antigen	Nature	Prevalence in Scleroderma	Associations
Hep-2 cell nuclei	Classic ANA	70%–90%	Numerous autoimmune diseases
Scl-70	DNA topoisomerase 1	70% Diffuse 13% Limited	High incidence of pulmonary fibrosis
Centromere	Centromere proteins	8% Diffuse 57%–82% Limited	Rare pulmonary fibrosis, but high incidence of pulmonary hypertension
Th/To	Protein complexed with 7S and 8S RNA	1%–11% Diffuse 8%–19% Limited	Pulmonary fibrosis and pulmonary hypertension
U1-RNP	Spliceosome complex	2%–5%	Pulmonary hypertension
U3-RNP	Fibrillarin	5% Diffuse 10% Limited	Pulmonary fibrosis and pulmonary hypertension, may be missed on non-IIF ANAs
Pol-1, Pol-2, Pol-3	RNA polymerases	23%	Pol-3 associated with low incidence of pulmonary fibrosis

Data from Kumar V, Abbas AK, Fausto N, et al. Diseases of the immune system. In: Robbins and Cotran pathologic basis of disease. 8th edition. Philadelphia: Saunders Elsevier; 2010. p. 215; von Mühlen CA, Nakamura RM. Clinical and laboratory evaluation of systemic rheumatic diseases. In: McPherson RA, Pincus MR, editors. Henry's clinical diagnosis and management by laboratory methods. 21st edition. Philadelphia: Saunders Elsevier; 2007. p. 916–44; and Nakamura RM, Tan EM. Steen VD. Autoantibodies in systemic sclerosis. Semin Arth Rheum 2006;35(1):35–42.

from the observation that patients with rheumatoid arthritis had antibodies against filaggrin derived from human skin.[14] The target antigen in filaggrin was found to be citrulline, a modified arginine residue. The posttranslational conversion of arginine to citrulline is accomplished by the enzyme peptidylarginine deiminase (PAD).[15,16] PAD normally occurs in an inactive intracellular form. PAD may leak out of apoptotic cells in the synovium of patients with rheumatoid arthritis and become activated, causing citrullination of extracellular arginine. Anti-CCP antibodies seem to be more specific for rheumatoid arthritis than rheumatoid factors (**Table 4**).

The higher the titer of rheumatoid factor, the more specific it is. Monitoring titers of rheumatoid factor or anti-CCP antibodies generally has little value for indicating activity of disease. General markers of inflammation (acute-phase reactants)—thrombocytosis, the erythrocyte sedimentation rate, and antibodies to C-reactive protein—can indicate disease activity.

SJÖGREN SYNDROME

Antinuclear antibodies are seen in 50% to 80% of patients with Sjögren syndrome. Autoantibodies to SS-A/Ro are seen in greater than 60% to 95% of patients with Sjögren syndrome, and antibodies to SS-B/La are seen in 40% to 90%. The importance of these antibodies is attested by their inclusion as one of six criteria in the Revised International Criteria for Sjögren syndrome.[17] These antibodies are generally measured with enzyme immunoassay, but they are included in some of the multiplex bead assays.

Development of lymphoma occurs in up to 5% of patients with Sjögren syndrome. The development of lymphoma has been associated with low levels of complement C'4 and the presence of type II (mixed) cryoglobulins.[17]

MIXED CONNECTIVE TISSUE DISEASE

Mixed connective tissue disease (alternatively called *undifferentiated autoimmune rheumatic/connective tissue disorder*) is characterized by high titers of anti-RNP. Mixed connective tissue disease is characterized by combined features of systemic lupus erythematosus, scleroderma, and polymyositis. Anti-RNP antibodies are usually measured with enzyme immunoassay or multiplex bead assay. Anti-RNP antibodies may be seen in other autoimmune diseases, such as systemic lupus, rheumatoid arthritis, and systemic sclerosis.

Table 3
Autoantibodies in PM/D

Antigen	Nature	Prevalence in PM/D	Associations
Hep-2 nuclei	Anti-ANA	40%–50%	
Jo-1	tRNA synthetase	20%	High incidence of interstitial lung disease
EJ, OJ, PL-7, PL-12	tRNA synthetases	2%–3%	
Mi-2	Nuclear protein	15%–35% polymyositis 5%–9% dermatomyositis	
SRP	Signal recognition protein	5% polymyositis 0% dermatomyositis	
PM-Scl	Nucleolar protein complex	8% polymyositis 25% polymyositis/ scleroderma overlap	
U1nRNP	Spliceosome complex	4%–17%	
SS-A(Ro)	Protein associated with RNA	16%	Interstitial lung disease
Ku	DNA binding protein	1%	Dermatomyositis with overlap of Sjögren syndrome or SLE and pulmonary hypertension

Abbreviations: PM/D, polymyositis and dermatomyositis; SLE, systemic lupus erythematosus; SRP, signal recognition protein.

Data from von Mühlen CA, Nakamura RM. Clinical and laboratory evaluation of systemic rheumatic diseases. In: McPherson RA, Pincus MR, editors. Henry's clinical diagnosis and management by laboratory methods. 21st edition. Philadelphia: Saunders Elsevier; 2007. p. 916–44; Schnabel A, Reuter M, Biederer J. Interstitial lung disease in polymyositis and dermatomyositis: clinical course and response to treatment. Semin Arth Rheum 2003;32(5):273–84; Hang L, Nakamura RM. Autoimmune diseases of muscle: myasthenia gravis and autoimmune myositis. In: Nakamura RM, Keren DF, Bylund DJ, editors. Clinical and laboratory evaluation of human autoimmune diseases. Chicago: ASCP Press; 2002. p. 298–9.

ANCA-RELATED VASCULITIDES

The advent of ANCA testing in the 1980s contributed greatly to the diagnosis and understanding of Wegener's granulomatosis and microscopic polyangiitis.[18,19] Indirect immunofluorescence

Table 4
Autoantibodies in rheumatoid arthritis

Autoantibody	Sensitivity	Specificity
Rheumatoid factor (RF)	66%–85%	72%–82%
Anti-CCP	56%–74%	90%–92%
RF and anti-CCP	48%	96%

Data from Bas S, Genevay S, Meyer O, Gabay C. Anti-cyclic citrullinated peptide antibodies, IgM and IgA rheumatoid factors in the diagnosis and prognosis of rheumatoid arthritis. Rheumatology 2003;442:677–80; and von Mühlen CA, Nakamura RM. Clinical and laboratory evaluation of systemic rheumatic diseases. In: McPherson RA, Pincus MR, editors. Henry's clinical diagnosis and management by laboratory methods. 21st edition. Philadelphia: Saunders Elsevier; 2007. p. 922.

testing for ANCA is performed with ethanol-fixed neutrophils as the substrate, which may result in two patterns: cytoplasmic (C-ANCA) and perinuclear (P-ANCA). The serum is then tested against formalin-fixed neutrophils, on which both C-ANCA and P-ANCA give a cytoplasmic pattern. Indirect immunofluorescence for ANCA is shown in **Fig. 2**. The antigen responsible for C-ANCA is usually Proteinase-3 (Pr-3), whereas the antigen usually detected by P-ANCA is myeloperoxidase. Myeloperoxidase is transported to a perinuclear location during ethanol fixation, but stays in the cytoplasm during formalin fixation. Anti-Pr3 and anti-myeloperoxidase antibodies may be tested with enzyme immunoassay or multiplex bead assay. Some other antibodies give a positive reaction on ethanol fixation, but are negative or give only a weak smudgy appearance when tested against formalin fixed neutrophils. These are called atypical ANCAs. ANCAs without myeloperoxidase or Pr-3 specificity may be caused by autoantibodies against elastase, lactoferrin, lactoperoxidase, cathepsin G, lysozyme, bactericidal/permeability-increasing (BPI) protein, and

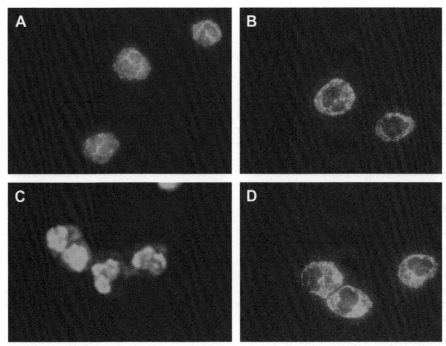

Fig. 2. ANCA patterns detected using indirect immunofluorescence. (*A*) A C-ANCA–positive serum placed on ethanol fixed neutrophils. (*B*) The same serum on formalin-fixed neutrophils. Both *A* and *B* show cytoplasmic labeling. (*C*) A P-ANCA–positive serum on ethanol-fixed neutrophils. (*D*) The same serum on formalin-fixed neutrophil. The P-ANCA antigen (myeloperoxidase) acquires a perinuclear localization during ethanol fixation but stays in the cytoplasm during formalin fixation.

azurocidin, and uncharacterized antigens. The clinical significance of non-myeloperoxidase, non-Pr3 ANCAs has not been established.

Two strategies for ANCA testing exist. The first is to perform indirect immunofluorescence screening, then, based on pattern, test for anti-Pr3 or myeloperoxidase (MPO). The indirect fluorescence is more sensitive and the antigen-specific testing is more specific. Like ANA testing, ANCA testing with indirect immunofluorescence is labor-intensive and subjective. The second strategy is to test for anti-MPO and anti-Pr3 using EIA, and then for ANCA using indirect fluorescence if indicated.

Table 5 shows the incidence of ANCA antibodies in Wegener granulomatosis, microscopic polyangiitis, and Churg-Strauss syndrome. There is an association of ANCA titers and activity of disease and relapse, but it is not strong enough to be very reliable.[20]

GOODPASTURE SYNDROME

Goodpasture syndrome is the presence of pulmonary hemorrhage and crescentic glomerulonephritis caused by the presence of antibodies to the glomerular basement membrane (anti-GBM). The anti-GBM antibodies can be shown in the

Table 5 Sensitivity of ANCAs in active vasculitis			
	C-ANCA/anti-Pr3	P-ANCA/anti-MPO	C-ANCA/Pr3 or P-ANCA/MPO
Wegener granulomatosis	56%–95%	5%–23%	85%–95%
Microscopic polyangiitis	8%–26%	49%–85%	67%–96%
Churg-Strauss syndrome	33%	33%	56%

Data from Hagen EC, Daha MR, Hermans J, et al. Diagnostic value of standardized assays for anti-neutrophil cytoplasmic antibodies in idiopathic systemic vasculitis. Kidney Int 1998;53:743–53; and Trevisin M, Pollock W, Dimech W, et al. Antigen specific ANCA ELISAs have different sensitivities for active and treated vasculitis and for nonvasculitic disease. Am J Clin Pathol 2008;129:42–53.

tissue using direct immunofluorescence, or in the serum using Western blot or enzyme immunoassay. Older tests using indirect immunofluorescence on normal renal tissue are unreliable and no longer clinically useful. The antigen in Goodpasture syndrome is the noncollagenous domain I type IV collagen. Western blot is more sensitive and specific than enzyme immunoassays,[21] but the enzyme immune assay is more suitable for use in the routine clinical laboratory. The EIA also allows for quantitation of the autoantibody, which may be used in following therapy.

SUMMARY

Autoantibody testing should only be performed in the context of the clinical workup of patients who have a reasonable likelihood of having the disease for which the testing is relevant. Otherwise, the predictive value of a positive test is too low. Particularly with ANA and ANCA testing, clinicians must know the methodology through which the tests are being performed, and should develop a relationship with the laboratory pathologist so that inconsistent or surprising results can be investigated.

REFERENCES

1. Kroshinsky D, Stone J, Bloch D, et al. Case 5-2009: a 47-year-old woman with a rash and numbness and pain in the legs. N Engl J Med 2009;360(7):711–20.
2. Tan EM, Feltkamp TEW, Smolen JS, et al. Range of antinuclear antibodies in "healthy" individuals. Arthritis Rheum 1997;40:1601–11.
3. Kumar V, Abbas AK, Fausto N, et al. Diseases of the immune system. In: Kumar V, Abbas AK, Fausto N, et al. Robbins and Cotran pathologic basis of disease. 8th edition. Philadelphia: Saunders Elsevier; 2010. p. 215.
4. Cheek W. Making sense of the ANA hodgepodge. CAP Today 2009;23(9):1–110.
5. von Mühlen CA, Nakamura RM. Guidelines for selecting and using laboratory test for autoantibodies to nuclear, nucleolar, and other related cytoplasmic antigens. In: Nakamura RM, Keren DF, Byland DJ, editors. Clinical and laboratory evaluation of autoimmune diseases. Chicago: ASCP Press; 2002. p. 183–98.
6. Nakamura RM, Tan EM. Clinical and laboratory evaluation of systemic lupus erythematosus and lupus-related disorders. In: Nakamura RM, Keren DF, Byland DJ, editors. Clinical and laboratory evaluation of autoimmune diseases. Chicago: ASCP Press; 2002. p. 111–39.
7. Isern RA, Yaneva M, Weiner E, et al. Autoantibodies in patients with primary pulmonary hypertension: association with anti-Ku. Am J Med 1992;93:307–12.
8. von Mühlen CA, Nakamura RM. Clinical and laboratory evaluation of systemic rheumatic diseases. In: McPherson RA, Pincus MR, editors. Henry's clinical diagnosis and management by laboratory methods. 21st edition. Philadelphia: Saunders Elsevier; 2007. p. 916–44.
9. Ho KT, Reveille JD. The clinical relevance of autoantibodies in scleroderma. Arthritis Res Ther 2003;5: 80–93.
10. Steen VD. Autoantibodies in systemic sclerosis. Semin Arthritis Rheum 2006;35(1):35–42.
11. Svengliati BS, Santillo M, Bevilacqua F, et al. Stimulatory autoantibodies to the PDGF receptor in systemic sclerosis. N Engl J Med 2006;354:2667–76.
12. Schnabel A, Reuter M, Biederer J. Interstitial lung disease in polymyositis and dermatomyositis: clinical course and response to treatment. Semin Arthritis Rheum 2003;32(5):273–84.
13. Wener MH. Rheumatoid factors. In: Rose NR, Hamilton RG, Detrick B, editors. Manual of clinical laboratory immunology. 6th edition. Washington, DC: American Society for Microbiology Press; 2002. p. 961–72.
14. Vincent C, de Keyser F, Masson-Bessiere C, et al. Anti-perinuclear factor compared with the so-called "antikeratin" antibodies and antibodies to human epidermis filaggrin, in the diagnosis of arthritides. Ann Rheum Dis 1999;58:42–8.
15. Vossenaar ER, vanVenrooij WJ. Citrullinated proteins: sparks that may ignite the fire in rheumatoid arthritis. Arthritis Res Ther 2004;6:107–11.
16. van Venrooij WJ, Prujin GJ. Citrullination, a small change for a protein with great consequences for rheumatoid arthritis. Arthritis Res 2000;2:249–51.
17. Mitsias D, Moutsopoulos M. Sjögren syndrome. In: Shoenfelk Y, Cervera R, Gershwin ME, editors. Diagnostic criteria in autoimmune disease. Totowa (NJ): Humana Press; 2008. p. 37–42.
18. Hagen EC, Daha MR, Hermans J, et al. Diagnostic value of standardized assays for anti-neutrophil cytoplasmic antibodies in idiopathic systemic vasculitis. Kidney Int 1998;53:743–53.
19. Trevisin M, Pollock W, Dimech W, et al. Antigen specific ANCA ELISAs have different sensitivities for active and treated vasculitis and for nonvasculitic disease. Am J Clin Pathol 2008;129:42–53.
20. Girard T, Mahr A, Noël L-H, et al. Are antineutrophil cytoplasmic antibodies a marker predictive of relapse in Wegener's granulomatosis? A prospective study. Rheumatology 2001;40:147–51.
21. Collins AB, Colvin RB. Kidney and lung disease mediated by anti-glomerular basement membrane antibodies: detection by Western blot analysis. In: Rose NR, Hamilton RG, Detrick B, editors. Manual of clinical laboratory immunology. 6th edition. Washington, DC: American Society for Microbiology Press; 2002. p. 1049–53.

Utility of Bronchoalveolar Lavage in Evaluation of Patients with Connective Tissue Diseases

Otylia Kowal-Bielecka, MD[a,*], Krzysztof Kowal, MD[b],
Elzbieta Chyczewska, MD[c]

KEYWORDS
- Bronchoalveolar lavage • Connective tissue diseases
- Lung pathology • Pulmonary complications

Connective tissue diseases (CTDs) comprise a group of systemic autoimmune disorders affecting a variety of body systems and organs. Pulmonary involvement is a frequent and severe manifestation of the CTDs. In patients with CTDs, namely rheumatoid arthritis (RA), systemic lupus erythematosus (SLE), systemic sclerosis (SSc), polymyositis (PM), dermatomyositis (DM), and Sjögren syndrome (SS), the lungs may be affected either primarily or due to complications of other CTD-related organ involvement.

Interstitial lung disease (ILD) is the best-known form of CTD-related lung involvement and a significant cause of increased mortality in this patient population. ILD can be subdivided histologically into nonspecific interstitial pneumonia (NSIP), usual interstitial pneumonia (UIP), organizing pneumonia, diffuse alveolar damage (DAD), and lymphocytic interstitial pneumonia (LIP).[1] Clinical presentation, prognosis, and response to therapy vary in CTD-associated ILD (CTD-ILD). In some CTD patients, ILD may progress leading to respiratory failure and, eventually, death. Major clinical problems in CTD-ILD have been discussed in detail in a recent review by Antoniou and colleagues.[2] In view of the highly variable clinical course of CTD-ILD and significant toxicity of immunosuppressive therapies used for treatment of CTD-ILD, identification of patients with a poor prognosis is of key importance, ideally before irreversible damage develops.

CTD-related involvement of pulmonary vessels includes different forms of pulmonary hypertension and pulmonary hemorrhages resulting from inflammation of pulmonary vessels.[2,3] Both are usually associated with a poor prognosis.

Lung pathology secondary to other organ involvement may also lead to serious morbidity and mortality. Weakness of pharyngeal and esophageal muscles caused by myositis or esophageal fibrosis predispose to development of aspiration pneumonia. Severe muscle weakness in PM/DM may cause hypoventilation, which in turn predisposes to and is frequently complicated by bronchopneumonia.[4,5] In addition, immunosuppressive therapies, which are a cornerstone of

a Department of Rheumatology and Internal Medicine, Medical University of Bialystok, Ul. M. Sklodowskiej-Curie 24A, Bialystok 15-276, Poland
b Department of Allergology and Internal Medicine, Medical University of Bialystok, Ul. M. Sklodowskiej-Curie 24A, Bialystok 15-276, Poland
c Department of Lung Diseases and Tuberculosis, Medical University of Bialystok, Ul. Zurawia 14, Bialystok 15-540, Poland
* Corresponding author.
E-mail address: otylia@umwb.edu.pl

Clin Chest Med 31 (2010) 423–431
doi:10.1016/j.ccm.2010.04.002

treatment of CTDs, may increase risk of opportunistic infection or lead to iatrogenic lung injury.

The wide spectrum of pulmonary involvement in CTD patients requires careful diagnostic workup, because different forms of lung involvement may overlap, causing similar clinical manifestations and similar radiological or functional impairment.

Bronchoalveolar lavage (BAL) is a method that makes it possible to investigate the lower respiratory tract through sampling of cellular and acellular (biochemical) components from bronchoalveolar lung units. BAL therefore appears to be a valuable source of information regarding the nature of lung pathology. Cytologic analysis of BAL fluid usually includes measurements of total and differential cell counts. In addition, evaluation of lymphocyte subsets and/or specific staining aimed at identification of particular cell types might also be performed. In healthy subjects the vast majority (95%–99%) of BAL cells consists of alveolar macrophages. Other leukocytes constitute a minority of BAL cells and, according to the recommendations of the European Respiratory Society and the American Thoracic Society, usually do not exceed 3% neutrophils, 2% eosinophils, and 15% lymphocytes.[6,7] The cytology of BAL fluid including macrophages, lymphocytes, and granulocytes is shown in **Fig. 1**. In addition, epithelial cells might also be present (**Fig. 2**).

Identification of microbiological agents in bronchoalveolar lavage fluid (BALF) is considered a method of choice in establishing the diagnosis of a pulmonary infection in patients with intrinsic lung disease and in those who are immunosuppressed. Also, analysis of smears of BALF revealing erythrocytes and hemosiderin-laden macrophages may confirm a diagnosis of pulmonary hemorrhage (**Fig. 3**).

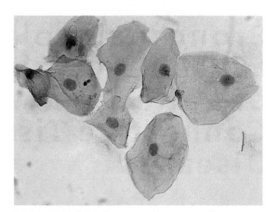

Fig. 2. Epithelial cells present in BAL cytology.

BALF analysis may also be helpful in the evaluation of the activity of the processes involved in the development of CTD-ILD, and therefore in identification of patients at risk of progressive lung fibrosis. An abnormally high number of BAL leukocytes, in particular granulocytes (neutrophils and eosinophils) or lymphocytes, have been found in patients with ILD; this is often referred to as "alveolitis" and reflects an inflammatory process of the lower respiratory tract in ILD. Moreover, studies of fluid recovered through BAL deliver information crucial for better understanding of the pathogenesis of CTD-ILDs and for identification of new therapeutic targets.

The purpose of this article is to review major findings concerning BAL analysis in the most frequent CTDs. The authors focus on the cytologic analysis of BALF, which has been studied most and is broadly accessible in clinical centers.

SYSTEMIC SCLEROSIS

Interstitial lung disease is the most frequent pulmonary complication and is a major cause of death in patients with SSc.[2,8] Sensitive diagnostic

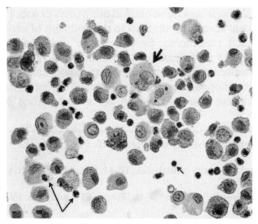

Fig. 1. BAL cytology showing macrophages (*thick arrow*), lymphocytes (*short arrow*), and granulocytes (*long arrows*).

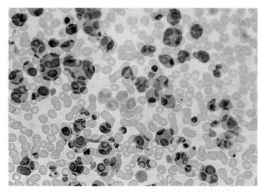

Fig. 3. BAL cytology showing presence of erythrocytes typical for pulmonary hemorrhage.

methods such as high-resolution computed tomography (HRCT) of the lungs reveal features of ILDs in more than 80% of patients with SSc. However, restrictive lung disease, which clinically is associated with increased mortality rates, develops in approximately 40% of SSc patients.[2,9] Studies evaluating lung biopsies revealed an NSIP pattern in the majority (68%–78%) of SSc-ILD patients and a UIP pattern in 8% to 26%. Unlike the idiopathic ILDs, there is no significant association between lung histopathology and survival.[10,11] Impaired lung function demonstrated by pulmonary function tests (PFTs) and fibrosis score on HRCT are associated with worse clinical prognosis in SSc-ILD, but these are already features of established lung disease.[2] Early identification of patients with progressive SSc-ILD is therefore of key importance.

Over the last 30 years several groups have investigated the role of cytologic analysis of BALF in evaluation of patients with SSc-ILD. The results of these studies have been summarized in a recent review.[12] An increased percentage of neutrophils, eosinophils, and/or lymphocytes were frequently found (range from 38% to 100%) in BALF from patients with SSc, irrespective of patient selection criteria, cut-off values applied for cytologic analysis, or technical aspects of BAL processing.[12] Although alveolitis might be present in SSc patients without clinically overt ILD, published reports almost unanimously indicate that an abnormal BAL cellular profile, in particular granulocytosis, is associated with more severe lung disease, as evaluated by PFTs or radiology.[12] Two independent studies did not show significant differences in BALF cytology and histopathological pattern (NSIP vs UIP) in SSc-ILD, except for an increased percentage of eosinophils in the SSc-NSIP group compared with the SSc-UIP group.[10,11]

Observational studies have demonstrated that increased proportions of granulocytes in BALF are associated with lung function deterioration in patients with SSc-ILD who did not receive immunosuppression[13,14] (reviewed in Ref.[12]). However, in 66 placebo-treated patients from the Scleroderma Lung Study, cytology of BALF had no additional value, compared with PFTs/HRCT, in predicting progression of SSc-ILD up to 12 months, as evaluated by forced vital capacity.[15] Of note, 3 retrospective studies indicate that BALF cytology might predict survival in patients with SSc-ILD.[10,14,16] In 2 of these studies, BAL neutrophilia and BAL eosinophilia were independent surrogate markers (after adjustment for lung disease severity) of mortality in an overall population of SSc-ILD patients[16] and in SSc-ILD patients

with a histologically proven NSIP pattern.[10] This result raises the hypothesis that granulocytosis in BALF might reflect other processes that are linked to survival in SSc-ILD patients. These observations are corroborated by the study of Kinder and colleagues,[17] who showed that the proportion of neutrophils in BALF is an independent predictor of early death in idiopathic pulmonary fibrosis, which is considered the prototypic ILD.

Studies evaluating the predictive value of BALF cytology with respect to response to immunosuppressive treatment in SSc-ILD have yielded contradictory results (reviewed in Ref.[12]). In a subgroup of 126 patients from the Scleroderma Lung Study in whom baseline BALF cytology and follow-up PFTs were available, the presence of alveolitis by cytologic analysis of BAL (neutrophils ≥3% and/or eosinophils ≥2%) was associated with a significantly higher probability in improvement or stabilization of lung function after treatment with cyclophosphamide as compared with patients with normal BALF cytology.[15] Because patients with alveolitis by BALF had more severe ILD and the severity of SSc-ILD was also shown to predict response to cyclophosphamide, the significance of BALF analysis for predicting treatment in SSc-ILD response remains unclear.

It should be noted that many population-related factors (smoking status, coexistence of infection or other respiratory diseases), influence of treatment, and technical discrepancies might influence BALF analysis (reviewed in Ref.[12]).

Although SSc patients are at high risk of pulmonary infections due to esophageal dysmotility-related reflux disease and/or immunosuppressive treatment used for controlling disease, there are only limited data concerning lung infections in patients with SSc. Two studies report on the microbiological analysis of BAL in patients with SSc-ILD.[18,19] The frequency of subclinical pulmonary infection, detected by BALF analysis, was 17% and 24%, respectively. In both studies no significant differences in BAL cytology could be found between patients with and without infections. In the study by De Santis and colleagues,[19] patients with infections detected by BAL deteriorated significantly compared with those without evidence of lung infection. Although there are no official upper limits of granulocytes in BALF, the authors' own experience indicates that a high percentage of neutrophils (usually exceeding 80%) is inevitably associated with the presence of bacteria in the lungs.

Thus, at present there is no sufficient evidence to support the utility of BALF analysis in routine clinical evaluation of SSc-ILD patients. However, BALF analysis might be helpful in highly selected patients in whom a clinical decision cannot be made based on staging of the severity of the SSc-ILD. BAL is also useful in the differential diagnosis of other entities that might overlap, such as infection or malignancy. Further studies should address the usefulness of BAL is assessing SSc-ILD.

RHEUMATOID ARTHRITIS

The prevalence of ILD in RA varies highly depending on the patient population and diagnostic methods.[2] In a recent analysis of 1429 RA patients, ILD was associated with a higher mortality rate, and was one of the most frequent causes of death in these patients.[20] Unlike in SSc and other CTDs, in RA-associated ILD (RA-ILD) a UIP pattern is found more frequently on HRCT and by histopathology, and a UIP pattern appears to be associated with a worse prognosis.[2,21]

The utility of BAL in evaluating RA-ILD has been studied less extensively than in SSc-ILD or the idiopathic ILDs. Published evidence indicates that an elevated percentage of neutrophils is frequently found in BALF from patients with RA.[22–25] In general, BAL neutrophilia appears to be associated with more severe RA-ILD, as evaluated by clinical symptoms, PFTs, or HRCT findings.[23,25–27] Lymphocytosis and eosinophilia were found less frequently in BALF of RA patients.[23] Unlike neutrophils, the percentage of lymphocytes is not associated with the presence of ILD on HRCT nor correlates with PFTs.[27] The results of BALF cytology often varies widely, and correlations with radiological or physiologic parameters are modest. It should, however, be recognized that the majority of studies included relatively low numbers of patients and most of these patients were receiving immunosuppressive treatments that could influence BALF cytology. Whether evaluation of BALF cytology could add important information in the evaluation of disease progression in RA-ILD requires further studies.

The prevalence of bronchiolar disease in RA varies from 8% to 65%, depending on the study. Bronchiolitis obliterans is characterized by airflow obstruction with or without radiological evidence of bronchiolitis or ILD on HRCT.[28] In a series of 12 patients with severe RA-associated bronchiolitis, BAL revealed increased leukocyte counts in 83%, with a predominant increase in neutrophils and lymphocytes as well as an absence of eosinophils. Of note, infectious pathogens including *Pseudomonas aeruginosa, Streptococcus pneumoniae, Staphylococcus aureus, Haemophilus influenzae*, and *Aspergillus* were identified by BAL in 9 patients.[28]

In RA patients presenting with dyspnea and radiological evidence of pulmonary infiltrates, infections and medication toxicity should be excluded.

In a study published in 2004 by Biederer and colleagues,[26] microbiological assessment of BALF, together with clinical and laboratory parameters, established a diagnosis of infectious pneumonia in 3 of 61 (5%) RA patients suspected to have ILD. It should be noted that the increasing usage of tumor necrosis factor (TNF)-α inhibitors for treatment of RA joint disease is associated with higher risk of infections, including potentially life-threatening respiratory system infections.

Necrobiotic nodules might be present in the lungs of RA patients and require differentiation with other granulomatous lung diseases, including infections and malignancies.[2] Potential complications of rheumatoid nodules in the lung include cavitation and colonization by *Aspergillus*.

Many drugs might induce interstitial lung reactions. Hypersensitivity pneumonitis has been described in association with methotrexate therapy, which is considered a gold standard therapy for RA joint disease, or with use of TNF-α inhibitors.[29,30] There are no specific BAL changes for drug-induced lung disease. However, BALF lymphocytosis with low CD4:CD8 ratio or striking eosinophilia (usually >25%) after excluding other reasons (parasites, Churg-Strauss syndrome, and so forth), in the context of a recent new drug exposure, supports the diagnosis of drug-induced lung disease.[31]

Patients with sarcoidosis, in addition to ILD, might present with inflammatory joint disease requiring differentiation with RA. Sarcoidosis has also been reported as a comorbidity in association with RA and other rheumatic disease or as a complication of anti–TNF-α therapy used for treatment of rheumatic disease (reviewed in Ref.[32]). A lymphocytosis with a high CD4:CD8 ratio in BALF is considered characteristic for pulmonary sarcoidosis. However, BALF neutrophilia has also been reported in patients with sarcoidosis and has been shown to correlate with more severe disease.[33]

Thus, in RA patients with lung involvement, BAL should be considered for excluding infections or other underlying lung pathology (eg, malignancy or sarcoidosis). BAL may also support the diagnosis of hypersensitivity pneumonitis and/or drug toxicity if a high proportion of eosinophils or lymphocytes is present.

SYSTEMIC LUPUS ERYTHEMATOSUS

By far the most frequent lung involvement in SLE patients is pleuritis, which reaches a prevalence of 36% in the clinical setting.[34] The frequency of respiratory lung involvement (excluding pleurisy) in SLE ranged from 7% to 14% in 3 large studies (Toronto n = 994, "Euro-Lupus" n = 1000, and University of South California n = 464).[35]

The prevalence and severity of ILD in SLE is considerably lower than that in other CTDs. Autopsy studies demonstrated signs of interstitial pneumonitis or fibrosis in as many as 13% of 120 cases studied, but clinical manifestations of chronic ILD disease is seen in only approximately 3% of SLE patients.[36,37] The course of chronic ILD in SLE is usually mild, slowly progressive with stabilization over time, and with little irreversible damage of the respiratory system.[37] Chronic interstitial pneumonitis is characterized by predominant lymphocytic infiltrates and dysfunction of alveolar macrophages.[38] The number of CD8[+] cells and natural killer cells in BALF are increased and correlate with an impairment of diffusion capacity of carbon monoxide.[39]

Acute lupus pneumonitis affects 1.4% to 4% of SLE patients.[2] In SLE-associated pneumonitis, a lower than normal CD4[+]/CD8[+] ratio was demonstrated in BAL fluid. However, this is also seen in patients with no respiratory symptoms, indicating that that finding is not specific for SLE pneumonitis but rather reflects general disturbances in the immune system of SLE patients.[40]

Acute pneumonitis is a rare complication of SLE and therefore it should be differentiated from other clinical conditions that present as lung infiltrates, including alveolar hemorrhage and infection or aspiration pneumonia.

Alveolar hemorrhage is also a relatively infrequent complication of SLE, being present in 1% to 5.4% of SLE patients.[3,41] Early bronchoscopy with BAL provides a reliable means of demonstrating alveolar hemorrhage. Increasing amount of blood in consecutive aliquots of BAL, gross blood, and/or hemosiderin-laden macrophages in the absence of infectious organisms favor alveolar hemorrhage.[42,43] In a study evaluating patients admitted to hospital because of complications of SLE over a period of 10 years, 17% of all cases were pulmonary complications and 3.7% alveolar hemorrhage.[44] In 15 patients suspected of alveolar hemorrhage, early bronchoscopy with BAL was performed. In all patients, lavage fluid was hemorrhagic. In another study of patients with clinical signs and symptoms of alveolar hemorrhage, hemosiderin-laden macrophages were demonstrated in BAL fluid.[3]

The rate of infection in SLE appears to exceed that in other autoimmune diseases and immunocompromised states by as much as 8-fold.[45] Accordingly, infection is the most common cause

of parenchymal lung disease and should always be considered in cases of new pulmonary infiltrates in patients with SLE. In patients with SLE, pulmonary infections are not only frequently encountered but also contribute substantially to morbidity and mortality, accounting for 30% to 50% of all deaths of SLE patients.[46,47] The great majority of infections (75%) are bacterial; however, mycobacteria, fungi, and viruses are responsible for 12%, 7%, and 5% of all infections, respectively.[48] Bacteria described in SLE lung infections include gram-positive cocci, gram-negative bacilli, and atypical bacteria such as *Chlamydia pneumoniae* and *Mycoplasma pneumoniae*. Opportunistic infections with *Pneumocystis carinii*, *Aspergillus*, *Nocardia*, and cytomegalovirus (CMV) have also been reported.[46,49] Infections of the respiratory tract are also frequent complications encountered in SLE patients with alveolar hemorrhage.[50] A prospective study of 13 SLE patients with pulmonary hemorrhage using BAL analysis demonstrated that infections could be documented within the first 48 hours after admission in 8 patients (61.5%).

Thus, in SLE patients with diffuse lung involvement, bronchoscopy with BAL is helpful in the differential diagnosis, confirming pulmonary hemorrhage due to SLE-related vasculitis and excluding other conditions that may coexist in SLE patients, such as infections.

POLYMYOSITIS AND DERMATOMYOSITIS

ILD is found in 5% to 64% of patients with PM/DM, depending on patient population and methods of diagnosis. In PM/DM, patients with ILD may progress rapidly (acute/subacute type, Hamman-Rich–like) or develop in a more chronic manner (chronic ILD).[2,4,5] Approximately 30% to 50% of patients improve with immunosuppressive therapy, while others may progress to respiratory failure and, possibly, death.

Several groups have reported elevated neutrophil and/or lymphocyte percentages in BALF from patients with PM/DM.[22,51-53] Neutrophilia and/or lymphocytosis were found in the majority (50%–100%) of PM/DM patients diagnosed with ILD, based on radiological examination and/or PFTs results, but also in up to 15% of PM/DM patients without radiological features of ILD on computed tomography scans.[52]

Two retrospective studies, each involving 20 patients with PM/DM-ILD and BAL, revealed associations between BALF neutrophilia and worse clinical prognosis. In the study by Schnabel and colleagues,[54] 10 patients with PM/DM-ILD who were not responding to treatment had a significantly higher percentage of neutrophils in BALF than 10 PM/DM-ILD patients who improved under immunosuppressive therapy. In another analysis, neutrophilia in BALF at initial evaluation was the only parameter, except for acute lung manifestations (Hamman-Rich–like syndrome), which was significantly associated with subsequent clinical deterioration. Patients with diminished lung diffusion capacity for carbon monoxide (DLCO; <45% of predicted) also experienced greater deterioration compared with those with higher DLCO values, but the difference was not significant. Because only 11 patients underwent lung biopsy, which revealed a variety of histopathologic patterns of lung involvement, reliable statistical analysis could not be performed to analyze the association between histopathologic pattern and clinical outcomes.[5]

In another study comparing patients with DM and PM, the percentages of lymphocytes and eosinophils in BALF were significantly higher in 9 patients with DM-ILD than in 9 patients with PM-ILD. The patients with DM-ILD had a significantly higher mortality than PM-ILD. The percentage of neutrophils in BALF tended to be higher in DM-ILD than in those with PM-ILD, but the difference was not statistically significant. It is noteworthy that when patients were compared according to the histopathological pattern on lung biopsy, 2 patients who died of DAD (both DM-ILD) had high neutrophil percentages in BALF (mean 31%) compared with patients with NSIP (2.4%) and those with UIP (4.2%). The low numbers of patients having both BALF cytology and lung biopsy precluded statistical evaluation.[55]

Several case series have shown that patients with ILD associated with PM/DM or the presence of anti–Jo-1 autoantibodies, which are characteristic for PM, have an increased proportion of CD8[+] cells in their BALF.[56,57] In another group of 22 patients with PM/DM-ILD, high proportions of BALF CD25[+]CD8[+] and CD25[+]CD4[+] lymphocytes were associated with resistance to steroid therapy.[58]

In conclusion, although some small studies suggest that high percentages of neutrophils in BALF are associated with more severe ILD in PM/DM, further studies involving greater numbers of patients are needed to clarify the role of BAL analysis in the evaluation of outcome in PM/DM-ILD.

Patients with PM/DM are particularly prone to lung infection because of muscle weakness, which leads to aspiration and/or hypoventilation. In a study by Dickey and Myers,[4] respiratory infections were the most common form of pulmonary disease and developed in 12 out of 42 (29%) PM/DM patients. Six of these (14.3% of all 42) had aspiration pneumonia, as diagnosed based on a clear history of aspiration, characteristic radiological picture, and consistent microbiological data. In another study involving 156 patients with PM/DM, aspiration pneumonia was found in 27 (17.3%) and respiratory insufficiency due to hypoventilation in 34 (22%).[5] The same group reported previously that all of 5 PM/DM patients with respiratory insufficiency due to generalized muscle weakness developed aspiration pneumonia.[52] One of these 5 patients died within 2 months after diagnosis of PM.

The association of PM/DM and malignancy has been well recognized. Marie and colleagues[5,52] identified malignancies (any) in approximately 16% to 17% of PM/DM patients. Primary pulmonary malignancy was identified in 2 of 55 (4%) PM/DM patients.[52] Of note, malignancies were found significantly less frequently in patients with PM/DM-ILD (5.6%) than in PM/DM patients without ILD (21.6%).[5]

BAL appears to be helpful in the differential diagnosis of lung involvement in PM/DM, particularly in excluding respiratory infection or malignancies.

SJÖGREN SYNDROME

The frequency of pulmonary involvement in patients with SS varies from 9% to 75% depending on the detection method, and consists of various forms of small airway disease and ILD.[59–62] Clinically significant ILD is rare in the course of primary SS and pulmonary fibrosis is uncommon.[59,63] Unlike in RA or SSc, the survival rate is similar in SS patients with and without ILD.[62]

The incidence of pneumonitis seems to be greater than generally assumed. In patients with SS, an abnormal BAL cytology was found is as many as 48% to 69%, and usually reveals an increased proportion of lymphocytes (in 44%–55% of patients). Neutrophilia is found infrequently in BALF from SS patients (range: 4%–17%).[22,64,65] No difference in the percentage of eosinophils was demonstrated.[64,66] Abnormal BAL findings were associated with more severe disease, as evaluated by extrapulmonary involvement, serum concentration of γ-globulins, rheumatoid factor, and autoantibodies.[64] Another 2-year prospective study evaluated 18 patients with documented alveolitis. There was no significant impairment of lung function tests demonstrated after 2 years of follow-up, despite features of alveolitis in BAL persisting in 57% of patients.[66]

An increased percentage of CD8[+] lymphocytes in BAL fluid was demonstrated in SS patients with associated BAL neutrophilia.[67] Reduced CD4[+]/CD8[+] ratio in BALF was associated with alterations of lung function, and clinically more severe

ILD was seen.[68] Moreover, natural killer cells displayed decreased activity and interleukin-2 production.[69] The clinical significance of those findings remains unclear.

Lymphocytic pneumonitis in SS is considered to represent a benign lymphoproliferation; however, an increased frequency of premalignant or malignant lymphoproliferative disorders has been demonstrated in patients with SS. Bronchoscopy with BAL and transbronchial biopsy is recommended in patients with symptoms of ILD and suspicion of malignancy.[33]

SUMMARY

The lungs are frequently involved in patients with CTDs. Different forms of pulmonary involvement and the highly variable course of CTD-related ILD, which is one of the major complications in CTDs, makes management of patients with CTD-associated lung disease especially challenging.

BAL, through sampling of cells and fluids from the lower respiratory tract, significantly contributes to revealing the nature of pulmonary complications. Specific findings in BAL allow definite diagnosis of certain pulmonary complications, for example, the high amount of erythrocytes accompanied by macrophages loaded with hemosiderin in pulmonary hemorrhages. BAL cellular profiles, together with clinical data, may help in establishing the diagnosis of hypersensitivity pneumonitis and drug toxicity.

Microbiological assessment of BALF plays a critical role in identification of respiratory tract infections and is considered a method of choice for the diagnosis of lung infections in patients with pulmonary diseases, including CTD-ILD.[33] Careful monitoring of respiratory infections seems particularly important in patients who are subjected to aggressive immunosuppressive therapy for coexisting autoimmune lung injury. Thus, in patients with CTD, BAL plays an important role in the differential diagnosis of coexisting infections of the respiratory tract.

At the moment, the role of BAL in assessing disease progression and outcome in CTD-ILD is controversial. Further controlled studies, including large populations with similar bronchoscopy technique and standardized performance of BAL and laboratory evaluations, are necessary to define the potential role of this technique in the evaluation of disease progression and outcome.

Except for lung biopsy, BAL is the only technique that allows direct insight into processes involved in injury of the lung interstitium. BAL is less invasive than biopsy, and may be applied more broadly and in a repeated manner.

Moreover, BAL enables sampling of a greater lung area compared with lung biopsy.

In conclusion, BAL is a useful technique in making a diagnosis of specific pulmonary complications in patients with CTD, such as infection or hemorrhage. At present, BAL is not recommended for routine clinical assessment of patients with CTD-ILD. In CTD-ILD, BAL is advocated to exclude coexisting infiltrating lung diseases (infections, hypersensitivity pneumonitis, malignancy) and might be helpful in highly selected cases when treatment decisions remain uncertain after analysis of clinical, functional, and radiological data. BAL, as a less invasive technique than lung biopsy enabling direct insight into lung pathology, is worthy of further studies with regard to its value in assessing activity of immune lung disease associated with CTD. Finally, although not discussed in detail in the present review, BAL is invaluable as a tool for receiving information on pathogenesis of CTD-associated ILD, which in turn is relevant for the development of new targeted therapies (reviewed in Ref.[70]).

REFERENCES

1. American Thoracic Society/European Respiratory Society. International multidisciplinary consensus classification of the idiopathic interstitial pneumonias. Am J Respir Crit Care Med 2002;165:277–304.
2. Antoniou KM, Margaritopoulos G, Economidou F, et al. Pivotal clinical dilemmas in collagen vascular diseases associated with interstitial lung involvement. Eur Respir J 2009;33:882–96.
3. Santos-Ocampo AS, Mandell BF, Fessler BJ. Alveolar hemorrhage in systemic lupus erythematosus. Chest 2000;118:1083–90.
4. Dickey BF, Myers AR. Pulmonary disease in polymyositis/dermatomyosistis. Semin Arthritis Rheum 1984;14:60–76.
5. Marie I, Hachulla E, Cherin P, et al. Interstitial lung disease in polymyositis and dermatomyositis. Arthritis Rheum 2002;47:614–22.
6. Technical recommendations and guidelines for bronchoalveolar lavage (BAL). Report of the European Society of Pneumology Task Group. Eur Respir J 1989;2:561–85.
7. Bronchoalveolar lavage constituents in healthy individuals, idiopathic pulmonary fibrosis, and selected comparison groups. The BAL Cooperative Steering Committee. Am Rev Respir Dis 1990;141:S169–202.
8. Steen VD, Medsger TA. Changes in causes of death in systemic sclerosis, 1972–2002. Ann Rheum Dis 2007;66:940–4.
9. Steen VD, Conte C, Owens GR, et al. Severe restrictive lung disease in systemic sclerosis. Arthritis Rheum 1994;37:1283–9.

10. Bouros D, Wells AU, Nicholson AG, et al. Histopath-ologic subsets of fibrosing alveolitis in patients with systemic sclerosis and their relationship to outcome. Am J Respir Crit Care Med 2002;165: 1581–6.

11. Kim DS, Yoo B, Lee JS, et al. The major histopatho-logic pattern of pulmonary fibrosis in scleroderma is nonspecific interstitial pneumonia. Sarcoidosis Vasc Diffuse Lung Dis 2002;19:121–7.

12. Kowal-Bielecka O, Kowal K, Highland KB, et al. Bronchoalveolar lavage fluid in scleroderma intersti-tial lung disease: technical aspects and clinical correlations: review of the literature. Semin Arthritis Rheum, in press.

13. Silver RM, Miller KS, Smith EA, et al. Evaluation and management of scleroderma lung disease using bronchoalveolar lavage. Am J Med 1990;88:470–6.

14. White B, Moore WC, Wigley FM, et al. Cyclophos-phamide is associated with pulmonary function and survival benefit in patients with scleroderma and alveolitis. Ann Intern Med 2000;132:947–54.

15. Strange C, Bolster MB, Roth MD, et al. Bronchoal-veolar lavage and response to cyclophosphamide in scleroderma interstitial lung disease. Am J Respir Crit Care Med 2008;177:91–8.

16. Goh NS, Veeraraghavan S, Desai SR, et al. Bron-choalveolar lavage cellular profiles in patients with systemic sclerosis-associated interstitial lung disease are not predictive of disease progression. Arthritis Rheum 2007;56:2005–12.

17. Kinder BW, Brown KK, Schwarz MI, et al. Baseline BAL neutrophilia predicts early mortality in idio-pathic pulmonary fibrosis. Chest 2008;133:226–32.

18. Clements PJ, Goldin JG, Kleerup EC, et al. Regional differences in bronchoalveolar lavage and thoracic high-resolution computed tomography results in dyspneic patients with systemic sclerosis. Arthritis Rheum 2004;50:1909–17.

19. De Santis M, Bosello S, La Torre G, et al. Functional, radiological and biological markers of alveolitis and infections of the lower respiratory tract in patients with systemic sclerosis. Respir Res 2005;6:96.

20. Young A, Koduri G, Batley M, et al. Early rheumatoid arthritis study (ERAS) group. Mortality in rheumatoid arthritis. Increased in the early course of disease, in ischaemic heart disease and in pulmonary fibrosis. Rheumatology (Oxford) 2007;46:350–7.

21. Kim EJ, Collard HR, King TE Jr. Rheumatoid arthritis-associated interstitial lung disease: the relevance of histopathologic and radiographic pattern. Chest 2009;136:1397–405.

22. Wallaert B, Hatron PY, Grosbois JM, et al. Subclinical pulmonary involvement in collagen vascular diseases assessed by bronchoalveolar lavage. Relationship between alveolitis and subsequent changes in lung function. Am Rev Respir Dis 1986; 133:574–80.

23. Gabbay E, Tarala R, Will R, et al. Interstitial lung disease in recent onset rheumatoid arthritis. Am J Respir Crit Care Med 1997;156:528–35.

24. Garcia JG, Parhami N, Killam D, et al. Bronchoalveo-lar lavage fluid evaluation in rheumatoid arthritis. Am Rev Respir Dis 1986;133:450–4.

25. Gilligan DM, O'Connor CM, Ward K, et al. Bron-choalveolar lavage in patients with mild and severe rheumatoid lung disease. Thorax 1990;45:591–6.

26. Biederer J, Schnabel A, Muhle C, et al. Correlation between HRCT findings, pulmonary function tests and bronchoalveolar lavage cytology in interstitial lung disease associated with rheumatoid arthritis. Eur Radiol 2004;14:272–80.

27. Garcia JG, James HL, Zinkgraf S, et al. Lower respi-ratory tract abnormalities in rheumatoid interstitial lung disease. Potential role of neutrophils in lung injury. Am Rev Respir Dis 1987;136:811–7.

28. Devouassoux G, Cottin V, Liote H, et al. Character-isation of severe obliterative bronchiolitis in rheuma-toid arthritis. Eur Respir J 2009;33:1053–61.

29. Zisman DA, McCune WJ, Tino G, et al. Drug-induced pneumonitis: the role of methotrexate. Sarcoidosis Vasc Diffuse Lung Dis 2001;18: 243–52.

30. Ostor AJ, Chilvers ER, Somerville MF, et al. Pulmonary complications of infliximab therapy in patients with rheumatoid arthritis. J Rheumatol 2006;33:622–8.

31. Costabel U, Uzaslan E, Guzman J. Bronchoalveolar lavage in drug-induced lung disease. Clin Chest Med 2004;24:25–35.

32. Torralba KD, Quismorio FP Jr. Sarcoidosis and the rheumatologist. Curr Opin Rheumatol 2009;2:62–70.

33. Bradley B, Branley HM, Egan JJ, et al. Interstitial lung disease guideline: the British Thoracic Society in collaboration with the Thoracic Society of Australia and New Zealand and the Irish Thoracic Society. Thorax 2008;63(Suppl V):v1–58.

34. Carvera R, Khamashta M, Font J, et al. Systemic lupus erythematosus: clinical and immunologic patterns of disease expression in a cohort of 1000 patients. Medicine 1993;72:113–24.

35. Gladman DD, Urowitz M. SLE clinical features. In: Hochberg MC, Silman AJ, Smolen JS, et al, editors. Rheumatology. 3rd edition. Philadelphia: Mosby Elsevier Ltd; 2003. p. 1359–79.

36. Haupt HM, Moore GW, Hutchins GM. The lung in systemic lupus erythematosus. Analysis in the path-ologic changes in 120 patients. Am J Med 1981;71: 791–8.

37. Weinrib L, Sharma OP, Quismorio FP Jr, et al. A long-term study of interstitial lung disease in systemic lupus erythematosus. Semin Arthritis Rheum 1990; 20:48–56.

38. Wallaert B, Aerts C, Bart F, et al. Alveolar macro-phage dysfunction in systemic lupus erythemato-sus. Am Rev Respir Dis 1987;136:293–7.

39. Groen H, Aslander M, Bootsma H, et al. Bronchoalveolar lavage cell analysis and lung function impairment in patients with systemic lupus erythematosus (SLE). Clin Exp Immunol 1993;94:127–33.

40. Paran D, Koifman B, Elkayam O, et al. Echocardiography, pulmonary function testing and induced sputum evaluation in systemic lupus erythematosus and the antiphospholipid syndrome. Lupus 2002;11:546.

41. Barile LA, Jara LJ, Medina-Rodriguez F, et al. Pulmonary hemorrhage in systemic lupus erythematosus. Lupus 1997;6:445–8.

42. Schwab EP, Schumacher HR, Freundlich B, et al. Pulmonary alveolar hemorrhage in systemic lupus erythematosus. Semin Arthritis Rheum 1993;23:8–15.

43. Orens JB, Martinez FJ, Lynch JP. Pleuropulmonary manifestations of systemic lupus erythematosus. Rheum Dis Clin North Am 1994;20:159–92.

44. Zamora MR, Warner ML, Tuder R, et al. Diffuse alveolar hemorrhage and systemic lupus erythematosus. Clinical presentation, histology, survival, and outcome. Medicine 1997;76:192–202.

45. Staples PJ, Gerding DN, Decker JL, et al. Incidence of infection in systemic lupus erythematosus. Arthritis Rheum 1974;17:1–10.

46. Zadman-Goddard G, Shoenfeld Y. Infections and SLE. Autoimmunity 2005;38:473–85.

47. Bernatsky S, Boivin JF, Joseph L, et al. Mortality of systemic lupus erythematosus. Arthritis Rheum 2006;54:2550–7.

48. Kinder BW, Freemer MM, King TE Jr, et al. Clinical and genetic risk factors for pneumonia in systemic lupus erythematosus. Arthritis Rheum 2007;56:2679–86.

49. Petri M. Infection in systemic lupus erythematosus. Rheum Dis Clin North Am 1998;24:423–56.

50. Rojas-Serrano J, Pedroza J, Regalado J, et al. High prevalence of infections in patients with systemic lupus erythematosus and pulmonary haemorrhage. Lupus 2008;17:295–9.

51. Grau JM, Miró O, Pedrol E, et al. Interstitial lung disease related to dermatomyositis. Comparative study with patients without lung involvement. J Rheumatol 1996;23:1921–6.

52. Marie I, Hatron PY, Hachulla E, et al. Pulmonary involvement in polymyositis and in dermatomyositis. J Rheumatol 1998;25:1336–43.

53. Komócsi A, Kumánovics G, Zibotics H, et al. Alveolitis may persist during treatment that sufficiently controls muscle inflammation in myositis. Rheumatol Int 2001;20:113–8.

54. Schnabel A, Reuter M, Biederer J, et al. Interstitial lung disease in polymyositis and dermatomyositis: clinical course and response to treatment. Semin Arthritis Rheum 2003;32:273–84.

55. Fujisawa T, Suda T, Nakamura Y, et al. Differences in clinical features and prognosis of interstitial lung diseases between polymyositis and dermatomyositis. J Rheumatol 2005;32:58–64.

56. Sauty A, Rochat T, Schoch OD, et al. Pulmonary fibrosis with predominant CD8 lymphocytic alveolitis and anti-Jo-1 antibodies. Eur Respir J 1997;10:2907–12.

57. Kourakata H, Takada T, Suzuki E, et al. Flowcytometric analysis of bronchoalveolar lavage fluid cells in polymyositis/dermatomyositis with interstitial pneumonia. Respirology 1999;4:223–8.

58. Kurasawa K, Nawata Y, Takabayashi K, et al. Activation of pulmonary T cells in corticosteroid-resistant and -sensitive interstitial pneumonitis in dermatomyositis/polymyositis. Clin Exp Immunol 2002;129:541–8.

59. Deheinzelin D, Capelozzi VL, Kairala RA, et al. Interstitial lung disease in primary Sjögren's syndrome: clinical pathological evaluation and response to treatment. Am J Respir Crit Care Med 1996;15:794–9.

60. Cain HC, Noble PW, Matthay RA. Pulmonary manifestations of Sjögren's syndrome. Clin Chest Med 1998;19:687–99.

61. Davidson BK, Kelly CA, Griffiths ID. Ten-year follow up of pulmonary function in patients with primary Sjögren's syndrome. Thorax 2000;59:709–12.

62. Ito I, Nagai S, Kitaichi M, et al. Pulmonary manifestations of primary Sjögren's syndrome: a clinical, radiologic and pathologic study. Am J Respir Crit Care Med 2005;171:632–8.

63. Strilman CV, Rosenow EC, Divertie MB, et al. Pulmonary manifestations of Sjögren's syndrome. Chest 1976;70:354–61.

64. Harton PY, Wallaert B, Gosset D, et al. Subclinical lung inflammation in primary Sjögren's syndrome. Arthritis Rheum 1987;30:1226–31.

65. Salaffi F, Subiaco S, Carotti M, et al. Bronchoalveolar lavage in primary Sjögren's syndrome. Eur J Intern Med 1995;6:109–16.

66. Salaffi F, Manganelli P, Carotti M, et al. A longitudinal study of pulmonary involvement in primary Sjögren's syndrome: relationship between alveolitis and subsequent lung changes on high-resolution computed tomography. Br J Rheumatol 1998;37:263–9.

67. Wallaert B, Prin L, Harton PY, et al. Lymphocyte subpopulations in bronchoalveolar lavage in Sjögren's syndrome. Evidence for an expansion of cytotoxic/suppressor subset in patients with alveolar neutrophilia. Chest 1987;92:1025–31.

68. Dalavanga YA, Constantopoulos SH, Galanopoulos V, et al. Alveolitis correlates with pulmonary involvement in primary Sjögren's syndrome. Chest 1991;99:1394–7.

69. Miyasaka N, Murota N, Sato K, et al. Interleukin-2 defect in the peripheral blood and the lung in patients with Sjögren's syndrome. Clin Exp Immunol 1986;65:497–505.

70. Silver RM, Wells AU. Histopathology and bronchoalveolar lavage. Rheumatology (Oxford) 2008;47(Suppl 5):v62–4.

Pulmonary Manifestations of Scleroderma and Mixed Connective Tissue Disease

Faye N. Hant, DO, MSCR[a],*, Laura B. Herpel, MD[b],
Richard M. Silver, MD[a]

KEYWORDS

- Systemic sclerosis • Scleroderma • Interstitial lung disease
- Mixed connective tissue disease
- Pulmonary arterial hypertension

CASE PRESENTATION

A 57-year-old white woman presents to your office with a 3- to 4-year history of progressive dyspnea on exertion. Her dyspnea occurs with walking up 1 flight of stairs. She has a cough that is variably nonproductive or productive of sputum. She has had a 13.6 kg weight loss during the past year, intermittent chest pain, orthopnea, and lower extremity edema. She reports that a recent cardiac workup was normal. Review of systems is notable for arthralgia, gastroesophageal reflux, skin rash, and Raynaud phenomenon (RP). She has a 20 pack-year history of tobacco use, but quit 12 years ago. Physical examination reveals a heart rate (HR) of 123 bpm, respiratory rate of 24/min, blood pressure (BP) 119/83, and O_2 saturation of 92% at rest breathing room air. She has widespread telangiectasias but no skin sclerosis. Chest examination reveals bibasilar dry inspiratory crackles. Cardiac examination reveals tachycardia without murmur, gallop, or rub, and there is no jugular venous distention. Edema is not present in the lower extremities. Data review shows a computed tomography (CT) scan with diffuse interstitial changes, bibasilar

honeycombing, and ground glass opacities (GGO). Pulmonary function tests (PFTs) reveal an forced vital capacity (FVC) of 1.76 L (61% predicted), forced expiratory volume in 1 second (FEV_1) 1.40 L (65% predicted), FEV_1/FVC 80%, total lung capacity (TLC) 2.27 L (52% predicted), diffusion capacity of carbon monoxide (DLCO) 8.7 mL/mm Hg/min (41% predicted), consistent with severe restriction and reduced diffusion capacity. During a 6-minute walk test, the patient walks 296 m and desaturates from a baseline of 96% to 92%. An abnormal cardiovascular response to exercise is noted with the HR increasing from 108 to 145 bpm with BP going from 102/70 to 100/60. Nailfold capillary microscopy is performed and reveals dilatated capillaries as well as capillary dropout. Laboratory studies show normal complete blood count (CBC), complete metabolic panel, and creatine kinase; brain natriuretic peptide (BNP) is 515 pg/mL (normal ≤ 100), and antinuclear antibody (ANA) is positive at titer of 1:1280 with a nucleolar pattern. Based on the clinical presentation, including RP, esophageal reflux, telangiectasias, interstitial lung disease (ILD), abnormal nailfold capillary morphology, and +ANA in the

[a] Division of Rheumatology and Immunology, Medical University of South Carolina, 96 Jonathan Lucas Street, Suite 912, Charleston, SC 29425-6370, USA
[b] Division of Pulmonary, Critical Care, Allergy and Sleep Medicine, Medical University of South Carolina, 96 Jonathan Lucas Street, Suite 812, Charleston, SC 29425, USA
* Corresponding author.
E-mail address: hant@musc.edu

Clin Chest Med 31 (2010) 433–449
doi:10.1016/j.ccm.2010.05.004
0272-5231/10/$ – see front matter © 2010 Elsevier Inc. All rights reserved.

setting of normal skin thickness, the patient is given a diagnosis of systemic sclerosis (SSc) sine scleroderma.

The respiratory system is frequently affected in the connective tissue diseases (CTDs) and contributes to significant morbidity and mortality. Involvement can occur in all aspects of the respiratory tract including, but not limited to, the blood vessels, airways, pleura, parenchyma, and musculature. As a diverse group of immunologically mediated disorders, the CTDs frequently overlap, making accurate diagnosis reliant on the clinical presentation, physical examination findings, and serologic markers. A systematic approach must be undertaken to evaluate the extent of organ involvement. Early detection of lung involvement is essential to improve outcomes. As illustrated in the case described earlier, a patient with CTD may sometimes present with the sole complaint of dyspnea or be found to have a lung disorder without other overt symptoms. This article discusses the pathogenesis, clinical presentation and evaluation of the patient with pulmonary disease related to SSc (also known as scleroderma) and mixed connective tissue disease (MCTD). In addition, various modalities and investigations to aid in diagnosis and treatment of these diseases are reviewed.

SSc

SSc is a rare autoimmune CTD of unknown cause, with an estimated annual incidence of 19.3 new cases per million adults per year.[1] SSc is characterized by 3 major processes: disease-specific autoantibodies, organ fibrosis, and small-vessel vasculopathy.[2] Organ fibrosis can involve several body systems, including the pulmonary, integument, cardiac, gastrointestinal, and renal systems.[2] The American College of Rheumatology classification criteria for SSc include the major criterion of skin thickening or induration proximal to the metacarpophalangeal or metatarsophalangeal joints, and 3 minor criteria of sclerodactyly, digital pitting, or loss of finger pad substance, and bibasilar pulmonary fibrosis (PF) not attributable to primary lung disease.[3] SSc is diagnosed when 1 major and 2 or more minor criteria are present.[3]

Mortality from scleroderma renal crisis has been significantly reduced with the use of angiotensin-converting enzyme inhibitors beginning in the 1980s, and lung disease has emerged as the leading cause of mortality. Pulmonary involvement is common (**Box 1**) and occurs in all SSc subsets, including limited cutaneous systemic sclerosis (lcSSc, formerly CREST syndrome), diffuse

---

> **Box 1**
> **Manifestations of SSc in the respiratory system**
>
> 1. ILD
>
> - Nonspecific interstitial pneumonia (NSIP)
> - Usual interstitial pneumonia (UIP)
> - Diffuse alveolar damage (DAD)
> - Cryptogenic organizing pneumonia (COP)
>
> 2. Pulmonary hypertension
> 3. Pleural involvement
> 4. Aspiration pneumonia
> 5. Alveolar hemorrhage
> 6. Small airways disease
> 7. Malignancy
> 8. Respiratory muscle weakness
> 9. Drug-induced toxicity
> 10. Spontaneous pneumothorax
> 11. Pneumoconiosis (silicosis)

---

cutaneous systemic sclerosis (dcSSc, formerly progressive systemic scleroderma), and SSc sine scleroderma.[4] Patients with lcSSc have skin involvement distal to the elbows and knees, whereas patients with dcSSc have truncal involvement and more proximal limb involvement. The face may be affected in lcSSc and dcSSc. ILD and pulmonary arterial hypertension (PAH) are now the leading causes of mortality in SSc.[5]

ILD

Inflammation or fibrosis involving the pulmonary interstitium denotes a group of disorders referred to as ILD. Because of the complexity of these disorders, the American Thoracic Society and European Respiratory Society published a consensus on the classification of the idiopathic interstitial pneumonias, and classified parenchymal lung disease related to CTD as diffuse parenchymal lung disease of known association.[6] ILD is the most common pulmonary manifestation in SSc, with 40% of patients having restrictive changes on PFTs and more than 90% of patients having evidence for ILD at autopsy.[7] Approximately 15% of patients who present with ILD have an underlying CTD, one of which might be SSc.[8]

PROGNOSTIC FACTORS

Restrictive lung disease is common in patients with limited or diffuse SSc. A retrospective cohort study found that patients who reached an FVC <55% predicted were most likely to do so in the first 5 years of disease.[9] This highlights the importance of close pulmonary function monitoring early in the course of disease. Although antibodies in SSc are not known to play a role in the pathogenesis of the disease, they may serve as markers of subsets of patients with distinct clinical features. There are at least 7 SSc-specific autoantibodies, and several have been shown to be associated with SSc-related ILD (SSc-ILD). Antitopoisomerase antibodies (Scl-70) are associated with increased risk of interstitial fibrosis, although they do not predict severity.[10] Several studies show that anticentromere antibodies (ACA) are negatively associated with severe ILD.[11,12] Other autoantibodies associated with increased risk of SSc-ILD are the nucleolar autoantibodies anti-Th/To and anti-U3 ribonucleoprotein (RNP).[13,14] Patients with the anti-RNA polymerase III autoantibody usually do not develop severe ILD.[14] Additional factors also seem to play a role in SSc-ILD. In a prospective study involving a multiethnic cohort of patients with SSc with less than 5 years of disease duration, several important independent associations portended early pulmonary involvement (eg, serum creatinine and creatine phosphokinase levels, skin score, African American ethnicity, cardiac involvement, and hypothyroidism).[15]

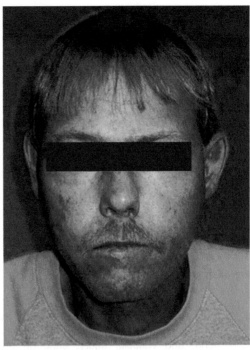

Fig. 2. Characteristic facial features in patient with SSc, with skin thickening and telangiectasias.

CLINICAL FEATURES

Patients may present with puffy fingers or sclerodactyly (thickening of skin over the digits), loss of the digital fat pads, pitting or ulceration of the digits, and RP (**Fig. 1**). Depending on the type of SSc, skin thickening may be limited to the digits and distal extremities (lcSSc), or may be more diffuse and involve most of the integument (dcSSc) (**Fig. 2**). Calcinosis, telangiectasias, poikiloderma, and other skin manifestations can also be clues to the diagnosis (**Fig. 3**). A small subset of patients

who have no skin tightening are in the SSc sine scleroderma category.

Patients with SSc-ILD may present in a variety of ways, making it essential that clinicians remain vigilant in monitoring and screening patients. Some patients with SSc-ILD are asymptomatic; however, the most common complaint is dyspnea on exertion, which may progress to symptoms at rest as the disease worsens. Cough that often is nonproductive, fatigue, and atypical chest pain may also be present. If productive cough,

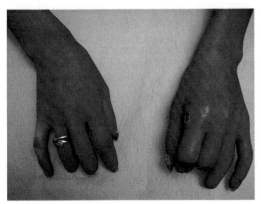

Fig. 1. Sclerodactyly, digital ulcerations, gangrene, and amputation in a patient with systemic sclerosis.

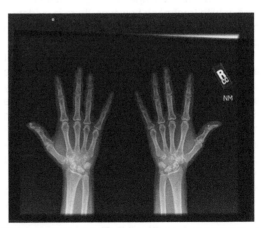

Fig. 3. Patient with SSc, and presence of calcinosis at the left first digit.

hemoptysis, or chest pain is present, infection, aspiration, neoplasm, alveolar hemorrhage, pleural and pericardial disease, cardiac abnormality, or bronchiectasis must be ruled out. Anemia, respiratory muscle weakness, cardiac disease, and deconditioning may contribute to the patient's breathlessness, thus complicating the evaluation of dyspnea.

Physical examination may be normal, but the most common finding is the presence of fine, inspiratory crackles with a Velcrolike sound, predominantly at the lung bases. Clubbing is rarely seen in SSc, contrary to other ILDs, possibly related to sclerodactyly. As ILD and related fibrosis progresses, cor pulmonale may ensue, with peripheral edema, right ventricular heave, cyanosis, and right-sided regurgitant murmurs.

PATHOGENESIS

The pathogenesis of ILD, including SSc-ILD, remains uncertain. There is a complex interplay between inflammatory activation, immunologic phenomena, and vascular injury, although the exact sequence of events remains elusive.

Although the analysis of bronchoalveolar lavage fluid (BALF) in diagnosis and management of SSc-ILD has recently been questioned,[16] it has provided insight into pathogenesis. Bronchoalveolar lavage provides an invaluable method of obtaining cultures and cells from the lower respiratory tract for investigation, and its merits from a research perspective were recently highlighted.[17] Silver and colleagues[18] first reported that, among patients with SSc and restrictive lung disease, a subset had increased levels of eosinophils or neutrophils (polymorphonuclear neutrophil leukocytes [PMNs]) in BALF. BALF cellularity does not seem to be independently associated with change in lung function over time or with treatment; however, there is evidence based on many studies for an imbalance between profibrotic and antifibrotic factors in BALF.

Myofibroblasts are distinctive fibroblasts that express α-smooth muscle actin (α-SMA) and are associated with a variety of fibrotic lesions. They seem to be the major cell responsible for the fibrosis seen in SSc-ILD and may evolve from multiple sources by numerous processes. BALF from patients with SSc-ILD contains myofibroblasts.[19,20] Patients with active ILD are believed to be those with increased cellularity in BALF, and are more likely to have an outgrowth of myofibroblasts.[19] Several factors found in BALF may play roles in the inflammatory and fibrosing process underlying SSc-ILD. There is overexpression of growth factors, cytokines, chemokines, coagulation factors, and eicosanoids in patients with SSc-ILD compared with normal controls. Increased amounts of fibrin, fibronectin, thrombin, and tumor necrosis factor-alpha (TNFα) are found, as well as transforming growth factor-β (TGF-β), connective tissue growth factor (CTGF, CCN2), platelet-derived growth factor, interleukin (IL)-1α, IL-8, IL-10 and macrophage inflammatory protein-1α (MIP-1 α).[19–23]

SSc lung fibroblasts express decreased levels of caveolin-1 protein (a scaffold for signaling molecules), compared with normal lung fibroblasts. Caveolin depletion seems to activate signaling molecules, leading to overexpression of collagen, α-SMA and tenascin-C.[24] In a murine model of SSc-ILD the in vivo fibrotic response was reduced by replacing caveolin-1 activity, and increased caveolin-1 levels reverses the scleroderma phenotype of SSc-ILD lung fibroblasts in vitro.[25,26] The antifibrotic factor, hepatocyte growth factor (HGF), was also recently shown to be deficient in some patients. Decreased HGF, as well as abnormalities in its antifibrotic signaling pathway, is seen in African Americans, an ethnic group known to have more severe SSc-ILD.[27]

Although the initiating event(s) in SSc-ILD remains unknown, there is accumulating evidence for alveolar epithelial cell and pulmonary capillary endothelial cell injury. Endothelial cell injury is widespread in SSc. Functional studies indicate the presence of pulmonary capillary endothelial dysfunction before the occurrence of PF.[28] 99mTc diethylenetriamine pentaacetate (99m-Tc-DTPA) clearance scans also show increased radionuclide clearance consistent with an abnormality at the alveolar epithelial cell barrier.[29] Ultrastructural analysis of SSc lung tissues shows epithelial and endothelial cell injury occurring together with interstitial edema and excess collagen deposition.[30] Histochemical studies of SSc-ILD tissues show alveolar epithelial cell injury characterized by increased expression of tissue factor and increased expression of surfactant protein.[31]

Genetic factors also play a critical role in the development of CTD in general, and recently several genetic susceptibility factors have been studied in SSc, including BANK-1, IRF5, and STAT4.[32–34] The type 1 interferon (IFN) signature has been characterized in the development of SSc, among other CTDs. Recently, STAT4 rs7574865, was studied and noted to be a new SSc genetic susceptibility factor with an odds ratio (OR) of 1.29, confidence interval (CI) 1.11 to 1.51, P = .001, and there was an additive effect with interferon regulatory factors (IRF) on susceptibility of disease and SSc-ILD.[33]

Dieudé and colleagues[32] showed a significant association between the IRF5 rs2004640 functional polymorphism and the development of SSc, with the TT genotype being associated with SSc-ILD (OR 1.02, CI 1.07–3.44, P = .029).

HISTOPATHOLOGY

A large retrospective study examined lung biopsies of 80 patients with SSc undergoing open or thoracoscopic lung biopsy.[35] The most frequent histopathologic pattern was NSIP (n = 62; 78%), with cellular NSIP (n = 15) and fibrotic NSIP (n = 47) occurring in 24% and 76%, respectively.[35] UIP (n = 6) and end-stage lung (ESL) (n = 6) made up 15% of patients, with other patterns comprising the remaining 6 patients.[35] Five-year survival did not differ significantly between the NSIP and UIP/ESL groups and was 91% and 82%, respectively. Mortality was associated with reduced initial DLCO (P = .004) and FVC (P = .007), although survival and trends in DLCO and FVC did not differ among NSIP cellular and fibrotic subsets.[35] Outcome did not seem to be related to histopathologic classification, thus the routine use of surgical lung biopsy is no longer necessary when imaging (ie, high-resolution computed tomography [HRCT]) findings are typical.[35]

Recently, de Carvalho and colleagues[36,37] described a unique histopathologic pattern of interstitial pneumonia termed centrilobular fibrosis (CLF), characterized by a prevalent bronchocentric distribution of lesions, bronchi containing intraluminal foreign bodies, and basophilic matter with occasional multinucleated giant cells. This underappreciated pattern of ILD has been causally linked to chronic aspiration. In a study by de Souza and colleagues[37] various clinical, histopathologic, and radiological attributes were found to support the link between aspiration and the development of SSc-ILD.

PFTs

Patients with SSc-ILD have a restrictive pulmonary physiology. TLC and FVC are used to measure severity of restriction and lung disease in ILD, with percentage of FVC (FVC%) predicted being the most commonly used outcome in clinical trials for SSc. FVC is highly reproducible, but performance of the test is effort dependent, and restriction can also be observed with muscle weakness, space-occupying abnormalities such as effusions and significant cardiomegaly, restricting chest wall or pleural abnormalities, and splinting because of pain. DLCO is decreased in SSc primarily as a result of parenchymal inflammation and fibrosis leading to thickening of the interstitium as seen in ILD, chronic hypoxemia leading to pulmonary vasoconstriction and loss of arterioles, or pulmonary artery (PA)/arteriole intimal hyperplasia and medial hypertrophy as seen in PAH. Changes in pulmonary function often occur before onset of significant symptoms; therefore, it is recommended that all patients with SSc undergo baseline PFT screening with spirometry and DLCO. Patients with dcSSc have been shown to have a greater risk of SSc-ILD and more rapid lung function decline than patients with lcSSc, and should undergo PFTs every 3 to 6 months for the first 5 years, or more frequently if pulmonary symptoms develop or ILD or PAH is present.[38,39] Patients with lcSSc have a higher risk of developing PAH, and should undergo testing every 6 to 12 months, even if the patient is asymptomatic and lung function is stable.[40] FVC less than 80% predicted has been reported to have a sensitivity of 80% and specificity of 72.4% (positive predictive value [PPV] 60%, negative predictive value [NPV] 87.5%) to predict a low TLC (<80% predicted) in patients with SSc, but sensitivity of only 70.8% and specificity of 86.3% to detect a low DLCO (<80% predicted) (PPV 85%, NPV 73%).[41] Prior studies have used a change in FVC% predicted of 10% or more from baseline or a change in DLCO% predicted of 15% or more from baseline as a clinically significant change in lung function with change in FVC% predicted proving to be the most reliable outcome measure.[42–44]

Progression of lung disease in SSc is variable and difficult to predict. However, pulmonary function measures early in the disease process may predict progression of ILD and mortality. Steen and colleagues[10] observed that during the first 2 years after SSc-ILD diagnosis, the rate of decline in FVC was 32% per year and decreased after 3 years to 3% per year. In a retrospective study of white patients with SSc-ILD without isolated PAH, patients who had a baseline decreased FVC of less than 80% predicted measured up to 3 years from disease onset were more likely to have a decline of 15 points or more of FVC% predicted and decreased DLCO of less than 40% predicted at 5 years compared with patients with SSc-ILD with a normal baseline FVC (25% vs 11% had FVC decline, P = .04 and 32% vs 11% had DLCO decline, P = .01).[45] In addition, the median time to DLCO decline to less than 70% predicted was 6 years for subjects with normal baseline FVC, versus 2 years for those with decreased baseline FVC of less than 80% predicted (P<.001).[45] Other studies have shown that FVC less than 70% predicted is the strongest predictor of pulmonary progression.[46]

The Genetics versus Environment in Scleroderma Outcome Study (GENISOS) is a prospective study assessing differences by ethnicity in multiple clinical and genetic parameters in subjects with SSc with similar average disease duration of 2.6 (±1.6) years. African Americans had more PF (25.5%) compared with white (12.3%) or Hispanic Americans (19.7%), and presented with lower FVC% predicted (75.8% ± 24.0% predicted) compared with white (88.1% ± 19.1% predicted) and Hispanic Americans (83.0% ± 23.7% predicted), as well as lower FEV$_1$ and DLCO (69% ± 21.4% vs 75.4% ± 24.8% and 79.5% ± 27.2% predicted, respectively).[15] Age-adjusted mortalities did not reveal increased mortality in African Americans in this study; however, FVC less than 50% predicted and DLCO less than 60% predicted were associated with increased mortality in the bivariate analysis with age.[47] A multivariate analysis in the same study, adjusting for age, body mass index (BMI), ACA, PF by radiograph, arrhythmia on electrocardiogram, and blood pressure, showed that FVC less than 50% predicted was associated with increased mortality with a hazard ratio (95% CI) of 4.8 (2.1–11.3), P<.001. When adding HLA genetics and race covariates, the mortality hazard ratio associated with FVC less than 50% predicted increased to 7.3 (2.8–19.1), P<.001.[47]

THE 6-MINUTE WALK TEST

Six-minute walk distance (6MWD) is frequently used as an outcome measure in clinical trials in ILD because of its high reproducibility and prognostic value.[48,49] In a multicenter study of 163 subjects with SSc-ILD with mean (±SD) FVC% predicted of 71% (±15.4%) and DLCO 46% (±12.4%) who had limited 6MWD less than 500 m because of dyspnea or walked 500 m or more but had oxygen desaturation during the walk, the mean 6MWD on 2 tests separated by less than 4 weeks was 396.6 (±84.6) m and 399.5 (±86.3) m (r = 0.95, P<.001). There were statistically significant but weak correlations of 6MWT with FVC% predicted (r = −0.19, P = .02) and Borg dyspnea index (r = −0.28, P<.001), and no correlation with DLCO.[50] Statistical correlation has been observed in SSc between a 6MWD of less than 400 m and oxygen desaturation of 4% or more during the walk. Both variables were associated with age 36 years or older, dyspnea index, fibrosis on chest radiography, and systolic pulmonary artery pressure (sPAP) 30 mm Hg or more measured by echocardiography. 6MWT oxygen desaturation of 4% or more was also associated with positive anti-Scl-70 autoantibody, FVC less

than 80% predicted, and presence of ground glass or reticular opacities on HRCT.[51] However, in the same study, multivariate logistic regression analysis showed only age 36 years or older, race, and dyspnea index were associated with 6MWD less than 400 m, whereas age 36 years or older, dyspnea index, anti-Scl-70 antibodies, and FVC less than 80% predicted were associated with oxygen desaturation during 6MWT. In SSc, there are multiple factors in addition to ILD that can influence the 6MWD, including musculoskeletal pain or weakness, peripheral vascular disease, and potential coexisting PAH; therefore, the specificity of 6MWT to follow progression of disease has been questioned. Garin and colleagues[52] reported that leg pain was the primary limitation in the 6MWD in 20% of subjects with SSc compared with 15% of subjects with idiopathic lung fibrosis (IPF), which may explain some of the lack of correlation with pulmonary function and 6MWD in SSc-ILD compared with IPF. In subjects with SSc overall, statistically significant correlations were observed between 6MWD and FVC when FVC is 60% predicted or less and 6MWD and PAP when sPAP is 45 mm Hg or more.[52]

IMAGING IN SCLERODERMA-RELATED ILD

HRCT is the most frequently used imaging modality for radiologic assessment of ILD. There is a correlation between findings on HRCT scans and chest radiographs; however, HRCT is more sensitive at detecting early ILD and more accurate at quantifying degree of interstitial fibrosis in patients with more progressive lung involvement.[53] The HRCT radiographic findings of NSIP can include GGO (increased lung attenuation believed to be associated with an active inflammatory process) and PF (reticular interstitial thickening with traction bronchiectasis or bronchiolectasis), both of which are typically bilateral, spatially uniform, and predominantly in the bases of the lungs (Fig. 4A).[54] Honeycomb cysts (HC; clustered air-filled cysts with visible walls) are more commonly associated with UIP (PPV 90%) and are typically present with reticular findings that are bilateral, spatially inhomogeneous, peripheral or subpleural, and occur predominantly in the bases of the lungs (see Fig. 4B). In the Scleroderma Lung Study (SLS), 91.2% of subjects had GGO, 92.9% had PF, and 37.2% had HC without significant difference between lcSSc and dcSSc for GGO, but greater PF seen in lcSSc and increased probability of HC in middle and upper lung zones at presentation. Overall, lower lung zones were more commonly affected and tended to have greater progression than middle

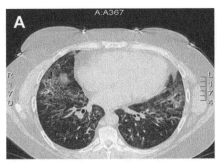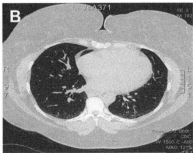

Fig. 4. (*A*) HRCT with mixture of GGO, honeycombing, traction bronchiectasis, and fibrosis consistent with NSIP pattern of ILD. (*B*) Lower lobe predominant peripheral honeycombing with absence of ground glass opacifications consistent with UIP pattern of ILD.

or upper lung zones (45% vs 30%). Only PF correlated with FVC and DLCO; and, unexpectedly, GGO correlated only weakly with active alveolitis as determined by BAL ($r = 0.28$, $P<.01$).[55] Intricate scoring systems have been developed for staging of ILD for research purposes and monitoring of disease progression; however, these methods require specific training and are typically performed at institutions with extensive research and clinical expertise in ILD. In the SLS study mentioned earlier,[55] the κ statistic for interobserver agreement was 0.72 for GGO, 0.61 for PF, and only 0.39 for HC. Therefore, CT densitometry, using a computer-generated scoring system to measure lung attenuation, has been evaluated. At least 1 study has shown increased intraoperator ($k = 0.97$) and interoperator ($k = 0.96$) reproducibility of mean lung attenuation using CT densitometry that were higher than those of a scoring system using visual assessment (intraobserver $k = 0.71$; interobserver $k = 0.69$), and CT densitometry mean lung attenuation better correlated with pulmonary function.[56] Goh and colleagues[57] developed a simplified staging system for SSc-ILD that combined HRCT analysis with PFT as a prediction for mortality and disease progression. Staging was determined by analysis of 5 levels of the HRCT for total disease extent, extent of reticulation, proportion of ground glass, and coarseness of reticulation, with disease extent defined as extensive (>20%), limited (<20%), or indeterminate. The indeterminate group was then classified based on PFT as extensive (FVC <70% predicted) or limited (FVC ≥70% predicted).[57] This combined staging system was a better predictor for mortality than either element alone, and the strongest predictor in multivariate models as well as in models including treatment or observation. In addition, this method of CT analysis had good interobserver agreement ($k = 0.64$) among physicians; less technical experience was needed

to master scoring, which suggests that this system could be used more broadly.

Sonographic imaging has recently been applied in conditions affecting the lung interstitium. This method is appealing because it is easily accessible and can be done at the bedside without incurring radiation exposure. The sonographic finding of ultrasound lung comets (ULCs), an echogenic image of multiple comet tails fanning out from the surface of the lung, arises from associated fibrosis or water-thickened interlobular septae.[58,59] In a recent study in which sonography was compared with the gold standard of HRCT, the presence of ULCs was found to correlate reasonably ($r = 0.72$, $P<.001$) with HRCT-derived assessment of lung fibrosis (Warrick scores), and ULCs scores were higher in patients with dcSSc versus lcSSc (73 ± 66 vs 21 ± 35, respectively, $P<.05$).[58] There was also a significant negative correlation between ULC number and DLCO ($r = -0.60$, $P<.05$).[58] Therefore, ultrasonography may have a potential role in the diagnosis and monitoring of SSc-ILD, and further study is warranted.

BIOMARKERS

There is a critical need for less invasive, clinically applicable biomarkers to improve the prospective evaluation of patients with SSc-ILD. Surfactant protein D (SP-D) and Krebs von den Lungen-6 (KL-6) are glycoproteins secreted by type II pneumocytes that have emerged as possible surrogates for ILD. Serum levels of SP-D increase when there is damage to the alveolar epithelium, such as in the alveolitis of SSc-ILD.[60–62] SP-D levels correlate with the presence of PF in SSc.[63] KL-6 directly reflects alveolar damage and inflammation and enters the circulation because of increased vascular and epithelial permeability, suggesting its use as a serologic marker to mirror the extent of alveolar damage.[64] We studied these

2 biomarkers in patients with SSc who were enrolled in the SLS, and found that serum levels of SP-D and KL-6 seem to indicate alveolitis in patients with SSc-ILD.[65] We found that SP-D had a sensitivity of 85% and specificity of 80%, and KL-6 had a sensitivity and specificity of 79% and 90%, respectively, for the diagnosis of active alveolitis.

Other possible markers of SSc-ILD that are actively being investigated as potential biomarkers include APRIL, a proliferation-inducing ligand, and a member of the TNF superfamily;[66] TNF-like weak inducer of apoptosis (TWEAK), another member of the TNF superfamily;[67] von Willebrand factor (vWf), serum levels of PMN elastase, exhaled nitric oxide (CA$_{NO}$), chemokine (C-C motif) ligand 13 (CCL13), and soluble E-selectin (sES).[68,69] The usefulness of using biomarkers to attempt to correlate and assess clinical response to treatment is a promising area, and more research is necessary to prove their true effectiveness in aiding in the diagnosis of SSc-ILD.

TREATMENT

The treatment of SSc-ILD is complicated by the many phenotypes seen in SSc. As each patient has a unique clinical, serologic, and radiographic picture, there is no single treatment that has been shown to work in all patients, and few randomized trials have been performed in this rare and enigmatic disease.

Immunosuppressive Agents

Because of the autoimmune nature of SSc, various therapeutic approaches targeting immune mechanisms are being evaluated. Several previous studies showed the promise of cyclophosphamide (CYC) as a treatment of SSc-ILD, despite its known toxicity and concerns about long-term safety. The first randomized double-blind placebo-controlled trial of CYC versus placebo in symptomatic SSc-ILD was not published until 2006 (SLS).[43] In this study, which included patients from 13 sites across the United States, 158 patients with symptomatic SSc-ILD were eligible to participate based on screening criteria; 145 completed at least 6 months of treatment and were included in the analysis.[43] CYC taken for 1 year had a modest, but significant, effect on improving lung function (changes in FVC and TLC), dyspnea (transitional dyspnea index scores), health-related quality of life (health transition and vitality), and skin scores (thickening).[43] CYC was associated with an increase in toxicity compared with placebo, although long-term effects are unknown, and safer, less toxic alternatives are

necessary. A follow-up analysis to the SLS was done to determine whether the effects of CYC treatment were sustained at 2 years. They found that, except for improvement in dyspnea, the effects on lung function, health-related quality of life, and skin scores were no longer apparent at 24 months.[70] Based on the SLS results, a current phase III trial is underway comparing CYC with mycophenolate mofetil (MMF) in the treatment of active SSc-ILD. The results of this trial are highly anticipated because MMF is considered to be a less toxic agent than CYC, although concerns about immunosuppressive therapies will always be raised.

Other therapies have also been evaluated, or at least have the potential to target SSc-associated fibrosis based on their various mechanisms of action and targets. IFN-α and -γ, pirfenidone, anti-TGF-β antibodies, anti-CTGF antibodies, halofuginone, and tyrosine kinase inhibitors (imatinib mesylate, dasatinib, nilotinib) may be useful, but further study is necessary and ongoing.[71]

Rituximab, a monoclonal antibody directed against the B cell CD20 antigen, has been proposed as a potential therapy in SSc-ILD. A recent small study was performed on 14 patients with SSc-ILD to assess the possible efficacy of rituximab.[72] They showed improvement in median FVC% predicted (10.25% vs 5.04%, $P = .002$) and DLCO% predicted (19.46% vs 7.5%, $P = .023$) in patients treated with rituximab compared with controls, respectively. Further randomized controlled trials should be considered.[72]

A recent review regarding therapeutics in SSc discussed compounds studied in vivo or in animal models with antifibrotic effects.[71] Some of these, such as human latency-associated peptide, SKL-2841, Src kinase inhibitors, CpG oligonucleotides, IL-12–encoding plasmid, campthothecin, histone deacetylase inhibitors, paclitaxel, and chondroitin sulfate, may lead to future drug therapeutics in SSc-related fibrosis.[71]

Lung Transplantation

In patients with SSc and end-stage pulmonary involvement unresponsive to available medical therapies, lung transplantation (LTX) should be considered, because previous studies have shown similar 2-year survival rates after LTX in patients with SSc-ILD compared with patients with IPF and idiopathic PA hypertension (IPAH).[73] A recent review of the literature examined LTX in 54 patients with SSc. They noted a mean age of 47.1 years with 59% of patients being women, and, of the 24 patients with preoperative lung data, 22 (92%) had PF and 17 (71%) had pulmonary hypertension

(PH).[74] Most patients (69%) underwent single-lung transplantation.[74] They determined that LTX was a suitable option in well-selected patients with SSc-ILD, because their series and those reported at single- and multicenter studies showed no differences in the early and late mortalities between patients receiving LTX for SSc versus other conditions.[74] Two- and 5-year survival rates for the 54 patients with SSc were 72% and 55%, respectively,[74] which is similar to rates reported by the International Society for Heart and Lung Transplantation for other conditions. That review suggested criteria for LTX in the SSc population that may serve to aid future studies regarding this area (**Table 1**).[74]

Stem Cell Transplantation

There have been several series studying the use of high-dose immunosuppression and autologous/allogenic hematopoietic stem cell transplantation in SSc. A phase I to II study (n = 6) showed improvement in skin scores and lung function with improved vital capacity and respiratory function.[75] It also reported, for the first time, a regression in GGO by HRCT, and no transplantation-related deaths occurred.[75] Two phase III trials are currently ongoing in Europe and the United States: Autologous Stem Cell Transplantation International Scleroderma trial (ASTIS) and Scleroderma Cyclophosphamide or Transplantation (SCOT), respectively. Both studies

have similar primary end points of event-free survival, but with different regimens for mobilization and conditioning, and their results will add vital knowledge to a promising therapeutic option in severe SSc.[71,76]

PAH

The other significant pulmonary complication commonly encountered in patients with SSc is PAH (**Box 2**). Detection and surveillance for PAH is vital in this patient population at high risk for this potentially fatal complication, especially because newer treatments have led to improved symptoms and function in patients with SSc-PAH.

The true prevalence of PAH in SSc is not known, but is estimated to be between 8% and 12%, when diagnosed by the gold standard, right heart catheterization (RHC).[77,78] PAH has been considered to occur as a late pulmonary manifestation in SSc, and more frequently in patients with lcSSc.[40,79] However, a recent retrospective study suggested that annual screening for PAH for patients with SSc should occur regardless of subtype. They categorized PAH as early or late based on PAH diagnosis within 5 years of the first non-RP symptom of SSc, and found that PAH occurred 6.3 (±6.6) years (mean ± SD, CI 2.88–6.0) after the diagnosis of SSc, with 55.1% and

Table 1
Suggested criteria for LTX in patients with SSc
1. Severe PF (FVC and DLCO <40%), unresponsive to medical treatment
2. Absence of severe pulmonary hypertension (mean PAP <45 mm Hg)
3. Absence of large pericardial effusion
4. Absence of severe small intestine, gastroparesis, rectal, and colorectal involvement
5. Absence of severe esophageal dysmotility and aspiration
6. Absence of severe skin involvement
7. Absence of significant cardiac conduction abnormalities (symptomatic bradycardia, atrial and ventricular tachycardia)
8. Creatinine clearance >50 mL/min

Data from Shitrit D, Amital A, Peled N, et al. Lung transplantation in patients with scleroderma: case series, review of the literature, and criteria for transplantation. Clin Transplant 2009;23(2):181.

Box 2
World Health Organization Diagnostic Classification of PH
1. PAH
Idiopathic
Familial
Associated with:
• CTD
• Congenital systemic-to-pulmonary shunts
• Portal hypertension
• Human immunodeficiency virus infection
• Drugs/toxins
• Other
2. PH as a result of left heart disease
3. PH as a result of hypoxemia or pulmonary disease
4. PH associated with chronic thromboembolism
5. PH caused by multifactorial mechanisms

Data from Simonneau G, Robbins I, Beghetti M, et al. Updated clinical classification of pulmonary hypertension. J Am Coll Cardiol 2009;54:S45.

44.9% of patients receiving a diagnosis of early onset PAH and late onset PAH, respectively.[80] Patients with early onset PAH (mean age, 58 ± 12.5 years) were generally older than those with late onset PAH (mean age 46.6 ± 12.9 years) (P = .0002), and PAH seemed to be more severe in early onset PAH with lower cardiac index and greater pulmonary resistance, although 3- and 5-year mortality did not differ between groups.[80] There did not seem to be differences in the SSc subtype (limited vs diffuse cutaneous), age at time of PAH diagnosis, or autoantibody status (anti-Scl-70 vs anticentromere), and early onset PAH occurred in approximately 50% of patients, as frequently in patients with dcSSc as with lcSSc.[80]

Histologically, the pulmonary vascular lesion in SSc-PAH resembles that of idiopathic PAH. In SSc, microvascular endothelial cell injury and death occurs, leading to small vessel alterations and organ malfunction.[81] Antiendothelial antibodies (AECA) are present in the serum of 40% to 50% of patients with SSc; moreover, AECA titers are inversely correlated with DLCO and positively correlated with PAH, suggesting a pathologic role of AECA contributing to vascular disease in SSc[82] Imbalanced endothelial vascular signals are also important. Endothelin production is amplified, and nitric oxide and prostacyclin release are impaired, leading to vasospasm as well as intimal proliferation, vascular fibrosis, and stiffness of vascular walls.[81] Activation of platelets and coagulation augmentation with decreased fibrinolysis also leads to fibrin deposition and then to luminal reduction and intimal proliferation.[81] These mechanisms leading to vascular change in SSc-PAH have served as the basis for therapeutic targets in clinical trials, as discussed later.

PH is defined as a mean pulmonary arterial pressure (mPAP) of 25 mm Hg or more at rest and a normal pulmonary capillary wedge pressure or left ventricular end diastolic pressure less than or equal to 15 mm Hg. In SSc, PH may occur as a primary event or secondary to ILD or cardiomyopathy with diastolic dysfunction. Mathai and colleagues[83] recently studied 39 patients with SSc-PAH and 20 patients with SSc-ILD–associated PH to see the effect of ILD on survival in these patients. Survival was significantly worse in patients with SSc-ILD–associated PH than in those with SSc-PAH, with 1-, 2-, and 3-year survival rates of 82%, 46%, and 39% compared with 87%, 79%, and 64%, respectively (P<.01).[83]

Clinical features of PAH are often absent early in the course of disease and progress without intervention, with more symptoms occurring in later stages. The earliest features may be a decreased exercise tolerance and a perception of dyspnea on exertion. In time, increased dyspnea on exertion may occur, with progression to shortness of breath at rest. Fatigue, chest pain, syncope, and near-syncope events may occur as a result of right ventricular angina and reduced cardiac reserve.[84] Physical examination is often normal early in the course of disease; late in the disease, a loud pulmonary second heart sound (P2), increased jugular venous pressure, lower extremity edema, ascites, and anasarca may be present. Once clinical symptoms occur and signs of right-sided heart failure are present, prognosis is poor with a median survival as brief as 12 months.[85,86]

Markers to aid in the diagnostic and prognostic assessment of patients with SSc-PAH are greatly needed. Williams and colleagues[87] studied 109 patients with SSc, 68 with SSc-PAH and 41 without PAH, to examine levels of N-terminal brain natriuretic peptide (N-TproBNP). N-TproBNP levels positively correlated with mean PAP (r = 0.62, P<.0001), pulmonary vascular resistance (PVR; r = 0.81, P<.0001), and negatively correlated with 6MWD (r = −0.46, P<.0001).[87] This study made several conclusions, including that raised N-TproBNP levels are directly related to the severity of PAH, and that baseline and longitudinal changes in N-TproBNP are predictive of survival, because they found that a tenfold increase in N-TproBNP while on therapy for PAH was associated with a greater than threefold increase in mortality.[87] They also suggested that, in screening patients with SSc, an N-TproBNP greater than 395 pg/mL is highly probable for having PAH in this patient population.[87]

ROLE OF PFTS AND 6-MINUTE WALK TESTING IN PAH

FVC% predicted and DLCO have been observed to be abnormal in PH associated with SSc, with DLCO often out of proportion with the extent of ILD as an indicator of PH. In a study of 114 patients with SSc, PH (defined as a right ventricular systolic pressure [RVSP] >40 mm Hg on echocardiography) was found in 33 (29%) patients, and was associated with higher prevalence of SSc-ILD on HRCT (64% vs 91%, P = .005 with OR 6.78, CI 1.54–29.9). FVC% predicted was lower in patients with PH compared with those without (82.9% ± 20.7% vs 73.9% ± 22.9% predicted, P = .044), and FVC less than 80% predicted was independently associated with PH (OR 3.03, CI 1.1–8.35), despite presence or absence of ILD. RP at least 3 years before onset of skin changes (OR 5.75, CI 1.9–17.41) was also an independent predictor of PH, whereas age, disease duration, disease subtype, and antibodies were not.[88]

The DLCO has been observed to be more significantly reduced in SSc-PH compared with IPAH cohorts even with absence of coexisting ILD (48.7% ± 2.4% vs 68.4% ± 3.4% predicted; $P<.001$).[89] In addition, DLCO has been shown to be significantly lower in SSc-ILD–associated PH compared with isolated SSc-PAH (31% ± 12% vs 51% ± 15% predicted, $P = .01$).[83] FVC% predicted/DLCO% predicted ratio of 2 or more has been used as a surrogate screening measure for the presence of SSc-PAH, but the sensitivity and specificity in SSc is not ideal, at 71% and 72% respectively.[90] This parameter was not significantly associated with mortality in SSc.[47]

Dyspnea on exertion is a common symptom in patients with PAH with eventual progression to dyspnea at rest. Although most measurements are performed at rest, a subset of individuals will only have PAH with exertion. In a study of 41 subjects with SSc, mean resting sPAP was 29.7 mm Hg, increasing to 41.4 mm Hg during exercise, and 26.8% had sPAP of more than 50 mm Hg and 19.5% more than 55 mm Hg. There was a significant correlation with sPAP and DLCO ($r = -0.4$, $P = .008$) and lower DLCO in the group with exercise-induced PAH with sPAP more than 55 mm Hg (78.9% vs 92.7% predicted, $P = .03$) with a DLCO of less than 72% predicted having 79.9% sensitivity and 76.3% specificity to detect exercise-induced PAH with sPAP more than 55 mm Hg. There were also significant correlations with BNP levels and increased prevalence of severe Raynaud phenomenon.[91]

ECHOCARDIOGRAPHY AND RHC IN SSC-PAH

RHC remains the gold standard for the detection of PAH in SSc. Echocardiography cannot measure mean PAP, but estimates RVSP as a measure of the tricuspid valve gradient or velocity of tricuspid regurgitation plus right atrial pressure. Recommendations for screening for SSc-PAH are echocardiographic examination every 6 to 12 months with validation by RHC.[92]

Estimates of sPAP obtained by echocardiography compared with RHC show that tricuspid valve gradient of 45 mm Hg or more has a low specificity of 47%, but a high sensitivity of 97% (PPV 98%) for identifying patients with PAH-SSc compared with a tricuspid valve gradient of 35 mm Hg or more (specificity 75%, sensitivity 66%, PPV 85%).[93] Alternatively, tricuspid valve gradient less than 40 mm Hg was associated with increased false-positive

diagnoses.[94] However, echocardiography seems to be the most accurate noninvasive method to screen for PAH. Magnetic resonance imaging measurement of PA diameter is being explored as another noninvasive modality.[90,92]

Echocardiographic findings in SSc-PAH compared with IPAH showed more left-sided abnormalities, despite normal left ventricular systolic function, including increased prevalence of left atrial dilatation (10.5% vs 28.6%, $P = .04$), left ventricular hypertrophy (13.2% vs 34.7%, $P = .02$), and diastolic dysfunction (13.2% vs 32.7%, $P = .04$). Pericardial effusions were more common in SSc-PAH than IPAH (34.7% vs 13.2%, $P = .02$) with increased mortality associated with presence of an effusion (HR 2.35, 95% CI 1.06–5.20, $P = .035$).[89]

TREATMENT

Discussion of therapeutics for PAH in SSc is beyond the scope of this article, but they include drugs that target specific pathways in PAH, namely the prostacylin, nitric oxide, and endothelin pathways. Some therapies exist outside the United States, but these are not discussed in this article. Prostanoids (epoprostenol, iloprost, treprostinil) are administered by a variety of routes, including intravenous, inhaled, and subcutaneous, and their complexity requires close monitoring by a PH expert. Phosphodiesterase-5 inhibitors (sildenafil and tadalafil) act via the nitric oxide pathway, mediated through cyclic guanosine monophosphate. Endothelin-1 receptor antagonists, nonselective type A and B (bosentan) and selective type A forms (ambrisentan) are also used, and target the receptor of the potent vasoconstrictor endothelin-1.[71]

Patients with SSc-PAH should also receive general medical treatments, when indicated, including receiving oxygen supplementation, diuretics, digoxin, anticoagulation, and up-to-date vaccinations, and avoidance of certain drugs, tobacco use, high altitudes, and pregnancy.[95]

MISCELLANEOUS PULMONARY MANIFESTATIONS
Malignancy

Studies have reported an increased frequency of neoplasm in patients with SSc, with lung carcinoma, especially bronchoalveolar carcinoma, being the most common.[96] In the Pittsburgh cohort, 14 of 262 (5%) patients with SSc developed a malignancy, and an increase in lung cancer was observed in the setting of chronic PF even in the absence of tobacco use.[97] In a study by

Peters-Golden and colleagues,[98] 71 patients with SSc were followed for a mean of 5 years, and 3 cases of lung cancer were observed with 8.6 cases/1000 persons/y post hoc incidence of lung cancer. This compared with an expected incidence ratio of 0.52 cases/1000 persons/y, leading them to calculate a relative risk ratio for lung cancer in SSc of 16.5. Each of the 3 cases of lung cancer had radiographic evidence of PF, but no definite association with tobacco use.[98] Because neoplasm may occur before, during, or years after the diagnosis of SSc, patients should be monitored for this, especially if they receive immunosuppression, or when they present with hemoptysis.

Drug-induced Pulmonary Disease

D-Penicillamine has long been used to treat SSc, although its use is not supported by the results of a randomized trial comparing low and high doses.[99] This drug has been associated with bronchiolitis obliterans and Goodpasture syndrome. Other medications used in the treatment of SSc-ILD (including the standard of care therapy at this time, CYC) have been associated with pulmonary toxicity. CYC-induced lung toxicity is associated with an early onset pneumonitis felt to be reversible and amenable to treatment with corticosteroids, and a late-onset pneumonitis coupled with pleural thickening that is progressive and fairly unresponsive to corticosteroids.[100]

Aspiration Pneumonia

As a result of esophageal dysmotility and an incompetent lower esophageal sphincter, aspiration of gastric content occurs frequently in SSc. Direct aspiration may be a major mechanism involved in the pathogenesis of SSc-ILD. Aggressive antireflux treatment may be helpful to reduce pulmonary damage caused by aspiration in patients with SSc, because a direct correlation has been shown between reflux severity and PF severity.[101] Another more recent study emphasized the need for larger controlled studies to evaluate whether development of SSc-ILD can be prevented by preventing reflux.[102] Aspiration pneumonia should be suspected in any patient with SSc presenting with pneumonia or cough, especially if there is an overlap or related myositis that might increase the risk for aspiration.

Pleural Disease

Pleural disease occurs in SSc as a result of pleural effusions or fibrosis. Pleural effusions are rare in SSc, and their exact pathogenesis is not known. Association of pleural effusions with malignancy, vasculitis, infection, and heart failure need to be considered, and causation identified if possible.

Pneumoconiosis

There is a known association between inhalational silica exposure and SSc, and an entity linking SSc with exposure to silica particles, with or without the development of silicosis, is called the Erasmus syndrome.[103] Patients with silicosis in general are also noted to have alterations in immunity, with a recent article noting alterations in soluble interleukin 2 (sIL2) receptors in these patients.[104]

MCTD

Sharp and colleagues[105] in 1972 first described a new clinical entity termed MCTD, a disease process in which patients exhibit a combination of clinical features of SSc, systemic lupus erythematosus (SLE), and an inflammatory myopathy (polymyositis, PM, or dermatomyositis [DM]). Serologically, they often have high titers of speckled ANAs, and autoantibodies to uridine-rich small nuclear ribonucleoprotein (snRNP). These patients present clinically with a myriad of signs and symptoms, notably arthralgia/arthritis, RP, esophageal dysfunction, myalgia, muscle weakness, sclerodactyly, swollen hands, and lymphadenopathy. There is controversy regarding whether MCTD represents a distinct clinical entity. Classification criteria require 3 of the following: synovitis or myositis (1 must be present), hand edema, RP, acrosclerosis, and serologic evidence of positive anti-snRNP in at least a moderate titer.[105] Although initially not felt to involve the lung to a large degree, MCTD has several pulmonary disease associations (**Box 3**), a few of which are discussed in this article.

Because MCTD is a clinical combination of SLE, SSc, and PM/DM, the pulmonary manifestations of any of these disease processes may occur, and their discussion is beyond the scope of this article.

Box 3
Pulmonary manifestations of MCTD

1. ILD
2. Pleural effusion
3. Alveolar hemorrhage
4. Aspiration pneumonia/pneumonitis
5. PH
6. Pulmonary vasculitis
7. Thromboembolic disease
8. Infections
9. Obstructive airways disease
10. Diaphragmatic dysfunction

Prakash[106] described respiratory complications in the population of patients with MCTD and reported interstitial pneumonitis and fibrosis, pleural effusion, pleurisy, and PH as the major complications, comprising incidences of 20% to 65%, 50%, 20%, and 10% to 45%, respectively.

ILD

The prevalence and incidence of ILD in MCTD is not known. Clinical features are similar to those seen in patients with SSc. In a study comparing HRCT in MCTD with other specific CTDs (SLE, SSc, PM, DM), the CT findings in MCTD were a combination of the other CTDs.[107] A more recent retrospective study looking at HRCT findings in MCTD revealed that most patients with MCTD had intralobular reticular opacities, ground glass attenuation, and nonseptal linear opacities predominating in the lower and peripheral lung fields, although this was not correlated with histopathologic findings.[108] Another study showed that it was not possible to distinguish patients with MCTD from those with other CTDs based on routine PFTs.[109]

Pulmonary Vascular Disease

PAH is a manifestation of MCTD with high morbidity and mortality similar to SSc. The treatments are similar to SSc and may be helpful. Other potential complications are pulmonary vasculitis and pulmonary thromboembolic disease, which may respond to immunosuppression and anticoagulation, respectively.[110]

Pleural Disease

Pleural disease seems to be common in MCTD, with the overall incidence of pleural effusion estimated to be 50%.[111] Effusions are often exudates and transient in nature. Patients may also present with pleuritic chest pain.

Alveolar Hemorrhage

SLE is associated with alveolar hemorrhage and there are patients who can be classified as having MCTD who present with this life-threatening complication. The mechanism is not completely understood but may be related to immune complex deposition and a pulmonary capillaritis. Treatment involves corticosteroids and immunosuppressants.

SUMMARY

The CTDs, including SSc and MCTD, represent a heterogeneous, complex group of disorders that have important pulmonary manifestations.

Patients may present to the pulmonologist initially with only dyspnea as their chief complaint. The astute clinician must recognize the importance of screening for CTD in any patient presenting with ILD or PAH.

REFERENCES

1. Mayes MD, Lacey JV Jr, Beebe-Dimmer J, et al. Prevalence, incidence, survival, and disease characteristics of systemic sclerosis in a large US population. Arthritis Rheum 2003;48(8):2246–55.
2. Mayes MD, Reveille JD. Epidemiology, demographics and genetics. In: Clements PJ, Furst DE, editors. Systemic sclerosis. 2nd edition. Philadelphia: Lippincott Williams and Wilkins; 2004. p. 1–15.
3. Preliminary criteria for the classification of systemic sclerosis (scleroderma). Subcommittee for scleroderma criteria of the American Rheumatism Association diagnostic and therapeutic criteria committee. Arthritis Rheum 1980;23(5):581–90.
4. LeRoy EC, Black C, Fleischmajer R, et al. Scleroderma (systemic sclerosis): classification, subsets and pathogenesis. J Rheumatol 1988;15(2):202–5.
5. Steen VD, Medsger TA. Changes in causes of death in systemic sclerosis, 1972-2002. Ann Rheum Dis 2007;66(7):940–4.
6. American Thoracic Society/European Respiratory Society International Multidisciplinary Consensus Classification of the Idiopathic Interstitial Pneumonias. This joint statement of the American Thoracic Society (ATS), and the European Respiratory Society (ERS) was adopted by the ATS board of directors, June 2001 and by the ERS Executive Committee, June 2001. Am J Respir Crit Care Med 2002;165(2):277–304.
7. Varga J. Systemic sclerosis: an update. Bull NYU Hosp Jt Dis 2008;66(3):198–202.
8. Strange C, Highland KB. Interstitial lung disease in the patient who has connective tissue disease. Clin Chest Med 2004;25(3):549–59, vii.
9. Steen VD, Medsger TA Jr. Severe organ involvement in systemic sclerosis with diffuse scleroderma. Arthritis Rheum 2000;43(11):2437–44.
10. Steen VD, Conte C, Owens GR, et al. Severe restrictive lung disease in systemic sclerosis. Arthritis Rheum 1994;37(9):1283–9.
11. Kane GC, Varga J, Conant EF, et al. Lung involvement in systemic sclerosis (scleroderma): relation to classification based on extent of skin involvement or autoantibody status. Respir Med 1996; 90(4):223–30.
12. Steen VD, Powell DL, Medsger TA Jr. Clinical correlations and prognosis based on serum autoantibodies in patients with systemic sclerosis. Arthritis Rheum 1988;31(2):196–203.

13. Steen VD. Autoantibodies in systemic sclerosis. Bull Rheum Dis 1996;45(6):6–8.

14. Steen VD. Autoantibodies in systemic sclerosis. Semin Arthritis Rheum 2005;35(1):35–42.

15. McNearney TA, Reveille JD, Fischbach M, et al. Pulmonary involvement in systemic sclerosis: associations with genetic, serologic, sociodemographic, and behavioral factors. Arthritis Rheum 2007;57(2):318–26.

16. Strange C, Bolster MB, Roth MD, et al. Bronchoalveolar lavage and response to cyclophosphamide in scleroderma interstitial lung disease. Am J Respir Crit Care Med 2008;177(1):91–8.

17. Kowal-Bielecka O, Kowal K, Highland KB, et al. Bronchoalveolar lavage fluid in scleroderma interstitial lung disease: technical aspects and clinical correlations: review of the literature. Semin Arthritis Rheum 2009. [Epub ahead of print].

18. Silver RM, Metcalf JF, Stanley JH, et al. Interstitial lung disease in scleroderma. Analysis by bronchoalveolar lavage. Arthritis Rheum 1984;27(11):1254–62.

19. Ludwicka A, Trojanowska M, Smith EA, et al. Growth and characterization of fibroblasts obtained from bronchoalveolar lavage of patients with scleroderma. J Rheumatol 1992;19(11):1716–23.

20. Kinsella MB, Smith EA, Miller KS, et al. Spontaneous production of fibronectin by alveolar macrophages in patients with scleroderma. Arthritis Rheum 1989;32(5):577–83.

21. Ludwicka A, Ohba T, Trojanowska M, et al. Elevated levels of platelet derived growth factor and transforming growth factor-beta 1 in bronchoalveolar lavage fluid from patients with scleroderma. J Rheumatol 1995;22(10):1876–83.

22. Bolster MB, Ludwicka A, Sutherland SE, et al. Cytokine concentrations in bronchoalveolar lavage fluid of patients with systemic sclerosis. Arthritis Rheum 1997;40(4):743–51.

23. Bogatkevich GS, Tourkina E, Silver RM, et al. Thrombin differentiates normal lung fibroblasts to a myofibroblast phenotype via the proteolytically activated receptor-1 and a protein kinase C-dependent pathway. J Biol Chem 2001;276(48):45184–92.

24. Tourkina E, Gooz P, Pannu J, et al. Opposing effects of protein kinase Calpha and protein kinase Cepsilon on collagen expression by human lung fibroblasts are mediated via MEK/ERK and caveolin-1 signaling. J Biol Chem 2005;280(14):13879–87.

25. Tourkina E, Richard M, Gooz P, et al. Antifibrotic properties of caveolin-1 scaffolding domain in vitro and in vivo. Am J Physiol Lung Cell Mol Physiol 2008;294(5):L843–61.

26. Wang XM, Zhang Y, Kim HP, et al. Caveolin-1: a critical regulator of lung fibrosis in idiopathic pulmonary fibrosis. J Exp Med 2006;203(13):2895–906.

27. Bogatkevich GS, Ludwicka-Bradley A, Highland KB, et al. Impairment of the antifibrotic effect of hepatocyte growth factor in lung fibroblasts from African Americans: possible role in systemic sclerosis. Arthritis Rheum 2007;56(7):2432–42.

28. Orfanos SE, Psevdi E, Stratigis N, et al. Pulmonary capillary endothelial dysfunction in early systemic sclerosis. Arthritis Rheum 2001;44(4):902–11.

29. Nakano A, Yamaguchi E, Naitoh S, et al. [Assessment of alveolar epithelial permeability in progressive systemic sclerosis (PSS) using 99mTc-DTPA (diethylene triamine penta acetate) aerosol inhalation]. Nihon Kyobu Shikkan Gakkai Zasshi 1992;30(1):45–50 [in Japanese].

30. Harrison NK, Myers AR, Corrin B, et al. Structural features of interstitial lung disease in systemic sclerosis. Am Rev Respir Dis 1991;144(3 Pt 1):706–13.

31. Imokawa S, Sato A, Hayakawa H, et al. Tissue factor expression and fibrin deposition in the lungs of patients with idiopathic pulmonary fibrosis and systemic sclerosis. Am J Respir Crit Care Med 1997;156(2 Pt 1):631–6.

32. Dieudé P, Guedj M, Wipff J, et al. Association between the IRF5 rs2004640 functional polymorphism and systemic sclerosis: a new perspective for pulmonary fibrosis. Arthritis Rheum 2009;60(1):225–33.

33. Dieude P, Guedj M, Wipff J, et al. STAT4 is a genetic risk factor for systemic sclerosis having additive effects with IRF5 on disease susceptibility and related pulmonary fibrosis. Arthritis Rheum 2009;60(8):2472–9.

34. Dieude P, Wipff J, Guedj M, et al. BANK1 is a genetic risk factor for diffuse cutaneous systemic sclerosis and has additive effects with IRF5 and STAT4. Arthritis Rheum 2009;60(11):3447–54.

35. Bouros D, Wells AU, Nicholson AG, et al. Histopathologic subsets of fibrosing alveolitis in patients with systemic sclerosis and their relationship to outcome. Am J Respir Crit Care Med 2002;165(12):1581–6.

36. de Carvalho ME, Kairalla RA, Capelozzi VL, et al. Centrilobular fibrosis: a novel histological pattern of idiopathic interstitial pneumonia. Pathol Res Pract 2002;198(9):577–83.

37. de Souza RB, Borges CT, Capelozzi VL, et al. Centrilobular fibrosis: an underrecognized pattern in systemic sclerosis. Respiration 2009;77(4):389–97.

38. Clements PJ, Roth MD, Elashoff R, et al. Scleroderma lung study (SLS): differences in the presentation and course of patients with limited versus diffuse systemic sclerosis. Ann Rheum Dis 2007;66(12):1641–7.

39. Gilson M, Zerkak D, Wipff J, et al. Prognostic factors for lung function in systemic

sclerosis: prospective study of 105 cases. Eur Respir J 2010;35(1):112–7.

40. Chang B, Schachna L, White B, et al. Natural history of mild-moderate pulmonary hypertension and the risk factors for severe pulmonary hypertension in scleroderma. J Rheumatol 2006;33(2): 269–74.

41. Quadrelli SA, Molinari L, Ciallella LM, et al. Patterns of pulmonary function in smoking and nonsmoking patients with progressive systemic sclerosis. Rheumatol Int 2009;29(9):995–9.

42. Ioannidis JP, Vlachoyiannopoulos PG, Haidich AB, et al. Mortality in systemic sclerosis: an international meta-analysis of individual patient data. Am J Med 2005;118(1):2–10.

43. Tashkin DP, Elashoff R, Clements PJ, et al. Cyclophosphamide versus placebo in scleroderma lung disease. N Engl J Med 2006;354(25):2655–66.

44. Wells AU, Behr J, Silver R. Outcome measures in the lung. Rheumatology (Oxford) 2008;47(Suppl 5):v48–50.

45. Plastiras SC, Karadimitrakis SP, Ziakas PD, et al. Scleroderma lung: initial forced vital capacity as predictor of pulmonary function decline. Arthritis Rheum 2006;55(4):598–602.

46. Marie I, Ducrotte P, Denis P, et al. Oesophageal mucosal involvement in patients with systemic sclerosis receiving proton pump inhibitor therapy. Aliment Pharmacol Ther 2006;24(11–12):1593–601.

47. Assassi S, Del Junco D, Sutter K, et al. Clinical and genetic factors predictive of mortality in early systemic sclerosis. Arthritis Rheum 2009;61(10): 1403–11.

48. Eaton T, Young P, Milne D, et al. Six-minute walk, maximal exercise tests: reproducibility in fibrotic interstitial pneumonia. Am J Respir Crit Care Med 2005;171(10):1150–7.

49. Lederer DJ, Arcasoy SM, Wilt JS, et al. Six-minute-walk distance predicts waiting list survival in idiopathic pulmonary fibrosis. Am J Respir Crit Care Med 2006;174(6):659–64.

50. Buch MH, Denton CP, Furst DE, et al. Submaximal exercise testing in the assessment of interstitial lung disease secondary to systemic sclerosis: reproducibility and correlations of the 6-min walk test. Ann Rheum Dis 2007;66(2):169–73.

51. Villalba WO, Sampaio-Barros PD, Pereira MC, et al. Six-minute walk test for the evaluation of pulmonary disease severity in scleroderma patients. Chest 2007;131(1):217–22.

52. Garin MC, Highland KB, Silver RM, et al. Limitations to the 6-minute walk test in interstitial lung disease and pulmonary hypertension in scleroderma. J Rheumatol 2009;36(2):330–6.

53. Pignone A, Matucci-Cerinic M, Lombardi A, et al. High resolution computed tomography in systemic sclerosis. Real diagnostic utilities in the assessment of pulmonary involvement and comparison with other modalities of lung investigation. Clin Rheumatol 1992;11(4):465–72.

54. Elliot TL, Lynch DA, Newell JD Jr, et al. High-resolution computed tomography features of nonspecific interstitial pneumonia and usual interstitial pneumonia. J Comput Assist Tomogr 2005;29(3): 339–45.

55. Goldin JG, Lynch DA, Strollo DC, et al. High-resolution CT scan findings in patients with symptomatic scleroderma-related interstitial lung disease. Chest 2008;134(2):358–67.

56. Camiciottoli G, Orlandi I, Bartolucci M, et al. Lung CT densitometry in systemic sclerosis: correlation with lung function, exercise testing, and quality of life. Chest 2007;131(3):672–81.

57. Goh NS, Desai SR, Veeraraghavan S, et al. Interstitial lung disease in systemic sclerosis: a simple staging system. Am J Respir Crit Care Med 2008; 177(11):1248–54.

58. Gargani L, Doveri M, D'Errico L, et al. Ultrasound lung comets in systemic sclerosis: a chest sonography hallmark of pulmonary interstitial fibrosis. Rheumatology (Oxford) 2009;48(11):1382–7.

59. Picano E, Frassi F, Agricola E, et al. Ultrasound lung comets: a clinically useful sign of extravascular lung water. J Am Soc Echocardiogr 2006; 19(3):356–63.

60. Honda Y, Kuroki Y, Matsuura E, et al. Pulmonary surfactant protein D in sera and bronchoalveolar lavage fluids. Am J Respir Crit Care Med 1995; 152(6 Pt 1):1860–6.

61. Greene KE, Wright JR, Steinberg KP, et al. Serial changes in surfactant-associated proteins in lung and serum before and after onset of ARDS. Am J Respir Crit Care Med 1999;160(6):1843–50.

62. Kuroki Y, Takahashi H, Chiba H, et al. Surfactant proteins A and D: disease markers. Biochim Biophys Acta 1998;1408(2–3):334–45.

63. Asano Y, Ihn H, Yamane K, et al. Clinical significance of surfactant protein D as a serum marker for evaluating pulmonary fibrosis in patients with systemic sclerosis. Arthritis Rheum 2001;44(6): 1363–9.

64. Kohno N, Awaya Y, Oyama T, et al. KL-6, a mucin-like glycoprotein, in bronchoalveolar lavage fluid from patients with interstitial lung disease. Am Rev Respir Dis 1993;148(3):637–42.

65. Hant FN, Ludwicka-Bradley A, Wang HJ, et al. Surfactant protein D and KL-6 as serum biomarkers of interstitial lung disease in patients with scleroderma. J Rheumatol 2009;36(4): 773–80.

66. Matsushita T, Fujimoto M, Hasegawa M, et al. Elevated serum APRIL levels in patients with systemic sclerosis: distinct profiles of systemic

sclerosis categorized by APRIL and BAFF. J Rheumatol 2007;34(10):2056–62.

67. Yanaba K, Yoshizaki A, Muroi E, et al. Elevated circulating TWEAK levels in systemic sclerosis: association with lower frequency of pulmonary fibrosis. J Rheumatol 2009;36(8):1657–62.

68. Kumanovics G, Minier T, Radics J, et al. Comprehensive investigation of novel serum markers of pulmonary fibrosis associated with systemic sclerosis and dermato/polymyositis. Clin Exp Rheumatol 2008;26(3):414–20.

69. Yanaba K, Yoshizaki A, Muroi E, et al. CCL13 is a promising diagnostic marker for systemic sclerosis. Br J Dermatol 2010;162(2):332–6.

70. Tashkin DP, Elashoff R, Clements PJ, et al. Effects of 1-year treatment with cyclophosphamide on outcomes at 2 years in scleroderma lung disease. Am J Respir Crit Care Med 2007;176(10):1026–34.

71. Bournia VK, Vlachoyiannopoulos PG, Selmi C, et al. Recent advances in the treatment of systemic sclerosis. Clin Rev Allergy Immunol 2009;36(2–3): 176–200.

72. Daoussis D, Liossis SN, Tsamandas AC, et al. Experience with rituximab in scleroderma: results from a 1-year, proof-of-principle study. Rheumatology (Oxford) 2010;49(2):271–80.

73. Schachna L, Medsger TA Jr, Dauber JH, et al. Lung transplantation in scleroderma compared with idiopathic pulmonary fibrosis and idiopathic pulmonary arterial hypertension. Arthritis Rheum 2006; 54(12):3954–61.

74. Shitrit D, Amital A, Peled N, et al. Lung transplantation in patients with scleroderma: case series, review of the literature, and criteria for transplantation. Clin Transplant 2009;23(2):178–83.

75. Tsukamoto H, Nagafuji K, Horiuchi T, et al. A phase I-II trial of autologous peripheral blood stem cell transplantation in the treatment of refractory autoimmune disease. Ann Rheum Dis 2006;65(4): 508–14.

76. van Laar JM, Farge D, Tyndall A. Autologous Stem cell Transplantation International Scleroderma (ASTIS) trial: hope on the horizon for patients with severe systemic sclerosis. Ann Rheum Dis 2005; 64(10):1515.

77. Mukerjee D, St George D, Coleiro B, et al. Prevalence and outcome in systemic sclerosis associated pulmonary arterial hypertension: application of a registry approach. Ann Rheum Dis 2003; 62(11):1088–93.

78. Hachulla E, Gressin V, Guillevin L, et al. Early detection of pulmonary arterial hypertension in systemic sclerosis: a French nationwide prospective multicenter study. Arthritis Rheum 2005; 52(12):3792–800.

79. Steen V, Medsger TA Jr. Predictors of isolated pulmonary hypertension in patients with systemic sclerosis and limited cutaneous involvement. Arthritis Rheum 2003;48(2):516–22.

80. Hachulla E, Launay D, Mouthon L, et al. Is pulmonary arterial hypertension really a late complication of systemic sclerosis? Chest 2009;136(5):1211–9.

81. Kahaleh B. The microvascular endothelium in scleroderma. Rheumatology (Oxford) 2008; 47(Suppl 5):v14–5.

82. Kahaleh B. Vascular disease in scleroderma: mechanisms of vascular injury. Rheum Dis Clin North Am 2008;34(1):57–71, vi.

83. Mathai SC, Hummers LK, Champion HC, et al. Survival in pulmonary hypertension associated with the scleroderma spectrum of diseases: impact of interstitial lung disease. Arthritis Rheum 2009; 60(2):569–77.

84. Denton C, Black C. Pulmonary vascular involvement in systemic sclerosis. In: Clements P, Furst DE, editors. Systemic sclerosis. 2nd edition. Philadelphia: Lippincott Williams and Wilkins; 2004. p. 184–93.

85. Kawut SM, Taichman DB, Archer-Chicko CL, et al. Hemodynamics and survival in patients with pulmonary arterial hypertension related to systemic sclerosis. Chest 2003;123(2):344–50.

86. Koh ET, Lee P, Gladman DD, et al. Pulmonary hypertension in systemic sclerosis: an analysis of 17 patients. Br J Rheumatol 1996;35(10): 989–93.

87. Williams MH, Handler CE, Akram R, et al. Role of N-terminal brain natriuretic peptide (N-TproBNP) in scleroderma-associated pulmonary arterial hypertension. Eur Heart J 2006;27(12):1485–94.

88. Plastiras SC, Karadimitrakis SP, Kampolis C, et al. Determinants of pulmonary arterial hypertension in scleroderma. Semin Arthritis Rheum 2007; 36(6):392–6.

89. Fisher MR, Mathai SC, Champion HC, et al. Clinical differences between idiopathic and scleroderma-related pulmonary hypertension. Arthritis Rheum 2006;54(9):3043–50.

90. Hsu VM, Moreyra AE, Wilson AC, et al. Assessment of pulmonary arterial hypertension in patients with systemic sclerosis: comparison of noninvasive tests with results of right-heart catheterization. J Rheumatol 2008;35(3):458–65.

91. Callejas-Rubio JL, Moreno-Escobar E, de la Fuente PM, et al. Prevalence of exercise pulmonary arterial hypertension in scleroderma. J Rheumatol 2008;35(9):1812–6.

92. Badesch DB, Abman SH, Simonneau G, et al. Medical therapy for pulmonary arterial hypertension: updated ACCP evidence-based clinical practice guidelines. Chest 2007;131(6):1917–28.

93. Mukerjee D, St George D, Knight C, et al. Echocardiography and pulmonary function as screening tests for pulmonary arterial hypertension in

systemic sclerosis. Rheumatology (Oxford) 2004; 43(4):461–6.

94. Denton CP, Cailes JB, Phillips GD, et al. Comparison of Doppler echocardiography and right heart catheterization to assess pulmonary hypertension in systemic sclerosis. Br J Rheumatol 1997;36(2): 239–43.

95. Highland KB. Pulmonary arterial hypertension. Am J Med Sci 2008;335(1):40–5.

96. Talbott JH, Barrocas M. Carcinoma of the lung in progressive systemic sclerosis: a tabular review of the literature and a detailed report of the roentgenographic changes in two cases. Semin Arthritis Rheum 1980;9(3):191–217.

97. Roumm AD, Medsger TA Jr. Cancer and systemic sclerosis. An epidemiologic study. Arthritis Rheum 1985;28(12):1336–40.

98. Peters-Golden M, Wise RA, Hochberg M, et al. Incidence of lung cancer in systemic sclerosis. J Rheumatol 1985;12(6):1136–9.

99. Clements PJ, Furst DE, Wong WK, et al. High-dose versus low-dose D-penicillamine in early diffuse systemic sclerosis: analysis of a two-year, double-blind, randomized, controlled clinical trial. Arthritis Rheum 1999;42(6):1194–203.

100. Malik SW, Myers JL, DeRemee RA, et al. Lung toxicity associated with cyclophosphamide use. Two distinct patterns. Am J Respir Crit Care Med 1996;154(6 Pt 1):1851–6.

101. Johnson DA, Drane WE, Curran J, et al. Pulmonary disease in progressive systemic sclerosis. A complication of gastroesophageal reflux and occult aspiration? Arch Intern Med 1989;149(3): 589–93.

102. Savarino E, Ghio M, Marabotto E, et al. [Possible connection between gastroesophageal reflux and interstitial pulmonary fibrosis in patients with systemic sclerosis]. Recenti Prog Med 2009; 100(11):512–6 [in Italian].

103. Ajlani H, Meddeb N, Sahli H, et al. [Erasmus syndrome: case report]. Rev Pneumol Clin 2009; 65(1):16–22 [in French].

104. Hayashi H, Maeda M, Murakami S, et al. Soluble interleukin-2 receptor as an indicator of immunological disturbance found in silicosis patients. Int J Immunopathol Pharmacol 2009;22(1):53–62.

105. Sharp GC, Irvin WS, Tan EM, et al. Mixed connective tissue disease–an apparently distinct rheumatic disease syndrome associated with a specific antibody to an extractable nuclear antigen (ENA). Am J Med 1972;52(2):148–59.

106. Prakash UB. Respiratory complications in mixed connective tissue disease. Clin Chest Med 1998; 19(4):733–46, ix.

107. Saito Y, Terada M, Takada T, et al. Pulmonary involvement in mixed connective tissue disease: comparison with other collagen vascular diseases using high resolution CT. J Comput Assist Tomogr 2002;26(3):349–57.

108. Kozuka T, Johkoh T, Honda O, et al. Pulmonary involvement in mixed connective tissue disease: high-resolution CT findings in 41 patients. J Thorac Imaging 2001;16(2):94–8.

109. Derderian SS, Tellis CJ, Abbrecht PH, et al. Pulmonary involvement in mixed connective tissue disease. Chest 1985;88(1):45–8.

110. Prakash UB. Lungs in mixed connective tissue disease. J Thorac Imaging 1992;7(2):55–61.

111. Bull TM, Fagan KA, Badesch DB. Pulmonary vascular manifestations of mixed connective tissue disease. Rheum Dis Clin North Am 2005;31(3): 451–64, vi.

Pulmonary Manifestations of Rheumatoid Arthritis

Danielle Antin-Ozerkis, MD[a],*, Janine Evans, MD[b],
Ami Rubinowitz, MD[c], Robert J. Homer, MD, PhD[d],
Richard A. Matthay, MD[e]

KEYWORDS

- Rheumatoid arthritis • Pulmonary disease
- Pulmonary function tests
- Pleuroparenchymal complications

Rheumatoid arthritis (RA) is a chronic inflammatory disease typically involving the small joints of the hands and feet in a symmetric fashion. RA can involve any synovial lined joint.[1] The American Rheumatism Association proposed diagnostic criteria for RA in 1987 (**Table 1**). However, many patients do not fulfill these criteria at diagnosis. The diagnostic criteria for RA are likely to change as our understanding of risk factors and molecular markers evolves.[2] For example, the presence of anticyclic citrullinated peptide (CCP) antibodies is as sensitive but more specific for the diagnosis than the presence of rheumatoid factor (RF), and is now used for early diagnosis and subcategorization of patient groups.[2]

RA likely results from a complex interaction between genetic susceptibility and environmental exposures that induces an abnormal immune response. The worldwide prevalence of RA suggests that various exposures and genetic backgrounds can initiate the autoimmune cascade of RA. Some of the causative environmental factors are inhaled antigens, especially cigarette smoke, a fact that supports the critical role of the lung in the disorder.[2]

The incidence of RA in the United States is approximately 30 per 100,000, with a prevalence of 0.5% to 1%; women are 2 to 3 times more likely to be affected than men.[3,4] The age at time of diagnosis is typically between 35 and 50 years. Overall survival is decreased in patients with RA as compared with the general population, primarily as a result of cardiovascular disease and the extra-articular manifestations of RA.[5]

Pulmonary disease, which is a major source of morbidity and mortality in RA, manifests most commonly as interstitial lung disease (ILD), airways disease, rheumatoid nodules, and pleural effusions (**Box 1**).[3] Respiratory manifestations usually become more prevalent as RA progresses, but they may present simultaneously with joint symptoms or even predate joint involvement.[6] Many pulmonary manifestations are directly linked to RA itself and may be a result of underlying defects in immunity and chronic inflammation.[7] Some are due to exposures and to the treatment

[a] Yale Interstitial Lung Disease Program, Internal Medicine - Pulmonary & Critical Care Division, Yale University School of Medicine, PO Box 208057, 300 Cedar Street, LCI 101B, New Haven, CT 06520-8057, USA
[b] Internal Medicine - Rheumatology Division, Yale University School of Medicine, PO Box 208031, 300 Cedar Street, TAC S-425D, New Haven, CT 06520-8031, USA
[c] Department of Diagnostic Imaging, Yale University School of Medicine, PO Box 208042, New Haven, CT 06520-8042, USA
[d] Department of Pathology, Yale University School of Medicine, PO Box 208023, 310 Cedar Street, LH 108, New Haven, CT 06520-8023, USA
[e] Internal Medicine – Pulmonary & Critical Care Division, Yale University School of Medicine, PO Box 208057, 300 Cedar Street, New Haven, CT 06520-8057, USA
* Corresponding author.
E-mail address: danielle.antin-ozerkis@yale.edu

Clin Chest Med 31 (2010) 451–478
doi:10.1016/j.ccm.2010.04.003

chestmed.theclinics.com

Table 1
American Rheumatism Association revised criteria, 1987

1. Morning stiffness for at least 1 hour
2. Arthritis of 3 or more joint areas, simultaneously
3. Hand arthritis (wrist, metacarpophalangeal, or proximal interphalangeal joint)
4. Symmetric joint involvement
5. Subcutaneous rheumatoid nodules
6. Presence of rheumatoid factor
7. Radiographic erosion or bony decalcification of involved joints

At least 4 of 7 must be present; the first 4 must have been present for at least 6 weeks.
　Data from Arnett FC, et al. The American Rheumatism Association 1987 revised criteria for the classification of rheumatoid arthritis. Arthritis Rheum 1988;31(3):315–24.

Box 1
Respiratory involvement in rheumatoid arthritis

Interstitial lung disease
　Nonspecific interstitial pneumonia (NSIP)
　Usual interstitial pneumonia (UIP)
　Follicular bronchiolitis
　Lymphoid interstitial pneumonitis (LIP)
　Diffuse alveolar damage (DAD)
　Organizing pneumonia (OP)
Pleural disease
　Pleuritis
　Pleural effusion
　Empyema
　Pneumothorax
　Bronchopleural fistula
Airways disease
　Upper airways
　　Cricoarytenoid arthritis
　　Rheumatoid nodules
　Lower airways
　　Small airway obstruction
　　Bronchiectasis
　　Bronchiolitis obliterans
　　Follicular bronchiolitis
Solitary and multiple lung nodules
　Rheumatoid nodules
　Caplan syndrome
　Lung cancer
Drug-related lung disease
　Gold
　D-Penicillamine
　Anti-inflammatory drugs
　Antimetabolites
　Biologics
Infection
　Opportunistic
　Bacterial
　Mycobacterial (tuberculosis)
Pulmonary vascular disease
　Vasculitis
　Pulmonary hemorrhage
　Pulmonary hypertension
Miscellaneous
　Respiratory muscle weakness
　Fibrobullous disease
　Amyloidosis

of RA with disease-modifying antirheumatic drugs (DMARDs).[8,9] Evaluation and management of RA-associated pulmonary disease frequently necessitates a multidisciplinary approach involving pulmonologists, rheumatologists, radiologists, and pathologists. This review emphasizes the approach to pleuroparenchymal complications of RA.

INTERSTITIAL LUNG DISEASE
Epidemiology

The association between interstitial lung disease and RA was first described in 1948.[10] Additional reports of RA patients with ILD, many presenting with cough, dyspnea, and chest radiograph abnormalities, supported this association.[10–12] Early series, using chest radiograph alone, found fewer than 5% of patients with RA to have RA-associated ILD (RA-ILD).[13] Subsequent studies using measurements of pulmonary function, particularly diffusing capacity of the lung for carbon monoxide (DL_{CO}), diagnosed RA-ILD in 33% to 41% of RA patients.[14,15] High-resolution computed tomography (HRCT) of the chest, which was introduced in the 1980s, is a less invasive and highly sensitive test for detection of parenchymal abnormalities.[16] Among unselected RA patients examined with HRCT, radiographic abnormalities have been detected in 20% to 63%.[17–20] Similar estimates have been obtained from autopsy series of patients with advanced RA, in which more than a third of patients had evidence of ILD.[17,21] The lower incidence (6.3% to 9.4%) of clinically significant RA-ILD found in retrospective population-based studies suggests that radiographic and pulmonary function test (PFT) abnormalities may not lead in all cases to progressive disease.[22,23] However, early clinical RA-ILD may not have been recognized or early mortality among patients with RA-ILD may have prevented development of clinically significant lung disease.[22]

Risk factors for the development of RA-ILD include older age, male sex, and a history of cigarette smoking.[24] One recent study proposes methotrexate therapy as a risk factor for disease progression, although the numbers of patients studied were small, and methods of detecting methotrexate toxicity were unclear.[19] The role of DMARDs in the pathogenesis or progression of ILD among RA patients is uncertain.

In general, ILD occurs in patients with well-established RA.[25] However, up to 20% of patients have onset of ILD before the diagnosis of RA.[24] Some patients with idiopathic ILD have been found to have RA-related autoantibodies (RF and CCP) but no articular findings of RA; some of these patients eventually develop clinical RA.[26] The delay between presentation of lung and joint symptoms can be as long as 6 years.[24,27]

Clinical Manifestations

The main symptom of patients with RA-ILD is progressive dyspnea, predominantly due to exertional hypoxemia and increased dead space ventilation. In late disease, dyspnea is related to high static recoil of the lung with increased work of breathing.[28] In advanced pulmonary fibrosis, pulmonary hypertension may develop, leading to right ventricular strain and cor pulmonale. Patients with RA-ILD are often asymptomatic until lung function is significantly impaired. Diagnosis is further delayed when patients attribute mild dyspnea to being deconditioned. Limited functional status in patients with advanced joint disease may also contribute to late diagnosis. Patients with cough may be evaluated earlier for ILD. Pleuritic chest pain does occasionally occur.[29]

Physical examination findings are often nonspecific but may include bibasilar fine, dry, "velcro" crackles. Late signs of RA-ILD may include digital clubbing and evidence of right heart failure.

Pulmonary Function Tests

PFTs typically show restrictive physiology and diffusion impairment. A defect in DL_{CO} is often the earliest PFT finding in RA-ILD.[14,15] Exercise testing is rarely used for screening; however, it is important to ambulate patients with RA-ILD because resting oximetry may be falsely reassuring.[30] Oxygen desaturation on 6-minute walk testing is predicted by abnormalities in lung function.[31]

There are 2 major mechanisms for exertional hypoxemia in ILD. First, an inappropriate decrease in DL_{CO} during exercise due to inadequate pulmonary capillary recruitment leads to a relatively smaller capillary blood volume and subsequently reduced time available for gas exchange.[32,33] Second, patients with ILD have a reduced mixed venous oxygen content due to areas of ventilation/perfusion mismatch and intrapulmonary shunt.[32] Late in disease, fibrosis and pulmonary vascular obliteration lead to severe diffusion abnormalities, with resting arterial hypoxemia and profound exertional desaturation. Correction of exertional hypoxemia with supplemental oxygen improves exercise endurance.[34]

Radiology

Although RA-ILD may be diagnosed from an abnormal chest radiograph (**Fig. 1**), affected patients often have no abnormalities on plain radiograph.[13] Particularly in early disease, HRCT is an important tool. Common features on HRCT include ground-glass opacities (hazy areas of increased parenchymal density that do not obscure the underlying vasculature), reticulation (a pattern of criss-crossing lines resulting in a weblike pattern), bronchiectasis, and micronodules.[35–37] Reticulation occurs predominantly at the periphery of the lung and is frequently associated with other signs of fibrosis, such as architectural distortion, traction bronchiectasis, and honeycombing. HRCT findings in RA-ILD are indistinguishable from those of the idiopathic interstitial pneumonias, and must be correlated with clinical and histopathologic features for diagnosis.[38] The differential diagnosis includes usual interstitial

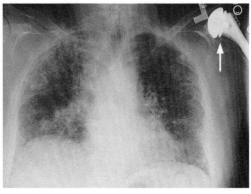

Fig. 1. A 76-year-old man with rheumatoid arthritis and progressive shortness of breath. Chest radiograph shows reduced lung volumes with peripheral, coarse interstitial markings as well as cystic changes due to traction bronchiectasis and honeycombing. Note is also made of a left shoulder prosthesis (*arrow*), which was placed due to severe erosive arthritis at this site.

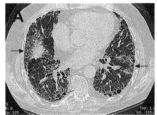
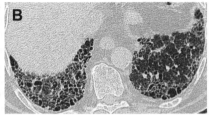

Fig. 2. A 71-year-old man with usual interstitial pneumonia secondary to rheumatoid arthritis. High-resolution (1.25-mm thick sections) CT images at the level of the mid (*A*) and lower (*B*) thorax show peripheral and basilar predominant reticular markings with architectural distortion, traction bronchiectasis (*white arrows*), and subpleural cysts/honeycombing (*black arrows*).

pneumonia (UIP), nonspecific interstitial pneumonia (NSIP), desquamative interstitial pneumonia (DIP), and organizing pneumonia (OP). Mixed or unclassifiable patterns are often present. Biopsy specimens may show end-stage fibrosis ("honeycombing"), which is a nonspecific pattern.

Among patients with idiopathic ILD, certain HRCT features predict the histopathologic findings of UIP, which is the histopathologic hallmark of idiopathic pulmonary fibrosis (IPF).[35,39] The most helpful features are bilateral subpleural reticulation and honeycombing (**Fig. 2**).[40] Several small studies suggest that the correlation between radiographic and pathologic findings for UIP occurs also in patients with RA-ILD.[41] A radiographic NSIP pattern has also been described, which includes bilateral, patchy areas of ground-glass opacities involving the lower lobes, subpleural sparing, areas of consolidation, irregular linear opacities, thickening of bronchovascular bundles, and bronchiectasis, but without honeycombing (**Fig. 3**).[42–45] Correlation between this radiographic pattern and the histopathologic pattern of NSIP is poor.[43] Despite the poor performance of radiology in predicting an NSIP patter, in routine practice most patients with RA do not undergo surgical

lung biopsy for histologic classification. It is often assumed that ground glass reflects active alveolitis without significant established fibrosis and thereby predicts corticosteroid responsiveness, although these findings often reflect "fine fibrosis" below the resolution capability of the HRCT.[42,46] On the other hand, worsening prognosis does correlate with higher fibrosis scores on chest CT.[47]

Other radiographic patterns in RA include "tree-in-bud" opacities (secondary to infectious or follicular bronchiolitis), traction bronchiectasis (secondary to underlying fibrosis), and ground-glass nodules (seen with follicular bronchiolitis or OP). The typical HRCT appearance of OP is diffuse, patchy, ground-glass, and alveolar opacities, which tend to have a peripheral distribution and may contain air bronchograms (**Fig. 4**). In general, radiographic evidence of fibrosis is absent, though OP can be present in conjunction with underlying fibrosis. In RA, it is common to see several histopathologic and/or radiographic patterns simultaneously, for example, the presence of airways disease or rheumatoid nodules in conjunction with ILD. When observed serially, HRCT manifestations in RA-ILD may include either acute exacerbations of disease, characterized by the onset of

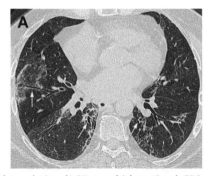
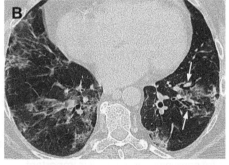

Fig. 3. High-resolution (1.25-mm thick sections) CT images obtained through the mid-lower thorax (*A* and *B*) in a 58-year-old woman with rheumatoid arthritis who presented with shortness of breath. Images show bilateral areas of ground-glass opacity with a subpleural and peribronchovascular distribution. Also seen are reticular markings and traction bronchiectasis (*arrows*). Surgical lung biopsy revealed nonspecific interstitial pneumonia (NSIP).

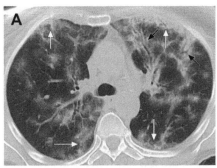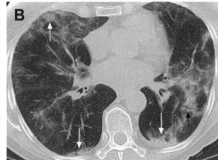

Fig. 4. A 75-year-old woman with organizing pneumonia secondary to rheumatoid arthritis. Axial CT images through the upper (A) and mid (B) thorax demonstrate multifocal ground-glass opacities with a patchy, peripheral (white arrows), and peribronchovascular distribution (black arrows).

diffuse ground-glass opacities, or progressive fibrosis, characterized by increasing reticularity and honeycombing.[48]

Bronchoalveolar Lavage

The role of bronchoalveolar lavage (BAL) in connective tissue disease-associated ILD (CTD-ILD) is discussed in detail in the article by Kowal-Bielecka and colleagues elsewhere in this issue. In RA-ILD, BAL has not proven useful for diagnosis.[49,50] Nonetheless, BAL is important in the evaluation of radiographic abnormalities, primarily in the evaluation of alternative diagnoses to RA-ILD, including drug reaction, diffuse alveolar hemorrhage, and opportunistic infection.[51–53] Bronchoscopy with BAL should be considered in the evaluation of new infiltrates in any RA patient receiving immunosuppressive therapy.

Pathology

Surgical lung biopsy is not commonly obtained in RA patients. However, specific pathologic patterns may help determine prognosis and response to treatment. The pathologic patterns observed in RA-ILD are similar to those in the idiopathic interstitial pneumonias. However, certain findings, such as lymphoid hyperplasia and plasma cell infiltration, are more common in RA-ILD.[54] One notable feature of RA-ILD is that more than one pathologic process, and often several, may occur in the same biopsy specimen, making comparison among series particularly difficult.[55,56] UIP and NSIP are the most common histopathologic patterns in RA. In other connective tissue diseases, particularly scleroderma and polymyositis/dermatomyositis, the NSIP pattern is the most common form of ILD.[57,58] By contrast, in RA, UIP is more common than NSIP.[59] Other histopathologic patterns in RA may include follicular bronchiolitis (FB), lymphoid interstitial pneumonitis (LIP), OP, and diffuse alveolar damage (DAD).[55]

UIP is characterized by a heterogeneous pattern in which areas of normal lung are interspersed with areas of active fibrosis (known as fibroblastic foci), interstitial inflammation, and honeycombing (**Fig. 5**).[60] The changes are usually most pronounced in the subpleural lung. UIP demonstrates "temporal heterogeneity" in that new, active areas of fibrosis can be found adjacent to areas of more advanced fibrosis and honeycombing in a pattern reflective of ongoing, repetitive lung damage.[61]

The features of NSIP, by contrast, are diffuse and spatially homogeneous.[43] There are 2 forms of NSIP: cellular NSIP, which is characterized by lymphocytic and plasma cell infiltrates with minimal fibrosis; and fibrotic NSIP, which is characterized by fibrotic changes, either alone or in combination with patchy areas of inflammation (**Fig. 6**). The amount of inflammation may range from a diffuse, mononuclear cell infiltrate to collagen deposition with minimal inflammation.

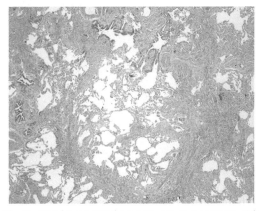

Fig. 5. Usual interstitial pneumonia in a patient with rheumatoid arthritis. Heterogeneous fibrosis and fibroblastic foci are present. (Hematoxylin and eosin staining; Original magnification ×2).

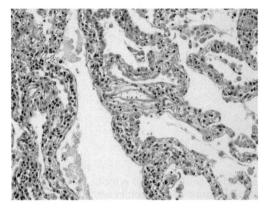

Fig. 6. Cellular nonspecific interstitial pneumonia in a patient with rheumatoid arthritis. A diffuse lymphocytic and plasma cell infiltrate involves the alveolar septae. (Hematoxylin and eosin staining; Original magnification ×40).

Areas of OP or features typical for UIP, such as fibroblastic foci, are infrequent and if present, not the dominant pattern. Advanced fibrotic NSIP can be difficult to differentiate from UIP.[62]

OP is the primary pattern on biopsy in 10% to 22% of cases and is a secondary component in a significant number of RA-ILD cases.[35,54,56,63,64] This pattern may be primarily due to RA but can be caused by drug hypersensitivity, having been reported in association with methotrexate, etanercept, rituximab, and sulfasalazine.[65–68] Pathologic findings in OP consist of plugs of granulation tissue called Masson bodies extending into lumens of the bronchioles and alveoli and obstructing the airways (**Fig. 7**). The plugs of tissues are composed of inflammatory cells, debris, fibrin, myofibroblasts, and immature connective tissue.[69]

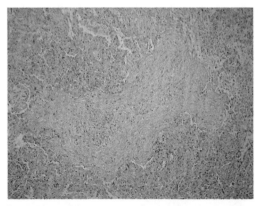

Fig. 7. Organizing pneumonia pattern in a patient with rheumatoid arthritis. Organizing pneumonia with plugs of organizing fibroblastic tissue in the distal bronchioles. Chronic inflammatory cells are present. (Hematoxylin and eosin staining; Original magnification ×20).

Prognosis

In general, RA-ILD tends to be either mild or very slowly progressive, and autopsy reports show that fewer than 10% of patients die of respiratory failure.[21] However, patients may experience spontaneous resolution of ground-glass opacities, progressive fibrosis with worsening lung function, and episodes of sudden deterioration.[48] Radiographic progression in RA-ILD has been observed over short-term follow-up, although there are few data regarding long-term outcomes after the detection of early disease.[19] The effect of RA therapy on progression of ILD has not been adequately studied.

A DL_{CO} less than 54% of predicted has been suggested as a sensitive and specific marker for worsening disease.[48] If respiratory disease becomes severe enough to warrant hospitalization, mortality estimates are very high, with a mean survival of 3.5 years and a 5-year survival rate of 39%.[70]

Prognosis in idiopathic interstitial pneumonias is closely linked to histopathologic pattern. UIP (IPF) has a poor prognosis, with median survival from time of diagnosis of less than 3 years.[30] NSIP, in contrast, has a significantly better prognosis.[71,72] Despite the similar radiographic and pathologic features to the idiopathic interstitial pneumonias, CTD-ILD has been found to carry a better prognosis than idiopathic ILD.[38,73,74] Studies suggesting no difference between the 2 groups have had a predominance of RA-ILD in the CTD-ILD group, suggesting a possible link between RA-ILD and poorer prognosis.[75] In fact, recent data suggest that the course of UIP in RA-ILD may be similar to that of idiopathic UIP (IPF).[76]

Treatment

Many asymptomatic patients with RA-ILD have radiographic evidence of lung disease, and it is unclear whether treatment alters their course. In particular, it is unclear whether RA-ILD with a UIP pattern responds as poorly to pharmacologic therapy as does idiopathic UIP (IPF).[7] In general, RA-ILD with NSIP and OP patterns are felt to be responsive to corticosteroids and other immunosuppressive therapy.[41] However, there are no controlled studies to guide the choice of drug or to clarify whether morbidity or mortality is improved with the use of immunosuppressive therapy.

Despite this lack of clarity on therapy, progressive lung disease is typically treated aggressively, because there are reports of therapeutic responses to therapy with corticosteroids, azathioprine, cyclosporine, and cyclophosphamide.[77,78]

Rapidly progressive or extensive disease with arterial hypoxemia is often treated with either daily oral or monthly intravenous cyclophosphamide in combination with corticosteroids.[79] Prophylaxis for *Pneumocystis jirovecii* pneumonia should be routinely given. Milder, but still progressive disease is often treated with azathioprine and prednisone.[79] If there is no response, therapy can be tapered and then discontinued to avoid unnecessary toxicity. Mycophenolate has recently been reported in small case series to have a beneficial effect on CTD-ILD, and may be considered in this setting.[80,81] Rituximab is used in the treatment of RA joint disease refractory to other therapy, but data regarding its use in RA-ILD are lacking. Some case reports suggest that tumor necrosis factor α (TNF-α) inhibitors may be effective in RA-ILD, but there are other reports suggesting pulmonary toxicity of these agents in patients with underlying ILD.[82–84]

In general, patients with progressive RA-ILD, particularly if accompanied by typical findings of inflammatory disease on radiographs, should be considered for immunosuppressive therapy. Patients with severe, fibrotic lung disease should be considered for referral for lung transplantation.

PLEURAL DISEASE
Epidemiology

Pleural involvement in RA includes pleurisy, pleural effusions, pleural thickening, and pneumothorax.[85–88] Micronodular involvement of the pleura has been described and is one cause of pleural effusions in RA.[89] Other potential causes include (1) prior infection, (2) local production of immune complexes, (3) chronic inflammation with cytokine release and activation of fibrosis, (4) impaired resorption of fluid due to its high protein content, and (5) the rupture of subpleural nodules leading to inflammation-induced capillary leak and obstruction of lymphatic drainage.[78,90]

Pleural manifestations of RA are more common in older patients and more common in men than in women.[91] Men with high serum levels of RF are at increased risk for pleural involvement.[86,90] In addition, men with certain HLA/Dw3 HLA antigens, late-onset disease, high RF levels, and low serum complement may reflect a subset of patients predisposed to developing pleural effusions.[92]

The most common finding in RA pleural disease is pleural thickening and scarring, which were detected in up to 73% of patients at autopsy in the pre-antibiotic era.[93] Subsequent studies have confirmed that the sequelae of pleurisy, including pleural thickening and scarring, occur in nearly 19% of all patients and 24% of males.[91] In contrast, pleural effusion has an estimated incidence in most studies ranging between 3% and 5%, though with some estimates as high as 22%.[86] Pleural effusion has a strong male preponderance, with more than 80% of cases reported in men.[85,86,91,94]

Diagnostic thoracentesis is often necessary in the evaluation of pleural effusion (**Table 2**). Many RA patients with effusion have a history of cigarette smoking, making evaluation for malignancy important. Empyema may be relatively common among RA patients.[95] Among patients treated with anti–TNF-α therapy, risk for disseminated tuberculosis is increased, and tuberculous empyema has been reported.[96] More benign, inflammatory conditions have been reported as well, such as a lupus-like syndrome among patients receiving anti–TNF-α therapy, which results in serositis.[97]

Clinical Features

More than 20% of patients with RA have a history of pleurisy, although most pleural effusions in RA are asymptomatic.[86] In addition to chest pain, symptoms include dyspnea and fever; patients with fever should be evaluated for underlying infection.[86] Cough often indicates the presence of underlying lung disease, which is present in up to one-third of patients.[98]

Pleural effusion may be present early in the course of RA and may be its presenting manifestation.[99,100] Effusion can present at any point in the course of RA, however, and may be associated with flares of joint symptoms.[90] Effusions are most commonly unilateral, but bilateral or migratory effusions have been reported.[90] Effusions are usually small to moderate-sized, but large effusions with respiratory compromise have been reported.[101] On rare occasions rupture of a rheumatoid nodule can lead to a pleural effusion, pneumothorax, bronchopleural fistula, or empyema.[98] One report of pneumothorax after the initiation of methotrexate therapy suggested a relationship between worsening nodular disease and the initiation of therapy.[87]

Diagnostic Approach

Imaging
The initial evaluation of RA pleural effusion typically includes chest radiograph, which may show blunting of the costophrenic angle. Smaller effusions may be detected with lateral and decubitus films. Chest CT is a more sensitive means of

Table 2
Pleural effusion characteristics in rheumatoid arthritis

Appearance	Comment
Greenish yellow	Typical
Clear	Typical
Straw colored	Typical
Milky with opalescent sheen	Suggests pseudochylothorax with elevated cholesterol levels
Bloody	Uncommon; malignancy or tuberculosis should be suspected
Purulent	Empyema should be suspected; rarely may be sterile
Laboratory values	
LDH	High, often >700 U/L
Total protein	High, often >3.5 g/dL
pH	Low, usually <7.2
Glucose	Low, usually <50 mg/dL
Cholesterol	High, often >1000 mg/dL
RF titer	High
Cell count	High, often >10,000/μL (polymorphonuclear or lymphocytic)

Abbreviations: LDH, lactate dehydrogenase; RF, rheumatoid factor.

detecting a small pleural effusion, resulting in some effusions being found incidentally in the evaluation for ILD or other parenchymal lesions (**Fig. 8**) Ultrasound is useful to evaluate the characteristics of the fluid, which may be loculated and complex, and to guide needle aspiration.[90,102]

Pleural fluid appearance

The pleural fluid in RA typically appears milky or greenish-yellow; however it may be clear, creamy, or straw-colored.[88] The milky appearance, sometimes with opalescent sheen, is due to pseudochylothorax, with elevated cholesterol levels (often above 1000 mg/dL) without the elevation in triglyceride levels typical of true chylothorax.[88] Cholesterol crystals are also observed on microscopy.[103] The cause for cholesterol elevation is unclear.[103,104] Bloody pleural fluid is uncommon in RA effusions and should prompt an evaluation for such causes as tuberculosis or malignancy.[98,105]

The presence of pus in the pleural space strongly suggests infectious empyema. In some cases, pyopneumothorax may develop as a result of rupture of a rheumatoid nodule into the pleural space.[106] Sterile purulent effusions with leukocyte counts greater than 50,000/μL have been described and are thought to be secondary to inflammation.[106] However, infection may be present even in well-appearing patients because RA patients with infectious empyema who have been chronically receiving corticosteroids can be remarkably asymptomatic.[107]

Pleural fluid laboratory values

Rheumatoid pleural effusions are generally exudative, with very high levels (>700 UI/L) of lactate dehydrogenase (LDH) and total protein (>3.5 g/dL).[88,90,108] The fluid pH is typically lower than 7.2, occasionally as low as 7.0. Mechanisms proposed for the low pH include increased cellular metabolism and lactate production due to the inflammatory process, as well as a decreased

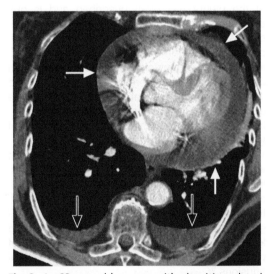

Fig. 8. An 83-year-old woman with pleuritis and pericarditis secondary to rheumatoid arthritis. Axial contrast-enhanced CT image shows small bilateral pleural effusions (*open arrows*) and a moderate-size pericardial effusion (*white arrows*) due to serositis.

efflux of carbon dioxide from the pleural space.[109,110]

Pleural fluid glucose levels may be normal but more commonly are quite low, particularly in long-standing effusions. More than 40% of rheumatoid effusions have a glucose level of less than 10 mg/dL; in more than 80%, the glucose level is less than 50 mg/dL.[88] The low glucose is thought to be the result of impaired glucose transport from blood to pleural space, in contrast to the increased glucose consumption that occurs in empyema or malignancy.[110,111]

Cholesterol crystals and lecithin-globulin complexes are helpful in distinguishing chylous from pseudochylous effusions.[90] Cholesterol-rich effusions may be due to rheumatoid or tuberculous effusions and may be seen with or without pleural thickening.[112]

Rheumatoid effusions are frequently characterized by high RF levels, often higher than serum levels. In some cases, evidence for synthesis of RF by pleural tissue and pleural fluid mononuclear cells in the absence of the synthesis of RF by peripheral blood mononuclear cells has been documented.[113] This finding suggests that rheumatoid pleural effusions are an extra-articular immune complex disease.

Other diagnostic tests have been suggested for distinguishing rheumatoid effusions from other causes of pleural effusion. Elevations in pleural fluid complement pathway products, ferritin concentration, β2-microglobulin, angiotensin-converting enzyme, hyaluronan, and cytokines including TNF-α and interleukin-1β (IL-1β), have all been described.[90] None has been shown to be specific for rheumatoid effusion, and several have also been noted in tuberculous and malignant effusions.[114,115] Adenosine deaminase has been suggested as a test specific for tuberculous effusions, but it is elevated in both rheumatoid and tuberculous effusions, and therefore cannot distinguish the 2 disorders.[116]

Cytology

Leukocyte counts are generally unhelpful in the evaluation of rheumatoid effusion.[98,117] The count is usually less than 10,000/μL, but extremely high cell counts may be observed, even in the absence of infection.[106] The cellular differential may include polymorphonuclear cells or lymphocytes. Granular polymorphonuclear leukocytes known as "RA-cells" or "ragocytes," characterized by cytoplasmic inclusion bodies thought to represent phagocytosed RF complexes, have been proposed as characteristic of rheumatoid effusions.[118,119] However, these cells may be found in tuberculous and malignant effusions as well.[120,121] Typical cytologic

findings in RA include multinucleated giant cells and elongated macrophages on a background of eosinophilic, granular necrotic material, particularly with a lack of mesothelial cells.[118,122]

Pleural biopsy

Pleural biopsy may be indicated if thoracentesis is not definitive, in particular when tuberculosis or malignancy is suspected. Pseudochylous and bloody effusions may prompt further evaluation. In general, transthoracic needle biopsy of the pleura is nondiagnostic in the case of rheumatoid effusions.[90] Thoracoscopy can be helpful and can be safely performed by experienced operators under local anesthesia.[89] The appearance of the parietal pleura is described as "gritty" or "frozen" with numerous small vesicles or granules of about 0.5 mm in diameter.[89] The visceral pleura is typically uninvolved or demonstrates nonspecific inflammatory changes. On biopsy, pathologic features include the lack of a normal mesothelial cell covering on the pleura, with replacement by a pseudostratified layer of epithelioid cells with focal multinucleated and foreign body (non-Langerhans) giant cells.[89]

Treatment

The treatment of pleural effusions in RA has not been well studied. For small, asymptomatic rheumatoid effusions, many experts recommend no specific intervention in the absence of features suggesting an alternative diagnosis.[98,108] If another diagnosis, such as infection or malignancy, is suspected because of the patient's smoking history, the presence of fever, or immunosuppressive therapy, the fluid should be sampled.

Many effusions resolve spontaneously within several weeks without sequelae, but up to 50% of patients have persistent effusion.[123] Long-standing pleural effusions may lead to pleural thickening, trapped lung, and infection.[123,124] For large, symptomatic effusions, therapy may consist of therapeutic thoracentesis alone, instillation of intrapleural corticosteroids or fibrinolytic agents, and augmentation of systemic immunosuppression, including oral corticosteroids.[89,90,125,126] No single method has been shown to produce superior outcomes.[90]

Surgical intervention for refractory effusions can include mechanical or chemical pleurodesis. Pleural fibrosis with lung entrapment may require decortication for the relief of dyspnea due to restrictive lung disease, although this procedure carries significant morbidity and mortality.[127] Surgical intervention may also be required in the event of a bronchopleural fistula. It has been recently suggested that the typical management of bronchopleural fistulae, which includes video-assisted thoracoscopic surgical (VATS) pleurodesis, may not be successful in rheumatoid pleural disease.[128] The presence of underlying rheumatoid nodules may hamper local healing, making early direct closure via thoracotomy worthy of consideration.

True infective empyema is often polymicrobial, and should be treated aggressively with both antibiotics and drainage of the pleural space.[90] Underlying necrotic subpleural nodules have been described in most patients with empyema.[129] A search for this source of bronchopleural fistula should be considered in patients with empyema, as continuous seeding from this source may occur. Tube thoracostomy is the preferred method of drainage for early-stage empyema without significant loculations and fibrosis, with later options including VATS or an open surgical procedure.[130]

AIRWAYS DISEASE
Upper Airway Disease

Upper airway involvement by RA can result in both disabling chronic disease and life-threatening airway emergencies. Close attention to the larynx should be paid, particularly in the perioperative setting. The most common form of upper airway RA is cricoarytenoid arthritis.

The cricoarytenoid joints function to abduct and adduct the vocal cords during speech. RA involving these joints was first described in 1955.[131] Early studies estimated an incidence of 26%.[132] In a group of 22 unselected RA patients, radiographic evidence of erosive arthritis of the cricoarytenoid joint was present in 45%, and when indirect laryngoscopy findings were included, 55% of patients were affected.[133] Subsequent studies have found an incidence of abnormal findings at laryngoscopy and on CT of the neck ranging between 52% and 75%, although these results may reflect referral bias.[134,135] Females are more commonly affected than males.[133] Abnormalities of the joints include cricoarytenoid erosion, cricoarytenoid subluxation, cricoarytenoid prominence, and abnormal position of the true vocal cord.[135] Flow volume loops may also suggest a variable or fixed upper airway obstruction, though these changes are not sensitive enough to reliably exclude laryngeal RA. Although most vocal cord paralysis is due to cricoarytenoid joint arthritis, cervicomedullary compression due to occipito-atlanto-axial arthritis with subluxation can occur.[136] The presence of myelopathy and neck pain are clues to cervicomedullary compression.

Symptoms of upper airway involvement include voice changes, sore throat, foreign body sensation, throat fullness, aspiration, and choking.[135] Dyspnea, pain radiating to the ears, stridor, dysphagia, odynophagia, and pain with speech have also been described.[137] Careful history may reveal airway symptoms in two-thirds of patients and up to 30% may have hoarseness.[135,138] Patients with sore throat and difficulty during inspiration are more likely to have mucosal and functional abnormalities, including vocal cord paralysis, as seen on indirect laryngoscopy.[134] For chronic, symptomatic upper airway disease, systemic or intra-articular corticosteroids have some benefit.[139] Surgical management, including tracheostomy, arytenoidectomy, or arytenoidopexy, may be necessary if progressive airway obstruction occurs despite medical treatment.[137]

In addition to the chronic symptoms of upper airway obstruction, cricoarytenoid arthritis may present acutely, with severe stridor requiring emergent airway management.[138,140–143] This event may represent a decompensation of chronic disease, in which manipulation of the larynx causes local edema superimposed on chronically immobile, adducted vocal cords.[138] An awareness of potential airway complications in the perioperative setting may prevent many such emergencies. Smaller endotracheal tubes are recommended in this setting.[138] Fiberoptic intubation may result in fewer complications than routine intubation.[140] Use of laryngeal mask airway has been reported to exacerbate laryngeal disease in RA.[144] Avoidance of intubation, with the use of local anesthesia, may be preferable in the case of severe disease. Once airway obstruction has occurred, emergent tracheostomy may be required.[142] RA patients may have cervical spine instability due to inflammatory arthritis of the atlanto-axial joint, leading to further difficulties in airway management.[145]

There are other head and neck manifestations of RA. Rheumatoid nodules can present as vocal cord nodules and submucosal masses, even mimicking squamous cell carcinoma.[137] Subluxation of the atlanto-axial joint and arthritis of the temporomandibular joint can lead to obstructive sleep apnea.[137,146] A high index of suspicion for upper airway manifestations of RA must be maintained. Through aggressive therapy, symptoms may be dramatically improved and preventative evaluation may be life-saving.[147,148]

Bronchiectasis

The prevalence of bronchiectasis in RA ranges from 30% to 58% when detected by HRCT.[149,150] HRCT is more sensitive than respiratory symptoms, PFTs, or chest radiograph for the presence of bronchiectasis (**Fig. 9**).[100,150] Both cylindrical and traction bronchiectasis occur and may accompany RA-ILD. Clinically evident bronchiectasis is much less frequent (1%–5% of RA patients) and may precede the onset of the articular symptoms and the diagnosis of RA.[151,152] The high prevalence of bronchiectasis in RA may be the result of defects in humoral immunity, with increased susceptibility to respiratory infections, and subsequent structural damage to the airways.[153,154] Genetic predisposition may also play a role. Heterozygosity for the ΔF508 cystic fibrosis transmembrane conductance regulator (*CFTR*) gene has been found in association with bronchiectasis in RA, and some DR haplotypes are more commonly observed.[155,156] It has also been hypothesized that a reverse association occurs, with bronchiectasis itself as a risk factor for RA.[157]

When bronchiectasis is symptomatic, clinical manifestations include productive cough, recurrent infections, dyspnea, and hemoptysis. Overall survival may be decreased in RA patients with bronchiectasis, predominantly due to infections and acute respiratory failure.[158,159] Bronchiectasis tends to develop late in RA, particularly in women with RF seropositive and nodular disease, although there is a subset of patients in whom bronchiectasis precedes the articular disease and in whom joint symptoms and overall severity of disease is less.[159] Symptomatic bronchiectasis in RA is managed like other forms of bronchiectasis, with aggressive airway clearance, early treatment of pulmonary infections, and bronchodilator therapy.

Airway Obstruction

Airway obstruction as determined by spirometry is present in up to 60% of patients with RA in some

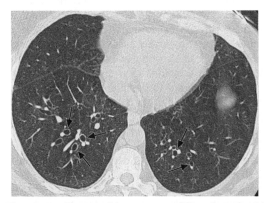

Fig. 9. A 58-year-old woman with rheumatoid arthritis and bronchiectasis. Axial CT image through the lower thorax shows cylindrical bronchiectasis (*arrows*) in both lower lobes.

studies.[160] Even when controlling for smoking history, the prevalence of airflow obstruction is higher in RA patients than in controls.[161,162] HRCT may be more sensitive than PFTs for the detection of small airways disease, with findings including air trapping, heterogeneous lung attenuation, and bronchiectasis.[150] Bronchial hyperreactivity may be increased among RA patients, as demonstrated by higher rates of responsiveness to methacholine challenge.[163]

The occurrence of airways disease in RA may be the result of recurrent respiratory infections or genetic susceptibility. Many patients have a history of smoking, and defects in α1-antitrypsin production have been observed.[164] Symptoms of airways disease include cough, wheezing, and sputum production, and may be treated with inhaled corticosteroids and bronchodilators.

Bronchiolitis Obliterans

Bronchiolitis obliterans (BO) is disorder of the small airways, pathologically characterized by obliterative bronchiolitis with circumferential narrowing, ulceration, and scarring of the terminal and respiratory bronchioles. BO is characterized clinically by progressive dyspnea accompanied by dry cough.[69] On examination, inspiratory crackles and squeaks are heard.[24]

PFTs show the rapid onset and progression of irreversible airflow limitation as demonstrated by a reduction in forced expiratory volume in 1 second (FEV_1) and in the ratio of FEV_1 to forced vital capacity (FVC). In addition, hyperinflation and air trapping may be present, although in later stages of disease, both restrictive and obstructive physiology due to the severity of the air trapping may be observed. HRCT may be more sensitive than PFTs for detecting small airways disease.[150] The radiographic appearance is that of moderate to severe air trapping, as demonstrated by a mosaic pattern of patchy or segmental regions of decreased lung attenuation that are accentuated on expiratory images (**Fig. 10**).[165] At times, the clinical presentation and radiographic findings may be difficult to distinguish from those in chronic obstructive pulmonary disease (COPD), and may be accompanied by RA-ILD.[166]

The diagnosis of BO is usually made indirectly, using clinical, physiologic, and radiographic criteria.[69] Other causes of small airways disease, such as significant tobacco use, should not be present. When surgical biopsy is obtained the pathologic appearance is as described above, with fibrotic obliteration of the small airways, often accompanied by a lymphoplasmacytic infiltrate.[24] The lesions tend to be patchy and must be sought

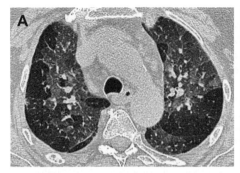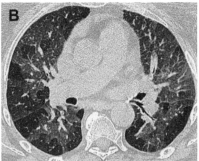

Fig. 10. A 67-year-old woman with shortness of breath and bronchiolitis obliterans secondary to rheumatoid arthritis. High-resolution (1.25-mm thick sections) CT images at the level of the upper (*A*) and mid (*B*) thorax performed during expiration demonstrate moderate multifocal lucent areas of air trapping.

with serial sectioning and trichrome stains, often requiring a large piece of tissue.[167]

BO was first described in 1977 in 6 patients, 5 of whom had RA.[168] Three of these patients had been treated with D-penicillamine, raising concern that BO might be related to medications used to treat RA. Subsequent reports suggested an association with both D-penicillamine and gold salts.[69] In a recent series of 25 RA patients with BO, most with minimal or no smoking history, 48% had been treated with D-penicillamine, 40% with gold salts, 52% with methotrexate, and nearly all with corticosteroids.[166] Of note, FEV_1 was lower in patients who had ever received D-penicillamine than in those who had not.[166] Other risk factors for BO include female sex and long-standing RA.[169] Most patients are RF-seropositive, a finding that does not help with the diagnosis of BO. Concomitant Sjögren syndrome has been suggested as a risk factor but has not been confirmed in all studies.[24,170,171]

BO generally has a poor prognosis, with inexorable progression and poor response to corticosteroids.[69] However, response to treatment with corticosteroids and other immunosuppressive medications has been reported, so a trial of such therapy is often attempted.[172,173] Macrolide antibiotics have been used for their anti-inflammatory properties in treatment of a similar syndrome of BO after lung transplantation, as well as in diffuse panbronchiolitis, with modest success.[174] There is one report of symptomatic, but not physiologic, improvement with low-dose erythromycin.[175] Therefore, therapy with azithromycin or erythromycin may be warranted.

Follicular Bronchiolitis

Follicular bronchiolitis is characterized pathologically by lymphocytic and plasmacytic infiltrate, with hyperplastic lymphoid follicles and reactive germinal centers distributed along and surrounding the bronchioles. This nonspecific histologic pattern is often seen in RA. Although follicular bronchiolitis affects the small airways, it often presents with HRCT findings more typical of an ILD, although there may be some overlap with BO.[69] Usual findings include ground-glass opacities as well as diffuse, small, centrilobular nodules.[176] Patients generally present with dyspnea, although fever and cough may be present. RF is usually present at very high levels. Pulmonary function testing may show a combination of restrictive and obstructive patterns with diffusion abnormalities. Response to corticosteroids and other immunosuppressive therapies varies. Therapy with erythromycin has been used in some patients.[175]

RHEUMATOID NODULES

Rheumatoid nodules, also called necrobiotic nodules, are common in patients with RA. Subcutaneous nodules are detected in approximately 20% of patients, although some reports estimate a frequency as high as 53%.[177–179] Rheumatoid nodules are more common in males than in females and are closely associated with RF seropositivity.[178] Most nodules are clinically asymptomatic, but subcutaneous nodules on pressure points or adherent to periosteum or tendons may become painful.[177] Nodules typically occur in patients with long-standing disease, but their time of onset varies and may even precede the diagnosis of RA.[180] On pathologic examination, the nodules consist of a central area of irregular fibrinoid necrosis surrounded by palisading mononuclear cells, with a peripheral area of chronic inflammatory cells and granulation tissue.[98] The pathogenesis of rheumatoid nodules is incompletely understood, but the inciting events are thought to include repetitive trauma or immune complex deposition, leading to focal vasculitis, complement activation, and cytokine release by local monocytes.[181,182] Anti-CCP antibodies may be an inciting factor in local tissue injury.[183] Proteinases, collagenases, and macrophage chemotactic factors contribute to the central necrosis and surrounding array of macrophages. Complex immunologic processes including both B and T lymphocytes contribute to further inflammation.[184] Recent evidence suggests that the nodule is a T_H1 granuloma.[185]

Rheumatoid nodules occur most commonly in the skin and subcutaneous tissue, but they may also occur in the lung, heart, and upper airway.[186–188] Initially, rheumatoid nodules were felt to be uncommon, as early reports, using chest radiography, found an incidence of approximately 2%.[86] However, small nodules may be more easily detected using more sensitive imaging modalities, and nodules with a characteristic appearance and location have been described in 22% of patients imaged with chest CT.[149] In one study of pathologic findings among patients sent for surgical lung biopsy, 32% had rheumatoid nodules.[56] Core needle biopsies should be interpreted carefully because the histology of the rheumatoid nodule has marked overlap with granulomatous infection and Wegener granulomatosis.[55]

In the lung multiple nodules are usually present, although solitary nodules are also found.[189] The nodules tend to be subpleural or septal and peripheral, although they may appear on the pleural surface.[125] Nodules may be as large as 7 cm in diameter.[11,189] The nodules may remain stable, regress spontaneously, or enlarge (**Fig. 11**). Cavitation may occur and occasionally leads to hemoptysis.[86] Due to their typical subpleural distribution, complications can include pneumothorax, empyema, pleural effusions, and bronchopleural fistula.[98] Both cutaneous and airway nodules have been reported to respond to corticosteroid injection.[190,191]

Nodules in an RA patient should be evaluated similarly to those in any other patient presenting with solitary or multiple pulmonary nodules, as nodules may reflect the presence of infection, malignancy, or other inflammatory diseases. The clinical situation may help guide the evaluation, as patients being treated with immunosuppressive agents are at particular risk for infection.[192,193] Depending on the clinical circumstances, serial radiographic follow-up, needle biopsy, or surgical resection of nodules may be required.

RA patients have increased risk for malignancies, including multiple myeloma and lymphoma, as well as primary lung cancer.[194–196] In one case series, 7 patients with seropositive RA and subcutaneous nodules with new pulmonary nodules were all found to have lung carcinomas at bronchoscopy or thoracotomy.[197] Similarly, documentation of one pathologically confirmed rheumatoid nodule does not ensure that other nodules in the same patient are benign.[198]

Rheumatoid Nodulosis

The presence of multiple nodules, involving the lung, skin, tendons, and other areas, is called rheumatoid nodulosis.[199] This condition, the pathogenesis of which is unknown, is generally benign and is associated with relatively minor joint disease. However, there have been reports of an accelerated variant of rheumatoid nodulosis in patients treated with methotrexate and etanercept.[200–202] The nodules are usually not painful, and therapy can be continued.[177] The nodulosis often regresses with discontinuation of the drug and can be specifically treated with hydroxychloroquine, D-penicillamine, colchicine, and sulfasalazine.[177]

Caplan Syndrome

Caplan syndrome, or rheumatoid pneumoconiosis, was initially described among Welsh coal miners in 1953.[203] It occurs in other occupations with exposure to silica, such as asbestos mining, production of roof tiles, and ceramics manufacturing.[204] The syndrome consists of the rapid onset of lung nodules, ranging in size from 0.5 to 5.0 cm, many of which are cavitary.[203] The nodules may appear at the time of onset of RA symptoms or in the presence of long-standing disease, and are described as "crops" of nodules, often appearing in conjunction with flares of joint disease.[205] In the initial report, most patients had mild pneumoconiosis but were not felt to have progressive massive fibrosis. The nodules in Caplan syndrome are similar histologically to necrobiotic nodules, although an additional layer of peripheral pigmented dust surrounds the lesion.[206] The relationship between RA and pneumoconiosis is poorly understood but may reflect autoimmunity induced by inhalational exposures.[207] Caplan syndrome is uncommon in the United States and now appears to be rare.[24,208]

DRUG-INDUCED LUNG DISEASE

Many of the drugs used to treat RA can cause pulmonary toxicity, but diagnosis of drug-induced lung disease in RA is complex. Distinguishing diagnostically between infection, drug reaction, and underlying RA-ILD can be problematic. The clinical features, pathology, and temporal

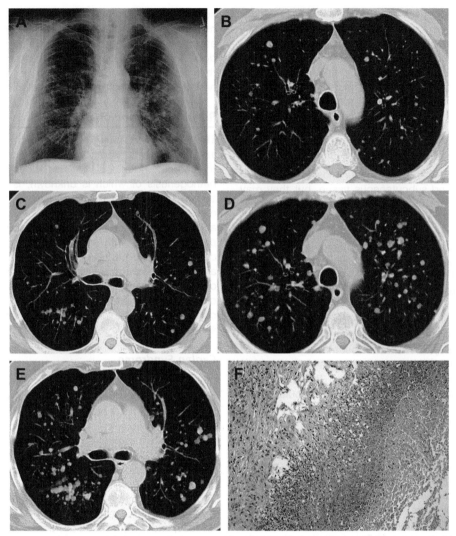

Fig. 11. A 66-year-old man with history of rheumatoid arthritis. Chest radiograph (*A*) is remarkable for the presence of multiple lung nodules bilaterally. CT images obtained through the upper (*B*) and mid (*C*) thorax demonstrate bilateral, multiple well-circumscribed lung nodules of varying sizes with a random distribution. Images from CT of the thorax 1 year later (*D* and *E*) at comparable levels to *B* and *C*, demonstrate an increase in both number and size of the lung nodules bilaterally. Surgical lung biopsy revealed necrobiotic (rheumatoid) nodules (*F*). (Hematoxylin and eosin staining; Original magnification ×20).

correlation with drug initiation may be useful, but the diagnosis often remains in question. The manifestations of drug-induced lung disease are comprehensively reviewed in the article by Meyer and colleagues elsewhere in this issue. A brief overview of therapies particularly used in RA is provided here.

Gold and D-Penicillamine

Drug-induced ILD in RA was first recognized with the use of gold and D-penicillamine, which are now rarely used for RA. Gold-induced pneumonitis manifests typically with rapid onset of cough, fever,

and dyspnea, usually within the first 6 months of therapy.[209] Radiographic findings are nonspecific and may include diffuse or patchy, peripheral ground-glass opacities. Histopathologic patterns include NSIP, eosinophilic pneumonia, and OP.[209] Corticosteroid therapy and withdrawal of the drug have been reported to improve outcomes.[210]

D-Penicillamine has been associated with ILD, BO, and a pulmonary-renal syndrome with alveolar hemorrhage.[98] Toxicity has been associated with peripheral blood eosinophilia and elevated serum IgE levels, and it tends to recur with reexposure to the drug.[211]

Anti-Inflammatory Drugs

Nonsteroidal anti-inflammatory drugs (NSAIDs) have been reported as a rare cause of eosinophilic lung disease, presenting with fever, cough, and dyspnea, with diffuse, patchy consolidations on chest radiograph.[78,212] The syndrome seen with sulfasalazine hypersensitivity is also rare and has similar clinical manifestations.[213] In addition, diffuse centrilobular ground-glass nodules, consistent with subacute hypersensitivity pneumonitis, have been described.[214] Therapy includes withdrawal of the drug and, in more severe cases, corticosteroid therapy. Response to therapy is typically good.[213]

Antimetabolites

Methotrexate

The mechanism of methotrexate-related pulmonary toxicity is unknown. However, it is thought to be an idiosyncratic or hypersensitivity reaction rather than being related to cumulative dose.[215] Although it is not possible to predict which patients will develop pulmonary toxicity, patients with underlying rheumatoid pleural or pulmonary disease may be at increased risk.[216] Some have advocated doing PFTs before the initiation of methotrexate therapy so that the drug can be avoided in patients with preexisting lung disease, and new respiratory symptoms could be better evaluated in treated patients.[217]

Several syndromes of methotrexate pulmonary toxicity have been described.[218] The most common is a hypersensitivity reaction, which presents subacutely with dyspnea (93%), dry cough (83%), and fever (69%), with diffuse interstitial infiltrates (**Fig. 12**).[215] Clinical presentations vary and may include the indolent onset of pulmonary fibrosis, acute lung injury with diffuse alveolar damage (DAD), rapidly progressive pulmonary fibrosis, pleuritis, pleural effusions, nodulosis, or bronchitis with airways hyperreactivity and cough.[78,218,219] Distinguishing methotrexate toxicity from infection and RA-ILD is difficult. Opportunistic infections should be considered, and most often a bronchoscopy with BAL is performed to evaluate for these pathogens. No specific findings on BAL can reliably predict or rule out methotrexate toxicity.[218,220,221] On surgical lung biopsy, several different pathologic patterns may be consistent with drug toxicity, including cellular interstitial infiltrates, granulomas, infiltration with eosinophils, and a DAD pattern with concomitant perivascular inflammation.[218,222]

Therapy is mainly supportive, usually starting with withdrawal of methotrexate therapy alone, although often empirical antibiotic therapy is also administered. In severe cases, corticosteroids may be used; for some patients, other immunosuppressive therapy, such as azathioprine or cyclophosphamide, may be required. Folinic acid to reverse the effects of methotrexate due to its long half-life has been recommended, although this has not been well studied.[217] Reinstitution of therapy with methotrexate after documented or strongly suspected pneumonitis is not recommended, as a 50% mortality rate has been reported.[215,219]

Leflunomide

Leflunomide, a pyrimidine synthesis inhibitor, is a DMARD that has been associated with fatal exacerbation of underlying lung disease.[223–225] The presence of prior ILD or methotrexate pneumonitis may be risk factors.[226,227] Current recommendations are to avoid leflunomide therapy in these patients and to consider screening at-risk populations with PFTs and/or HRCT before initiating therapy with leflunomide.[228] Leflunomide has also been linked with the development of rarer pulmonary syndromes, such as diffuse nodulosis, pulmonary alveolar proteinosis, and diffuse alveolar hemorrhage.[229–231]

Biologic Agents

Tumor necrosis factor-α inhibitors

Case reports implicate the TNF-α inhibitors etanercept, infliximab, and adalimumab with onset or exacerbation of ILD.[83,84,232] Although there are insufficient data to determine the safety of these medications, some investigators recommend avoidance of these drugs in patients with underlying RA-ILD.[79] Studies examining the incidence of ILD among patients treated with TNF-α inhibitors are hampered by a lack of comparison groups and the fact that some patients were receiving the agents as therapy for RA-ILD.[233,234] In fact, case reports suggest a beneficial effect of TNF-α inhibition for some patients with ILD.[82,235]

Abatacept

Abatacept inhibits T-lymphocyte activation by binding CD80 and CD86 on antigen-presenting cells. It is used in patients with moderate to severe, active RA who have not had adequate response to other DMARDs or TNF-α inhibitors.[236] Abatacept should be avoided in patients with underlying COPD, as exacerbations of underlying lung disease and other respiratory adverse events were more common in these patients.[237]

INFECTIONS

Patients with RA are at increased risk for infections, which are often severe.[238–240] The sites of highest risk for infection in RA are the joints,

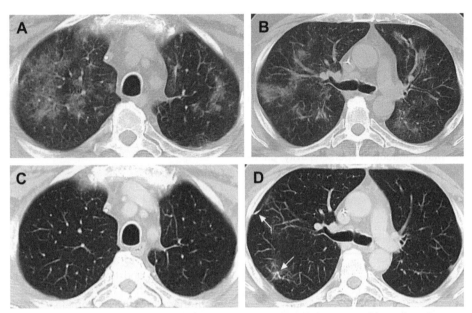

Fig. 12. A 62-year-old man with rheumatoid arthritis who developed shortness of breath and nonproductive cough while being treated with methotrexate. Axial CT images through the upper (A) and mid (B) thorax show bilateral, patchy ground-glass opacities. Surgical lung biopsy revealed organizing pneumonia, presumed secondary to methotrexate toxicity. Arrows in (D) denote surgical staples. The organizing pneumonia resolved (C and D) with discontinuation of methotrexate.

bone (osteomyelitis), and soft tissue.[241] The lung is also a common site for infection, with RA patients having nearly twice the rate of pneumonia as the general population.[241] Some portion of the increased mortality rates in RA is directly attributable to serious infections.[242,243] It is unclear how much of the increased frequency and severity of infection is due to a defect in immunity caused by RA itself and how much reflects the presence of underlying lung disease and therapy with immunomodulatory agents.[244]

Corticosteroid therapy is associated with a dose-dependent increase in the risk for pneumonia; the risk is most prominent with dosages greater than 10 mg per day.[241,245,246] The data for the newer biologic agents is inconsistent, but most biologic agents appear to confer some increased risk for serious infection.

Methotrexate therapy is associated with the development of severe systemic infections as well as opportunistic infections, such as *Pneumocystis jirovecii* pneumonia and disseminated histoplasmosis, even in the absence of concomitant corticosteroid use.[247,248] Most of these infections occur in the first 2 years of therapy.[247] However, large series have found no increased risk or only minimally increased risk for infections with long-term methotrexate use.[240,249–251] The underlying immune defect in RA may play a significant role, given the fact that opportunistic infections have

been reported in the absence of immunosuppressive therapy.[252] Some theorize that with long-term use, the anti-inflammatory effects of methotrexate allow return of immune defenses against infection.[247]

TNF-α is an important component of the immune defense against infection, and plays a key role in the systemic inflammatory response to infection and sepsis as well as in the defense against intracellular and mycobacterial infections.[253] Most of the early randomized controlled trials did not demonstrate an increased risk for infection in patients receiving anti–TNF-α therapy, although the studies were limited by small size and short follow-up time.[254] Larger studies, including one meta-analysis, have confirmed a significant increased risk for serious infections with these agents.[255–257] Coccidioidomycosis and histoplasmosis as well as infections due to *Listeria, Aspergillus, Nocardia,* and mycobacteria have all been reported.[258] The risk for serious infection appears to be particularly high during the first months of therapy.[254,255,259]

Anti–TNF-α therapy significantly increases the risk for mycobacterial infection, especially with *Mycobacterium tuberculosis* (**Fig. 13**).[258] TNF-α is critical in the formation and maintenance of granulomas, and blockade of this molecule leads to reactivation of latent disease. Of importance is that tuberculosis may have an unusual presentation in

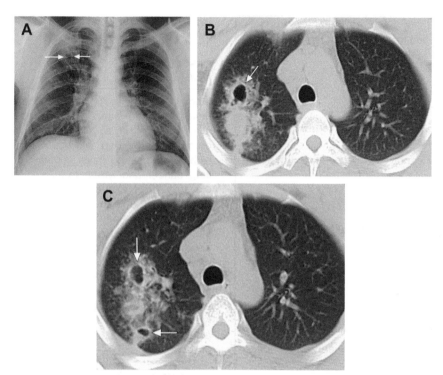

Fig. 13. A 20-year-old man with rheumatoid arthritis being treated with infliximab who developed a new productive cough and fever. Chest radiograph (*A*) shows consolidation in the right apex as well as a small cavity (*arrows*). Axial CT images obtained through the upper thorax (*B* and *C*) show consolidation and 2 small cavities (*arrows*) in the right upper lobe. Subsequent sputum cultures were positive for *Mycobacterium tuberculosis*.

patients treated with these agents, especially extrapulmonary or disseminated disease.[260]

Screening of patients for latent tuberculosis before use of these agents has significantly decreased the number of infections (**Box 2**).[258] Also, measures for tuberculosis prevention should be undertaken, including taking a detailed history for tuberculosis risk factors, as well as tuberculin skin testing (with induration <5 mm indicating a positive response).[261] A negative tuberculin skin test in an otherwise immunosuppressed patient may not reliably exclude latent infection. The use of interferon-γ release assays (such as the QuantiFERON TB Gold test) may be more sensitive that the tuberculin skin test, but it is unclear whether these assays perform accurately in immunosuppressed patients.[258] Patients with latent tuberculosis should be treated with isoniazid for 9 months before the start of therapy with anti–TNF-α agents. This strategy has been shown to decrease the frequency of tuberculosis infections with anti–TNF-α therapy.[262] Patients receiving these drugs should be closely monitored for signs and symptoms of infection.

Newer biologic agents used in therapy for RA include rituximab, tocilizumab, anakinra, and abatacept. Infections have been reported with these agents, but data are too sparse to draw definitive conclusions regarding their risk profiles as compared with methotrexate and anti-TNF agents. Screening for latent tuberculosis is recommended before initiating therapy with abatacept and tocilizumab, and should likely be considered before beginning therapy with any biologic agent.[254]

Distinguishing infection and noninfectious lung inflammation may be difficult. In particular, OP and other ILDs may have the appearance of infectious pneumonia. The differential diagnosis for pulmonary nodules includes not only rheumatoid nodules but also bacterial, fungal, and mycobacterial infections. In many cases invasive studies, including bronchoscopy and surgical biopsy, may need to be considered.

PULMONARY VASCULAR DISEASE

Diffuse alveolar hemorrhage (DAH) due to pulmonary capillaritis has been described in association with RA but is extremely rare.[263] Some milder cases of alveolar hemorrhage may go unrecognized because presenting signs and symptoms are nonspecific. Affected patients may present with shortness of breath, cough, and fever.[264]

Hemoptysis may also be present. HRCT features include diffuse ground-glass opacities and alveolar opacities, which are relatively nonspecific findings and can appear similar to pulmonary edema, diffuse infection, or a drug reaction. The diagnosis of DAH is confirmed in the correct clinical setting by bronchoscopy with BAL, in which progressively bloodier fluid is obtained on serial lavage specimens. Surgical lung biopsy may be required. Infliximab, leflunomide, and rituximab have all been reported to cause alveolar hemorrhage.[231,265,266]

Pulmonary artery hypertension is a frequent complication of many connective tissue diseases, particularly scleroderma and mixed connective tissue disease. Its incidence in RA, however, is believed to be low.[267] Secondary pulmonary hypertension due to advanced ILD may be more common but generally is not severe.[98]

MISCELLANEOUS
Malignancy

Many patients with RA are middle aged, a typical time of onset for cancer, making the diagnosis of a malignancy in a patient with RA relatively common.[268] Beyond this baseline risk, patients with RA appear to have increased risk for both lung cancer and lymphoma.[196,269] Whether this elevated risk is related to smoking history, chronic inflammation due to RA itself, RA therapy, or increased detection of malignancy due to higher interaction with the medical system is not clear.[270,271] In particular, whether the risk of cancer is elevated with use of the TNF-α inhibitors is still debated.[256,272] RA patients who smoke, like all smokers, should be counseled regarding smoking cessation. The presence of mediastinal lymphadenopathy or lung nodules should prompt a thorough evaluation, including direct sampling of tissue.

Myopathy and Muscle Weakness

Muscle weakness is common in RA, most often attributed to deconditioning and immobilization secondary to the joint disease.[273] Also common are muscle loss due to catabolic effects of generalized inflammation, muscle degeneration, changes in blood flow, and nerve function abnormalities.[274] Much of this type of muscle weakness can be improved through exercise and strength training.

Other clinically significant causes for muscle weakness include rheumatoid myositis, rheumatoid vasculitis, overlap with polymyositis, and medication toxicity.[273,275,276] Often in these situations, clinical markers of muscle inflammation, such as elevations in serum creatine kinase, are absent.[276] In particular, D-penicillamine and hydroxychloroquine have been implicated in drug-related toxicity. Hydroxychloroquine myopathy typically presents as a mild to moderate vacuolar myopathy; however, profound muscle weakness with respiratory failure has been described.[277] Myopathy due to corticosteroid use may also play a role.[278]

In the RA patient with progressive dyspnea, muscle weakness should be considered as a potential cause. When the cause for a patient's symptoms is unclear, cardiopulmonary exercise testing with expired gas analysis may indicate muscular sources of limitation. Further evaluation, including muscle biopsy, may be warranted.

Fibrobullous Disease

Apical fibrobullous disease has rarely been described in RA and is radiographically similar to that found in ankylosing spondylitis.[279] Cavitary necrobiotic nodules have been detected on pathologic evaluation, even in the absence of radiographically evident rheumatoid nodules.[280]

Amyloidosis

Secondary amyloidosis in RA may involve the lung. Single and multiple pulmonary nodules made up of amyloid deposits have been described.[281,282] Other reported manifestations include ILD and tracheobronchomalacia.[283,284]

SUMMARY

Pleuropulmonary involvement in RA is common. Although pulmonary disease is often asymptomatic, progressive disease is an important cause of morbidity and mortality in RA. The diagnostic assessment of respiratory abnormalities is complicated by underlying risk for infection, the use of drugs with known pulmonary toxicity, and the frequency of lung disease related to RA itself. Nevertheless, thorough evaluation should be undertaken because early intervention may be life-saving.

The role of screening with PFTs or chest radiographs among RA patients is unclear. Their use has been suggested in patients in whom therapy with DMARDs is being considered, but this practice has not been widely adopted. In the routine care of the patient with RA, a careful search for respiratory symptoms should be undertaken, with a low threshold for further testing if lung disease is suspected.

Much of the focus in RA is on aggressive therapy to prevent joint destruction and disability. It is clear that additional attention must be paid to the extra-articular manifestations of RA, particularly in the lung. More research is needed to assist in our understanding of the pathophysiology, diagnosis, and treatment of these diseases.

REFERENCES

1. Arnett FC, Edworthy SM, Bloch DA, et al. The American Rheumatism Association 1987 revised criteria for the classification of rheumatoid arthritis. Arthritis Rheum 1988;31(3):315–24.
2. Klareskog L, Catrina AI, Paget S. Rheumatoid arthritis. Lancet 2009;373(9664):659–72.
3. Gabriel SE, Michaud K. Epidemiological studies in incidence, prevalence, mortality, and comorbidity of the rheumatic diseases. Arthritis Res Ther 2009;11(3):229.
4. Spector TD. Rheumatoid arthritis. Rheum Dis Clin North Am 1990;16(3):513–37.
5. Gabriel SE, Crowson CS, Kremers HM, et al. Survival in rheumatoid arthritis: a population-based analysis of trends over 40 years. Arthritis Rheum 2003;48(1):54–8.
6. Mori S, Cho I, Koga Y, et al. A simultaneous onset of organizing pneumonia and rheumatoid arthritis, along with a review of the literature. Mod Rheumatol 2008;18(1):60–6.
7. Nannini C, Ryu JH, Matteson EL. Lung disease in rheumatoid arthritis. Curr Opin Rheumatol 2008; 20(3):340–6.
8. Saag KG, Kolluri S, Koehnke RK, et al. Rheumatoid arthritis lung disease. Determinants of radiographic and physiologic abnormalities. Arthritis Rheum 1996;39(10):1711–9.
9. Kinder AJ, Hassell AB, Brand J, et al. The treatment of inflammatory arthritis with methotrexate in clinical practice: treatment duration and incidence of adverse drug reactions. Rheumatology (Oxford) 2005;44(1):61–6.
10. Ellman P, Ball RE. Rheumatoid disease with joint and pulmonary manifestations. Br Med J 1948; 2(4583):816–20.
11. Christie GS. Pulmonary lesions in rheumatoid arthritis. Australas Ann Med 1954;3(1):49–58.
12. Dixon AS, Ball J. Honeycomb lung and chronic rheumatoid arthritis; a case report. Ann Rheum Dis 1957;16(2):241–5.
13. Stack BH, Grant IW. Rheumatoid interstitial lung disease. Br J Dis Chest 1965;59(4):202–11.
14. Frank ST, Weg JG, Harkleroad LE, et al. Pulmonary dysfunction in rheumatoid disease. Chest 1973; 63(1):27–34.
15. Popper MS, Bogdonoff ML, Hughes RL. Interstitial rheumatoid lung disease. A reassessment and review of the literature. Chest 1972;62(3): 243–50.
16. Fewins HE, McGowan I, Whitehouse GH, et al. High definition computed tomography in rheumatoid arthritis associated pulmonary disease. Br J Rheumatol 1991;30(3):214–6.
17. Dawson JK, Fewins HE, Desmond J, et al. Fibrosing alveolitis in patients with rheumatoid arthritis as assessed by high resolution computed tomography, chest radiography, and pulmonary function tests. Thorax 2001;56(8):622–7.
18. Gabbay E, Tarala R, Will R, et al. Interstitial lung disease in recent onset rheumatoid arthritis. Am J Respir Crit Care Med 1997;156(2 Pt 1):528–35.
19. Gochuico BR, Avila NA, Chow CK, et al. Progressive preclinical interstitial lung disease in rheumatoid arthritis. Arch Intern Med 2008; 168(2):159–66.

20. Bilgici A, Ulusoy H, Kuru O, et al. Pulmonary involvement in rheumatoid arthritis. Rheumatol Int 2005;25(6):429–35.

21. Suzuki A, Ohosone Y, Obana M, et al. Cause of death in 81 autopsied patients with rheumatoid arthritis. J Rheumatol 1994;21(1):33–6.

22. Turesson C, O'Fallon WM, Crowson CS, et al. Occurrence of extraarticular disease manifestations is associated with excess mortality in a community based cohort of patients with rheumatoid arthritis. J Rheumatol 2002;29(1): 62–7.

23. Cimmino MA, Salvarani C, Macchioni P, et al. Extra-articular manifestations in 587 Italian patients with rheumatoid arthritis. Rheumatol Int 2000;19(6): 213–7.

24. King MFAT. Connective tissue diseases. In: Schwarz TE, editor. Interstitial lung disease. London: BC Decker Inc; 2003. p. 535–98.

25. Brannan HM, Good CA, Divertie MB, et al. Pulmonary disease associated with rheumatoid arthritis. JAMA 1964;189:914–8.

26. Gizinski AM, Mascolo M, Loucks JL, et al. Rheumatoid arthritis (RA)-specific autoantibodies in patients with interstitial lung disease and absence of clinically apparent articular RA. Clin Rheumatol 2009;28(5):611–3.

27. Akira M, Sakatani M, Hara H. Thin-section CT findings in rheumatoid arthritis-associated lung disease: CT patterns and their courses. J Comput Assist Tomogr 1999;23(6):941–8.

28. O'Donnell DE, Ora J, Webb KA, et al. Mechanisms of activity-related dyspnea in pulmonary diseases. Respir Physiol Neurobiol 2009;167(1): 116–32.

29. Roschmann RA, Rothenberg RJ. Pulmonary fibrosis in rheumatoid arthritis: a review of clinical features and therapy. Semin Arthritis Rheum 1987;16(3):174–85.

30. Bjoraker JA, Ryu JH, Edwin MK, et al. Prognostic significance of histopathologic subsets in idiopathic pulmonary fibrosis. Am J Respir Crit Care Med 1998;157(1):199–203.

31. Chetta A, Aiello M, Foresi A, et al. Relationship between outcome measures of six-minute walk test and baseline lung function in patients with interstitial lung disease. Sarcoidosis Vasc Diffuse Lung Dis 2001;18(2):170–5.

32. O'Donnell D. Physiology of interstitial lung disease. In: Schwartz M, editor. Interstitial lung disease. Ontario: BC Decker; 2003. p. 54–74.

33. Hughes JM, Lockwood DN, Jones HA, et al. DLCO/Q and diffusion limitation at rest and on exercise in patients with interstitial fibrosis. Respir Physiol 1991;83(2):155–66.

34. Harris-Eze AO, Sridhar G, Clemens RE, et al. Oxygen improves maximal exercise performance in interstitial lung disease. Am J Respir Crit Care Med 1994;150(6 Pt 1):1616–22.

35. Tanaka N, Kim JS, Newell JD, et al. Rheumatoid arthritis-related lung diseases: CT findings. Radiology 2004;232(1):81–91.

36. Miller W. Diagnostic thoracic imaging. New York: McGraw-Hill; 2006.

37. Mori S, Cho I, Koga Y, et al. Comparison of pulmonary abnormalities on high-resolution computed tomography in patients with early versus long-standing rheumatoid arthritis. J Rheumatol 2008; 35(8):1513–21.

38. Kocheril SV, Appleton BE, Somers EC, et al. Comparison of disease progression and mortality of connective tissue disease-related interstitial lung disease and idiopathic interstitial pneumonia. Arthritis Rheum 2005;53(4):549–57.

39. Hunninghake GW, Zimmerman MB, Schwartz DA, et al. Utility of a lung biopsy for the diagnosis of idiopathic pulmonary fibrosis. Am J Respir Crit Care Med 2001;164(2):193–6.

40. Hunninghake GW, Lynch DA, Galvin JR, et al. Radiologic findings are strongly associated with a pathologic diagnosis of usual interstitial pneumonia. Chest 2003;124(4):1215–23.

41. Kim EJ, Collard HR, King TE Jr. Rheumatoid arthritis-associated interstitial lung disease: the relevance of histopathologic and radiographic pattern. Chest 2009;136(5):1397–405.

42. Kim TS, Lee KS, Chung MP, et al. Nonspecific interstitial pneumonia with fibrosis: high-resolution CT and pathologic findings. AJR Am J Roentgenol 1998;171(6):1645–50.

43. Kligerman SJ, Groshong S, Brown KK, et al. Nonspecific interstitial pneumonia: radiologic, clinical, and pathologic considerations. Radiographics 2009;29(1):73–87.

44. Travis WD, Hunninghake G, King TE Jr, et al. Idiopathic nonspecific interstitial pneumonia: report of an American Thoracic Society Project. Am J Respir Crit Care Med 2008;177(12): 1338–47.

45. Park JS, Lee KS, Kim JS, et al. Nonspecific interstitial pneumonia with fibrosis: radiographic and CT findings in 7 patients. Radiology 1995;195(3): 645–8.

46. Sumikawa H, Johkoh T, Ichikado K, et al. Nonspecific interstitial pneumonia: histologic correlation with high-resolution CT in 29 patients. Eur J Radiol 2009;70(1):35–40.

47. Shin KM, Lee KS, Chung MP, et al. Prognostic determinants among clinical, thin-section CT, and histopathologic findings for fibrotic idiopathic interstitial pneumonias: tertiary hospital study. Radiology 2008;249(1):328–37.

48. Dawson JK, Fewins HE, Desmond J, et al. Predictors of progression of HRCT diagnosed fibrosing

alveolitis in patients with rheumatoid arthritis. Ann Rheum Dis 2002;61(6):517–21.

49. Nagasawa Y, Takada T, Shimizu T, et al. Inflammatory cells in lung disease associated with rheumatoid arthritis. Intern Med 2009;48(14):1209–17.

50. Biederer J, Schnabel A, Muhle C, et al. Correlation between HRCT findings, pulmonary function tests and bronchoalveolar lavage cytology in interstitial lung disease associated with rheumatoid arthritis. Eur Radiol 2004;14(2):272–80.

51. Costabel U, Guzman J, Bonella F, et al. Bronchoalveolar lavage in other interstitial lung diseases. Semin Respir Crit Care Med 2007;28(5):514–24.

52. Schnabel A, Richter C, Bauerfeind S, et al. Bronchoalveolar lavage cell profile in methotrexate induced pneumonitis. Thorax 1997;52(4):377–9.

53. Ramirez P, Valencia M, Torres A. Bronchoalveolar lavage to diagnose respiratory infections. Semin Respir Crit Care Med 2007;28(5):525–33.

54. Kim DS. Interstitial lung disease in rheumatoid arthritis: recent advances. Curr Opin Pulm Med 2006;12(5):346–53.

55. Leslie KO, Trahan S, Gruden J. Pulmonary pathology of the rheumatic diseases. Semin Respir Crit Care Med 2007;28(4):369–78.

56. Yousem SA, Colby TV, Carrington CB. Lung biopsy in rheumatoid arthritis. Am Rev Respir Dis 1985; 131(5):770–7.

57. Kim DS, Yoo B, Lee JS, et al. The major histopathologic pattern of pulmonary fibrosis in scleroderma is nonspecific interstitial pneumonia. Sarcoidosis Vasc Diffuse Lung Dis 2002;19(2):121–7.

58. Douglas WW, Tazelaar HD, Hartman TE, et al. Polymyositis-dermatomyositis-associated interstitial lung disease. Am J Respir Crit Care Med 2001; 164(7):1182–5.

59. Lee HK, Kim DS, Yoo B, et al. Histopathologic pattern and clinical features of rheumatoid arthritis-associated interstitial lung disease. Chest 2005;127(6):2019–27.

60. Visscher DW, Myers JL. Histologic spectrum of idiopathic interstitial pneumonias. Proc Am Thorac Soc 2006;3(4):322–9.

61. Nicholson AG. Classification of idiopathic interstitial pneumonias: making sense of the alphabet soup. Histopathology 2002;41(5):381–91.

62. Nicholson AG, Addis BJ, Bharucha H, et al. Interobserver variation between pathologists in diffuse parenchymal lung disease. Thorax 2004;59(6): 500–5.

63. van Thiel RJ, van der Burg S, Groote AD, et al. Bronchiolitis obliterans organizing pneumonia and rheumatoid arthritis. Eur Respir J 1991; 4(7):905–11.

64. Ippolito JA, Palmer L, Spector S, et al. Bronchiolitis obliterans organizing pneumonia and rheumatoid arthritis. Semin Arthritis Rheum 1993;23(1):70–8.

65. Cordier JF. Cryptogenic organising pneumonia. Eur Respir J 2006;28(2):422–46.

66. Ulubas B, Sahin G, Ozer C, et al. Bronchiolitis obliterans organizing pneumonia associated with sulfasalazine in a patient with rheumatoid arthritis. Clin Rheumatol 2004;23(3):249–51.

67. Soubrier M, Jeannin G, Kemeny JL, et al. Organizing pneumonia after rituximab therapy: two cases. Joint Bone Spine 2008;75(3):362–5.

68. Cho SK, Oh IH, Park CK, et al. Etanercept induced organizing pneumonia in a patient with rheumatoid arthritis. Rheumatol Int.

69. White ES, Tazelaar HD, Lynch JP 3rd. Bronchiolar complications of connective tissue diseases. Semin Respir Crit Care Med 2003;24(5):543–66.

70. Hakala M. Poor prognosis in patients with rheumatoid arthritis hospitalized for interstitial lung fibrosis. Chest 1988;93(1):114–8.

71. Flaherty KR, Toews GB, Travis WD, et al. Clinical significance of histological classification of idiopathic interstitial pneumonia. Eur Respir J 2002; 19(2):275–83.

72. Riha RL, Duhig EE, Clarke BE, et al. Survival of patients with biopsy-proven usual interstitial pneumonia and nonspecific interstitial pneumonia. Eur Respir J 2002;19(6):1114–8.

73. Park JH, Kim DS, Park IN, et al. Prognosis of fibrotic interstitial pneumonia: idiopathic versus collagen vascular disease-related subtypes. Am J Respir Crit Care Med 2007;175(7):705–11.

74. Tansey D, Wells AU, Colby TV, et al. Variations in histological patterns of interstitial pneumonia between connective tissue disorders and their relationship to prognosis. Histopathology 2004;44(6): 585–96.

75. Hubbard R, Venn A. The impact of coexisting connective tissue disease on survival in patients with fibrosing alveolitis. Rheumatology (Oxford) 2002;41(6):676–9.

76. Kim EJ, Elicker BM, Maldonado F, et al. Usual interstitial pneumonia in rheumatoid arthritis-associated interstitial lung disease. Eur Respir J 2010;35(6):1322.

77. Chang HK, Park W, Ryu DS. Successful treatment of progressive rheumatoid interstitial lung disease with cyclosporine: a case report. J Korean Med Sci 2002;17(2):270–3.

78. Gauhar UA, Gaffo AL, Alarcon GS. Pulmonary manifestations of rheumatoid arthritis. Semin Respir Crit Care Med 2007;28(4):430–40.

79. Kelly C, Saravanan V. Treatment strategies for a rheumatoid arthritis patient with interstitial lung disease. Expert Opin Pharmacother 2008;9(18): 3221–30.

80. Saketkoo LA, Espinoza LR. Experience of mycophenolate mofetil in 10 patients with autoimmune-related interstitial lung disease demonstrates promising effects. Am J Med Sci 2009;337(5):329–35.

81. Saketkoo LA, Espinoza LR. Rheumatoid arthritis interstitial lung disease: mycophenolate mofetil as an antifibrotic and disease-modifying antirheumatic drug. Arch Intern Med 2008;168(15):1718–9.

82. Vassallo R, Matteson E, Thomas CF Jr. Clinical response of rheumatoid arthritis-associated pulmonary fibrosis to tumor necrosis factor-alpha inhibition. Chest 2002;122(3):1093–6.

83. Huggett MT, Armstrong R. Adalimumab-associated pulmonary fibrosis. Rheumatology (Oxford) 2006; 45(10):1312–3.

84. Tournadre A, Ledoux-Eberst J, Poujol D, et al. Exacerbation of interstitial lung disease during etanercept therapy: two cases. Joint Bone Spine 2008;75(2):215–8.

85. Horler AR, Thompson M. The pleural and pulmonary complications of rheumatoid arthritis. Ann Intern Med 1959;51:1179–203.

86. Walker WC, Wright V. Pulmonary lesions and rheumatoid arthritis. Medicine (Baltimore) 1968;47(6): 501–20.

87. Gotsman I, Goral A, Nusair S. Secondary spontaneous pneumothorax in a patient with pulmonary rheumatoid nodules during treatment with methotrexate. Rheumatology (Oxford) 2001; 40(3):350–1.

88. Lillington GA, Carr DT, Mayne JG. Rheumatoid pleurisy with effusion. Arch Intern Med 1971; 128(5):764–8.

89. Faurschou P, Francis D, Faarup P. Thoracoscopic, histological, and clinical findings in nine cases of rheumatoid pleural effusion. Thorax 1985;40(5): 371–5.

90. Balbir-Gurman A, Yigla M, Nahir AM, et al. Rheumatoid pleural effusion. Semin Arthritis Rheum 2006;35(6):368–78.

91. Jurik AG, Davidsen D, Graudal H. Prevalence of pulmonary involvement in rheumatoid arthritis and its relationship to some characteristics of the patients. A radiological and clinical study. Scand J Rheumatol 1982;11(4):217–24.

92. Hakala M, Tiilikainen A, Hameenkorpi R, et al. Rheumatoid arthritis with pleural effusion includes a subgroup with autoimmune features and HLA-B8, Dw3 association. Scand J Rheumatol 1986; 15(3):290–6.

93. Baggenstoss AH, Rosenberg EF. Visceral lesions associated with chronic infectious (rheumatoid) arthritis. Arch Pathol 1943;35:503.

94. Graham WR. Rheumatoid pleurisis. South Med J 1990;83(8):973–5.

95. Jones FL, Blodgett RC Jr. Empyema and rheumatoid pleuropulmonary disease. Ann Intern Med 1978;89(1):139–40.

96. Dixon WG, Hyrich KL, Watson KD, et al. Drug-specific risk of tuberculosis in patients with rheumatoid arthritis treated with anti-TNF therapy: results from the British Society for Rheumatology Biologics Register (BSRBR). Ann Rheum Dis 2010;69(3):522.

97. Wetter DA, Davis MD. Lupus-like syndrome attributable to anti-tumor necrosis factor alpha therapy in 14 patients during an 8-year period at Mayo Clinic. Mayo Clin Proc 2009;84(11):979–84.

98. Tanoue LT. Pulmonary manifestations of rheumatoid arthritis. Clin Chest Med 1998;19(4):667–85, viii.

99. Allan JS, Donahue DM, Garrity JM. Rheumatoid pleural effusion in the absence of arthritic disease. Ann Thorac Surg 2005;80(4):1519–21.

100. Metafratzi ZM, Georgiadis AN, Ioannidou CV, et al. Pulmonary involvement in patients with early rheumatoid arthritis. Scand J Rheumatol 2007;36(5): 338–44.

101. Pritikin JD, Jensen WA, Yenokida GG, et al. Respiratory failure due to a massive rheumatoid pleural effusion. J Rheumatol 1990;17(5):673–5.

102. Tsai TH, Yang PC. Ultrasound in the diagnosis and management of pleural disease. Curr Opin Pulm Med 2003;9(4):282–90.

103. Ferguson GC. Cholesterol pleural effusion in rheumatoid lung disease. Thorax 1966;21(6):577–82.

104. Hillerdal G. Chylothorax and pseudochylothorax. Eur Respir J 1997;10(5):1157–62.

105. Lee SS, Trimble RB. Rheumatoid arthritis with bloody and cholesterol pleural effusion. Arch Pathol Lab Med 1985;109(8):769–71.

106. Dieppe PA. Empyema in rheumatoid arthritis. Ann Rheum Dis 1975;34(2):181–5.

107. Sahn SA, Lakshminarayan S, Char DC. "Silent" empyema in patients receiving corticosteroids. Am Rev Respir Dis 1973;107(5):873–6.

108. Joseph J, Sahn SA. Connective tissue diseases and the pleura. Chest 1993;104(1):262–70.

109. Potts DE, Willcox MA, Good JT Jr, et al. The acidosis of low-glucose pleural effusions. Am Rev Respir Dis 1978;117(4):665–71.

110. Sahn SA, Kaplan RL, Maulitz RM, et al. Rheumatoid pleurisy. observations on the development of low pleural fluid pH and glucose level. Arch Intern Med 1980;140(9):1237–8.

111. Dodson WH, Hollingsworth JW. Pleural effusion in rheumatoid arthritis. Impaired transport of glucose. N Engl J Med 1966;275(24):1337–42.

112. Wrightson JM, Stanton AE, Maskell NA, et al. Pseudochylothorax without pleural thickening: time to reconsider pathogenesis? Chest 2009;136(4): 1144–7.

113. Halla JT, Schrohenloher RE, Koopman WJ. Local immune responses in certain extra-articular manifestations of rheumatoid arthritis. Ann Rheum Dis 1992;51(5):698–701.

114. Soderblom T, Nyberg P, Pettersson T, et al. Pleural fluid beta-2-microglobulin and angiotensin-converting enzyme concentrations in rheumatoid

arthritis and tuberculosis. Respiration 1996;63(5): 272–6.

115. Soderblom T, Pettersson T, Nyberg P, et al. High pleural fluid hyaluronan concentrations in rheumatoid arthritis. Eur Respir J 1999;13(3):519–22.

116. Pettersson T, Ojala K, Weber TH. Adenosine deaminase in the diagnosis of pleural effusions. Acta Med Scand 1984;215(4):299–304.

117. Avnon LS, Abu-Shakra M, Flusser D, et al. Pleural effusion associated with rheumatoid arthritis: what cell predominance to anticipate? Rheumatol Int 2007;27(10):919–25.

118. Nosanchuk JS, Naylor B. A unique cytologic picture in pleural fluid from patients with rheumatoid arthritis. Am J Clin Pathol 1968;50(3):330–5.

119. Carmichael DS, Golding DN. Rheumatoid pleural effusion with "R.A. cells" in the pleural fluid. Br Med J 1967;2(5555):814.

120. Faurschou P, Faarup P. Granulocytes containing cytoplasmic inclusions in human tuberculous pleuritis. Scand J Respir Dis 1973;54(6):341–6.

121. Faurschou P, Faarup P. Pleural granulocytes with cytoplasmic inclusions from patients with malignant lung tumours and mesothelioma. Eur J Respir Dis 1980;61(3):151–5.

122. Engel U, Aru A, Francis D. Rheumatoid pleurisy. Specificity of cytological findings. Acta Pathol Microbiol Immunol Scand A 1986;94(1):53–6.

123. Sahn SA. State of the art. The pleura. Am Rev Respir Dis 1988;138(1):184–234.

124. Yigla M, Simsolo C, Goralnik L, et al. The problem of empyematous pleural effusion in rheumatoid arthritis: report of two cases and review of the literature. Clin Rheumatol 2002;21(2):180–3.

125. Helmers R, Galvin J, Hunninghake GW. Pulmonary manifestations associated with rheumatoid arthritis. Chest 1991;100(1):235–8.

126. Chapman PT, O'Donnell JL, Moller PW. Rheumatoid pleural effusion: response to intrapleural corticosteroid. J Rheumatol 1992;19(3):478–80.

127. Yarbrough JW, Sealy WC, Miller JA. Thoracic surgical problems associated with rheumatoid arthritis. J Thorac Cardiovasc Surg 1975;69(3): 347–54.

128. Rueth N, Andrade R, Groth S, et al. Pleuropulmonary complications of rheumatoid arthritis: a thoracic surgeon's challenge. Ann Thorac Surg 2009;88(3):e20–1.

129. Jones FL Jr, Blodgett RC Jr. Empyema in rheumatoid pleuropulmonary disease. Ann Intern Med 1971;74(5):665–71.

130. Koegelenberg CF, Diaconi AH, Bolligeri CT. Parapneumonic pleural effusion and empyema. Respiration 2008;75(3):241–50.

131. Montgomery WW, Perone PM, Schall LA. Arthritis of the cricoarytenoid joint. Ann Otol Rhinol Laryngol 1955;64(4):1025–33.

132. Lofgren RH, Montgomery WW. Incidence of laryngeal involvement in rheumatoid arthritis. N Engl J Med 1962;267:193–5.

133. Jurik AG, Pedersen U. Rheumatoid arthritis of the crico-arytenoid and crico-thyroid joints: a radiological and clinical study. Clin Radiol 1984;35(3): 233–6.

134. Lawry GV, Finerman ML, Hanafee WN, et al. Laryngeal involvement in rheumatoid arthritis. A clinical, laryngoscopic, and computerized tomographic study. Arthritis Rheum 1984;27(8):873–82.

135. Brazeau-Lamontagne L, et al. Cricoarytenoiditis: CT assessment in rheumatoid arthritis. Radiology 1986;158(2):463–6.

136. Thompson Link D, Charlin B, Levesque RY, et al. Cervicomedullary compression: an unrecognized cause of vocal cord paralysis in rheumatoid arthritis. Ann Otol Rhinol Laryngol 1998;107(6):462–71.

137. Chen JJ, Branstetter BF, Myers EN. Cricoarytenoid rheumatoid arthritis: an important consideration in aggressive lesions of the larynx. AJNR Am J Neuroradiol 2005;26(4):970–2.

138. Segebarth PB, Limbird TJ. Perioperative acute upper airway obstruction secondary to severe rheumatoid arthritis. J Arthroplasty 2007;22(6): 916–9.

139. Dockery KM, Sismanis A, Abedi E. Rheumatoid arthritis of the larynx: the importance of early diagnosis and corticosteroid therapy. South Med J 1991;84(1):95–6.

140. Wattenmaker I, Concepcion M, Hibberd P, et al. Upper-airway obstruction and perioperative management of the airway in patients managed with posterior operations on the cervical spine for rheumatoid arthritis. J Bone Joint Surg Am 1994; 76(3):360–5.

141. Bengtsson M, Bengtsson A. Cricoarytenoid arthritis—a cause of upper airway obstruction in the rheumatoid arthritis patient. Intensive Care Med 1998;24(6):643.

142. Kolman J, Morris I. Cricoarytenoid arthritis: a cause of acute upper airway obstruction in rheumatoid arthritis. Can J Anaesth 2002;49(7):729–32.

143. Absalom AR, Watts R, Kong A. Airway obstruction caused by rheumatoid cricoarytenoid arthritis. Lancet 1998;351(9109):1099–100.

144. Miyanohara T, Igarashi T, Suzuki H, et al. Aggravation of laryngeal rheumatoid arthritis after use of a laryngeal mask airway. J Clin Rheumatol 2006; 12(3):142–4.

145. Bandi V, Munnur U, Braman SS. Airway problems in patients with rheumatologic disorders. Crit Care Clin 2002;18(4):749–65.

146. Redlund-Johnell I. Upper airway obstruction in patients with rheumatoid arthritis and temporomandibular joint destruction. Scand J Rheumatol 1988; 17(4):273–9.

147. Kumai Y, Murakami D, Masuda M, et al. Arytenoid adduction to treat impaired adduction of the vocal fold due to rheumatoid arthritis. Auris Nasus Larynx 2007;34(4):545–8.

148. Funk D, Raymon F. Rheumatoid arthritis of the cricoarytenoid joints: an airway hazard. Anesth Analg 1975;54(6):742–5.

149. Remy-Jardin M, Remy J, Cortet B, et al. Lung changes in rheumatoid arthritis: CT findings. Radiology 1994;193(2):375–82.

150. Perez T, Remy-Jardin M, Cortet B. Airways involvement in rheumatoid arthritis: clinical, functional, and HRCT findings. Am J Respir Crit Care Med 1998;157(5 Pt 1):1658–65.

151. Crestani B. The respiratory system in connective tissue disorders. Allergy 2005;60(6):715–34.

152. McMahon MJ, Swinson DR, Shettar S, et al. Bronchiectasis and rheumatoid arthritis: a clinical study. Ann Rheum Dis 1993;52(11):776–9.

153. Toussirot E, Despaux J, Wendling D. Increased frequency of HLA-DRB1*0401 in patients with RA and bronchiectasis. Ann Rheum Dis 2000;59(12):1002–3.

154. Snowden N, Moran A, Booth J, et al. Defective antibody production in patients with rheumatoid arthritis and bronchiectasis. Clin Rheumatol 1999;18(2):132–5.

155. Puechal X, Fajac I, Bienvenu T, et al. Increased frequency of cystic fibrosis deltaF508 mutation in bronchiectasis associated with rheumatoid arthritis. Eur Respir J 1999;13(6):1281–7.

156. Hillarby MC, McMahon MJ, Grennan DM, et al. HLA associations in subjects with rheumatoid arthritis and bronchiectasis but not with other pulmonary complications of rheumatoid disease. Br J Rheumatol 1993;32(9):794–7.

157. Kaushik VV, Hutchinson D, Desmond J, et al. Association between bronchiectasis and smoking in patients with rheumatoid arthritis. Ann Rheum Dis 2004;63(8):1001–2.

158. Swinson DR, Symmons D, Suresh U, et al. Decreased survival in patients with co-existent rheumatoid arthritis and bronchiectasis. Br J Rheumatol 1997;36(6):689–91.

159. Shadick NA, Fanta CH, Weinblatt ME, et al. Bronchiectasis. A late feature of severe rheumatoid arthritis. Medicine (Baltimore) 1994;73(3):161–70.

160. Collins RL, Turner RA, Johnson AM, et al. Obstructive pulmonary disease in rheumatoid arthritis. Arthritis Rheum 1976;19(3):623–8.

161. Klareskog L, Padyukov L, Alfredsson L. Smoking as a trigger for inflammatory rheumatic diseases. Curr Opin Rheumatol 2007;19(1):49–54.

162. Vergnenegre A, Pugnere N, Antonini MT, et al. Airway obstruction and rheumatoid arthritis. Eur Respir J 1997;10(5):1072–8.

163. Hassan WU, Keaney NP, Holland CD, et al. Bronchial reactivity and airflow obstruction in rheumatoid arthritis. Ann Rheum Dis 1994;53(8):511–4.

164. Mountz JD, Turner RA, Collins RL, et al. Rheumatoid arthritis and small airways function. Effects of disease activity, smoking, and alpha 1-antitrypsin deficiency. Arthritis Rheum 1984;27(7):728–36.

165. Padley SP, Adler BD, Hansell DM, et al. Bronchiolitis obliterans: high resolution CT findings and correlation with pulmonary function tests. Clin Radiol 1993;47(4):236–40.

166. Devouassoux G, Cottin V, Liote H, et al. Characterisation of severe obliterative bronchiolitis in rheumatoid arthritis. Eur Respir J 2009;33(5):1053–61.

167. Kelly K, Hertz MI. Obliterative bronchiolitis. Clin Chest Med 1997;18(2):319–38.

168. Geddes DM, Corrin B, Brewerton DA, et al. Progressive airway obliteration in adults and its association with rheumatoid disease. Q J Med 1977;46(184):427–44.

169. Schwarz MI, Lynch DA, Tuder R. Bronchiolitis obliterans: the lone manifestation of rheumatoid arthritis? Eur Respir J 1994;7(4):817–20.

170. Cooney TP. Interrelationship of chronic eosinophilic pneumonia, bronchiolitis obliterans, and rheumatoid disease: a hypothesis. J Clin Pathol 1981;34(2):129–37.

171. Schlesinger C, Veeraraghavan S, Koss MN. Constructive (obliterative) bronchiolitis. Curr Opin Pulm Med 1998;4(5):288–93.

172. Penny WJ, Knight RK, Rees AM, et al. Obliterative bronchiolitis in rheumatoid arthritis. Ann Rheum Dis 1982;41(5):469–72.

173. van de Laar MA, Westermann CJ, Wagenaar SS, et al. Beneficial effect of intravenous cyclophosphamide and oral prednisone on D-penicillamine-associated bronchiolitis obliterans. Arthritis Rheum 1985;28(1):93–7.

174. Gerhardt SG, McDyer JF, Girgis RE, et al. Maintenance azithromycin therapy for bronchiolitis obliterans syndrome: results of a pilot study. Am J Respir Crit Care Med 2003;168(1):121–5.

175. Hayakawa H, Sato A, Imokawa S, et al. Bronchiolar disease in rheumatoid arthritis. Am J Respir Crit Care Med 1996;154(5):1531–6.

176. Howling SJ, Hansell DM, Wells AU, et al. Follicular bronchiolitis: thin-section CT and histologic findings. Radiology 1999;212(3):637–42.

177. Sayah A, English JC 3rd. Rheumatoid arthritis: a review of the cutaneous manifestations. J Am Acad Dermatol 2005;53(2):191–209 [quiz 210–2].

178. Kaye BR, Kaye RL, Bobrove A. Rheumatoid nodules. Review of the spectrum of associated conditions and proposal of a new classification, with a report of four seronegative cases. Am J Med 1984;76(2):279–92.

179. Gordon DA, Stein JL, Broder I. The extra-articular features of rheumatoid arthritis. A systematic analysis of 127 cases. Am J Med 1973;54(4):445–52.

180. Lowney ED, Simons HM. "Rheumatoid" nodules of the skin: their significance as an isolated finding. Arch Dermatol 1963;88:853–8.

181. Ziff M. The rheumatoid nodule. Arthritis Rheum 1990;33(6):761–7.

182. Kato H, Yamakawa M, Ogino T. Complement mediated vascular endothelial injury in rheumatoid nodules: a histopathological and immunohistochemical study. J Rheumatol 2000;27(8):1839–47.

183. Kuhn KA, Kulik L, Tomooka B, et al. Antibodies against citrullinated proteins enhance tissue injury in experimental autoimmune arthritis. J Clin Invest 2006;116(4):961–73.

184. Highton J, Hessian PA, Stamp L. The rheumatoid nodule: peripheral or central to rheumatoid arthritis? Rheumatology (Oxford) 2007;46(9):1385–7.

185. Hessian PA, Highton J, Kean A, et al. Cytokine profile of the rheumatoid nodule suggests that it is a Th1 granuloma. Arthritis Rheum 2003;48(2):334–8.

186. Burrows FG. Pulmonary nodules in rheumatoid disease: a report of two cases. Br J Radiol 1967;40(472):256–61.

187. Kang H, Baron M. Embolic complications of a mitral valve rheumatoid nodule. J Rheumatol 2004;31(5):1001–3.

188. Friedman BA. Rheumatoid nodules of the larynx. Arch Otolaryngol 1975;101(6):361–3.

189. Case records of the Massachusetts General Hospital. Weekly clinicopathological exercises. Case 10-2001. A 53-year-old woman with arthritis and pulmonary nodules. N Engl J Med 2001;344(13):997–1004.

190. Baan H, Haagsma CJ, van de Laar MA. Corticosteroid injections reduce size of rheumatoid nodules. Clin Rheumatol 2006;25(1):21–3.

191. Voulgari PV, Papazisi D, Bai M, et al. Laryngeal involvement in rheumatoid arthritis. Rheumatol Int 2005;25(5):321–5.

192. Lin J, Ziring D, Desai S, et al. TNFalpha blockade in human diseases: an overview of efficacy and safety. Clin Immunol 2008;126(1):13–30.

193. Weinblatt ME, Abbott GF, Koreishi AF. Case records of the Massachusetts General Hospital. Case 13-2009. A 54-year-old woman with respiratory failure and a cavitary lesion in the lung. N Engl J Med 2009;360(17):1770–9.

194. Eriksson M. Rheumatoid arthritis as a risk factor for multiple myeloma: a case-control study. Eur J Cancer 1993;29(2):259–63.

195. Kelly C, Baird G, Foster H, et al. Prognostic significance of paraproteinaemia in rheumatoid arthritis. Ann Rheum Dis 1991;50(5):290–4.

196. Khurana R, Wolf R, Berney S, et al. Risk of development of lung cancer is increased in patients with rheumatoid arthritis: a large case control study in US veterans. J Rheumatol 2008;35(9):1704–8.

197. Jolles H, Moseley PL, Peterson MW. Nodular pulmonary opacities in patients with rheumatoid arthritis. A diagnostic dilemma. Chest 1989;96(5):1022–5.

198. Baruch AC, Steinbronn K, Sobonya R. Pulmonary adenocarcinomas associated with rheumatoid nodules: a case report and review of the literature. Arch Pathol Lab Med 2005;129(1):104–6.

199. Wisnieski JJ, Askari AD. Rheumatoid nodulosis. A relatively benign rheumatoid variant. Arch Intern Med 1981;141(5):615–9.

200. Toussirot E, Berthelot JM, Pertuiset E, et al. Pulmonary nodulosis and aseptic granulomatous lung disease occurring in patients with rheumatoid arthritis receiving tumor necrosis factor-alpha-blocking agent: a case series. J Rheumatol 2009;36(11):2421–7.

201. Patatanian E, Thompson DF. A review of methotrexate-induced accelerated nodulosis. Pharmacotherapy 2002;22(9):1157–62.

202. van Ede A, den Broeder A, Wagenaar M, et al. Etanercept-related extensive pulmonary nodulosis in a patient with rheumatoid arthritis. J Rheumatol 2007;34(7):1590–2.

203. Caplan A. Certain unusual radiological appearances in the chest of coal-miners suffering from rheumatoid arthritis. Thorax 1953;8(1):29–37.

204. Hunninghake GW, Fauci AS. Pulmonary involvement in the collagen vascular diseases. Am Rev Respir Dis 1979;119(3):471–503.

205. Kelly CA. Rheumatoid arthritis: classical rheumatoid lung disease. Baillieres Clin Rheumatol 1993;7(1):1–16.

206. Gough J, Rivers D, Seal RM. Pathological studies of modified pneumoconiosis in coal-miners with rheumatoid arthritis; Caplan's syndrome. Thorax 1955;10(1):9–18.

207. Otsuki T, Maeda M, Murakami S, et al. Immunological effects of silica and asbestos. Cell Mol Immunol 2007;4(4):261–8.

208. De Capitani EM, Schweller M, da Silva CM, et al. Rheumatoid pneumoconiosis (Caplan's syndrome) with a classical presentation. J Bras Pneumol 2009;35(9):942–6.

209. Tomioka R, King TE Jr. Gold-induced pulmonary disease: clinical features, outcome, and differentiation from rheumatoid lung disease. Am J Respir Crit Care Med 1997;155(3):1011–20.

210. Blancas R, Moreno JL, Martin F, et al. Alveolar-interstitial pneumopathy after gold-salts compounds administration, requiring mechanical ventilation. Intensive Care Med 1998;24(10):1110–2.

211. Zitnik RJ, Cooper JA Jr. Pulmonary disease due to antirheumatic agents. Clin Chest Med 1990;11(1):139–50.

212. Goodwin SD, Glenny RW. Nonsteroidal anti-inflammatory drug-associated pulmonary infiltrates with eosinophilia. Review of the literature and food and drug administration adverse drug reaction reports. Arch Intern Med 1992;152(7):1521–4.

213. Parry SD, Barbatzas C, Peel ET, et al. Sulphasalazine and lung toxicity. Eur Respir J 2002;19(4):756–64.

214. Woltsche M, Woltsche-Kahr I, Roeger GM, et al. Sulfasalazine-induced extrinsic allergic alveolitis in a patient with psoriatic arthritis. Eur J Med Res 2001;6(11):495–7.

215. Kremer JM, Alarcon GS, Weinblatt ME, et al. Clinical, laboratory, radiographic, and histopathologic features of methotrexate-associated lung injury in patients with rheumatoid arthritis: a multicenter study with literature review. Arthritis Rheum 1997;40(10):1829–37.

216. Alarcon GS, Kremer JM, Macaluso M, et al. Risk factors for methotrexate-induced lung injury in patients with rheumatoid arthritis. A multicenter, case-control study. Methotrexate-Lung Study Group. Ann Intern Med 1997;127(5):356–64.

217. Saravanan V, Kelly C. Drug-related pulmonary problems in patients with rheumatoid arthritis. Rheumatology (Oxford) 2006;45(7):787–9.

218. Cannon GW. Methotrexate pulmonary toxicity. Rheum Dis Clin North Am 1997;23(4):917–37.

219. Schnabel A, Dalhoff K, Bauerfeind S, et al. Sustained cough in methotrexate therapy for rheumatoid arthritis. Clin Rheumatol 1996;15(3):277–82.

220. Fuhrman C, Parrot A, Wislez M, et al. Spectrum of CD4 to CD8 T-cell ratios in lymphocytic alveolitis associated with methotrexate-induced pneumonitis. Am J Respir Crit Care Med 2001;164(7):1186–91.

221. Chikura B, Sathi N, Lane S, et al. Variation of immunological response in methotrexate-induced pneumonitis. Rheumatology (Oxford) 2008;47(11):1647–50.

222. Imokawa S, Colby TV, Leslie KO, et al. Methotrexate pneumonitis: review of the literature and histopathological findings in nine patients. Eur Respir J 2000;15(2):373–81.

223. Ito S, Sumida T. Interstitial lung disease associated with leflunomide. Intern Med 2004;43(12):1103–4.

224. Kamata Y, Nara H, Kamimura T, et al. Rheumatoid arthritis complicated with acute interstitial pneumonia induced by leflunomide as an adverse reaction. Intern Med 2004;43(12):1201–4.

225. Suissa S, Hudson M, Ernst P. Leflunomide use and the risk of interstitial lung disease in rheumatoid arthritis. Arthritis Rheum 2006;54(5):1435–9.

226. Sawada T, Inokuma S, Sato T, et al. Leflunomide-induced interstitial lung disease: prevalence and risk factors in Japanese patients with rheumatoid arthritis. Rheumatology (Oxford) 2009;48(9):1069–72.

227. Chikura B, Lane S, Dawson JK. Clinical expression of leflunomide-induced pneumonitis. Rheumatology (Oxford) 2009;48(9):1065–8.

228. Kelly C. Leflunomide and the lung. Rheumatology (Oxford) 2009;48(9):1017–8.

229. Rozin A, Yigla M, Guralnik L, et al. Rheumatoid lung nodulosis and osteopathy associated with leflunomide therapy. Clin Rheumatol 2006;25(3):384–8.

230. Wardwell NR Jr, Miller R, Ware LB. Pulmonary alveolar proteinosis associated with a disease-modifying antirheumatoid arthritis drug. Respirology 2006;11(5):663–5.

231. Carloni A, Piciucchi S, Giannakakis K, et al. Diffuse alveolar hemorrhage after leflunomide therapy in a patient with rheumatoid arthritis. J Thorac Imaging 2008;23(1):57–9.

232. Villeneuve E, St-Pierre A, Haraoui B. Interstitial pneumonitis associated with infliximab therapy. J Rheumatol 2006;33(6):1189–93.

233. Takeuchi T, Tatsuki Y, Nogami Y, et al. Postmarketing surveillance of the safety profile of infliximab in 5000 Japanese patients with rheumatoid arthritis. Ann Rheum Dis 2008;67(2):189–94.

234. Wolfe F, Caplan L, Michaud K. Rheumatoid arthritis treatment and the risk of severe interstitial lung disease. Scand J Rheumatol 2007;36(3):172–8.

235. Antoniou KM, Mamoulaki M, Malagari K, et al. Infliximab therapy in pulmonary fibrosis associated with collagen vascular disease. Clin Exp Rheumatol 2007;25(1):23–8.

236. Furst DE, Keystone EC, Kirkham B, et al. Updated consensus statement on biological agents for the treatment of rheumatic diseases, 2008. Ann Rheum Dis 2008;67(Suppl 3):iii2–25.

237. Weinblatt M, Combe B, Covucci A, et al. Safety of the selective costimulation modulator abatacept in rheumatoid arthritis patients receiving background biologic and nonbiologic disease-modifying antirheumatic drugs: a one-year randomized, placebo-controlled study. Arthritis Rheum 2006;54(9):2807–16.

238. Baum J. Infection in rheumatoid arthritis. Arthritis Rheum 1971;14(1):135–7.

239. Walker WC. Pulmonary infections and rheumatoid arthritis. Q J Med 1967;36(142):239–51.

240. Smitten AL, Choi HK, Hochberg MC, et al. The risk of hospitalized infection in patients with rheumatoid arthritis. J Rheumatol 2008;35(3):387–93.

241. Doran MF, Crowson CS, Pond GR, et al. Frequency of infection in patients with rheumatoid arthritis

compared with controls: a population-based study. Arthritis Rheum 2002;46(9):2287–93.

242. Mitchell DM, Spitz PW, Young DY, et al. Survival, prognosis, and causes of death in rheumatoid arthritis. Arthritis Rheum 1986;29(6):706–14.

243. Myllykangas-Luosujarvi R, Aho K, Kautiainen H, et al. Shortening of life span and causes of excess mortality in a population-based series of subjects with rheumatoid arthritis. Clin Exp Rheumatol 1995;13(2):149–53.

244. Doran MF, Gabriel SE. Infections in rheumatoid arthritis—a new phenomenon? J Rheumatol 2001; 28(9):1942–3.

245. Saag KG, Koehnke R, Caldwell JR, et al. Low dose long-term corticosteroid therapy in rheumatoid arthritis: an analysis of serious adverse events. Am J Med 1994;96(2):115–23.

246. Wolfe F, Caplan L, Michaud K. Treatment for rheumatoid arthritis and the risk of hospitalization for pneumonia: associations with prednisone, disease-modifying antirheumatic drugs, and anti-tumor necrosis factor therapy. Arthritis Rheum 2006;54(2):628–34.

247. Boerbooms AM, Kerstens PJ, van Loenhout JW, et al. Infections during low-dose methotrexate treatment in rheumatoid arthritis. Semin Arthritis Rheum 1995;24(6):411–21.

248. LeMense GP, Sahn SA. Opportunistic infection during treatment with low dose methotrexate. Am J Respir Crit Care Med 1994;150(1):258–60.

249. Bernatsky S, Hudson M, Suissa S. Anti-rheumatic drug use and risk of serious infections in rheumatoid arthritis. Rheumatology (Oxford) 2007;46(7): 1157–60.

250. Coyne P, Hamilton J, Heycock C, et al. Acute lower respiratory tract infections in patients with rheumatoid arthritis. J Rheumatol 2007;34(9):1832–6.

251. McLean-Tooke A, Aldridge C, Waugh S, et al. Methotrexate, rheumatoid arthritis and infection risk: what is the evidence? Rheumatology (Oxford) 2009;48(8):867–71.

252. Oien KA, Black A, Hunter JA, et al. *Pneumocystis carinii* pneumonia in a patient with rheumatoid arthritis, not on immunosuppressive therapy and in the absence of human immunodeficiency virus infection. Br J Rheumatol 1995;34(7):677–9.

253. Khraishi M. Comparative overview of safety of the biologics in rheumatoid arthritis. J Rheumatol Suppl 2009;82:25–32.

254. Martin-Mola E, Balsa A. Infectious complications of biologic agents. Rheum Dis Clin North Am 2009; 35(1):183–99.

255. Askling J, Dixon W. The safety of anti-tumour necrosis factor therapy in rheumatoid arthritis. Curr Opin Rheumatol 2008;20(2):138–44.

256. Bongartz T, Sutton AJ, Sweeting MJ, et al. Anti-TNF antibody therapy in rheumatoid arthritis and the risk of serious infections and malignancies: systematic review and meta-analysis of rare harmful effects in randomized controlled trials. JAMA 2006;295(19):2275–85.

257. Listing J, Strangfeld A, Kary S, et al. Infections in patients with rheumatoid arthritis treated with biologic agents. Arthritis Rheum 2005;52(11):3403–12.

258. Winthrop KL. Risk and prevention of tuberculosis and other serious opportunistic infections associated with the inhibition of tumor necrosis factor. Nat Clin Pract Rheumatol 2006;2(11):602–10.

259. Askling J, Fored CM, Brandt L, et al. Time-dependent increase in risk of hospitalisation with infection among Swedish RA patients treated with TNF antagonists. Ann Rheum Dis 2007;66(10):1339–44.

260. Keane J, Gershon S, Wise RP, et al. Tuberculosis associated with infliximab, a tumor necrosis factor alpha-neutralizing agent. N Engl J Med 2001; 345(15):1098–104.

261. Centers for Disease Control and Prevention (CDC). Tuberculosis associated with blocking agents against tumor necrosis factor-alpha—California, 2002-2003. MMWR Morb Mortal Wkly Rep 2004; 53(30):683–6.

262. Carmona L, Gomez-Reino JJ, Rodriguez-Valverde V, et al. Effectiveness of recommendations to prevent reactivation of latent tuberculosis infection in patients treated with tumor necrosis factor antagonists. Arthritis Rheum 2005;52(6): 1766–72.

263. Schwarz MI, Zamora MR, Hodges TN, et al. Isolated pulmonary capillaritis and diffuse alveolar hemorrhage in rheumatoid arthritis and mixed connective tissue disease. Chest 1998;113(6): 1609–15.

264. Ioachimescu OC, Stoller JK. Diffuse alveolar hemorrhage: diagnosing it and finding the cause. Cleve Clin J Med 2008;75(4):258 [260, 264–5 passim].

265. Panagi S, Palka W, Korelitz BI, et al. Diffuse alveolar hemorrhage after infliximab treatment of Crohn's disease. Inflamm Bowel Dis 2004;10(3): 274–7.

266. Heresi GA, Farver CF, Stoller JK. Interstitial pneumonitis and alveolar hemorrhage complicating use of rituximab: case report and review of the literature. Respiration 2008;76(4):449–53.

267. Hassoun PM. Pulmonary arterial hypertension complicating connective tissue diseases. Semin Respir Crit Care Med 2009;30(4):429–39.

268. Askling J. Malignancy and rheumatoid arthritis. Curr Rheumatol Rep 2007;9(5):421–6.

269. Smitten AL, Simon TA, Hochberg MC, et al. A meta-analysis of the incidence of malignancy in adult patients with rheumatoid arthritis. Arthritis Res Ther 2008;10(2):R45.

270. Baecklund E, Iliadou A, Askling J, et al. Association of chronic inflammation, not its treatment, with

increased lymphoma risk in rheumatoid arthritis. Arthritis Rheum 2006;54(3):692–701.

271. Kallberg H. Rheumatoid arthritis and lung cancer: you probably heard it before. J Rheumatol 2008; 35(9):1695–6.

272. Askling J, van Vollenhoven RF, Granath F, et al. Cancer risk in patients with rheumatoid arthritis treated with anti-tumor necrosis factor alpha therapies: does the risk change with the time since start of treatment? Arthritis Rheum 2009;60(11): 3180–9.

273. Chatterjee S, Kupsky WJ. Severe proximal myopathy and mononeuritis multiplex in rheumatoid arthritis: manifestations of rheumatoid vasculitis. J Clin Rheumatol 2005;11(1):50–5.

274. Hakkinen A. Effectiveness and safety of strength training in rheumatoid arthritis. Curr Opin Rheumatol 2004;16(2):132–7.

275. Halla JT, Koopman WJ, Fallahi S, et al. Rheumatoid myositis. Clinical and histologic features and possible pathogenesis. Arthritis Rheum 1984; 27(7):737–43.

276. Miro O, Pedrol E, Casademont J, et al. Muscle involvement in rheumatoid arthritis: clinicopathological study of 21 symptomatic cases. Semin Arthritis Rheum 1996;25(6):421–8.

277. Abdel-Hamid H, Oddis CV, Lacomis D. Severe hydroxychloroquine myopathy. Muscle Nerve 2008; 38(3):1206–10.

278. Schakman O, Gilson H, Thissen JP. Mechanisms of glucocorticoid-induced myopathy. J Endocrinol 2008;197(1):1–10.

279. Strohl KP, Feldman NT, Ingram RH Jr. Apical fibrobullous disease with rheumatoid arthritis. Chest 1979;75(6):739–41.

280. Yue CC, Park CH, Kushner I. Apical fibrocavitary lesions of the lung in rheumatoid arthritis. Report of two cases and review of the literature. Am J Med 1986;81(4):741–6.

281. Calatayud J, Candelas G, Gomez A, et al. Nodular pulmonary amyloidosis in a patient with rheumatoid arthritis. Clin Rheumatol 2007;26(10):1797–8.

282. Tokunaga T, Takeda S, Sawabata N, et al. Nodular pulmonary amyloidosis. Jpn J Thorac Cardiovasc Surg 2006;54(9):399–401.

283. Sumiya M, Ohya N, Shinoura H, et al. Diffuse interstitial pulmonary amyloidosis in rheumatoid arthritis. J Rheumatol 1996;23(5):933–6.

284. Turkstra F, Rinkel RN, Biermann H, et al. Tracheobronchomalacia due to amyloidosis in a patient with rheumatoid arthritis. Clin Rheumatol 2008; 27(6):807–8.

Pulmonary Manifestations of Systemic Lupus Erythematosus

Diane L. Kamen, MD, MSCR[a],*, Charlie Strange, MD[b]

KEYWORDS

• Lupus • Inflammation • Lung disease • Pulmonary

Systemic lupus erythematosus (SLE) is a potentially severe, frequently disabling autoimmune disease with multiorgan involvement and a typically waxing and waning course. SLE is often considered the prototypical autoimmune disease. It is characterized by the production of a vast array of autoantibodies and a variable clinical presentation that can include lung disease, although the more common early manifestations include arthritis, photosensitive rashes, immune-mediated cytopenias, and the development of glomerulonephritis.[1] The clinical symptoms and immunologic manifestations of SLE are diverse, and no two patients present the same way. Early diagnosis can be difficult and often delayed because of the insidious onset of predominantly nonspecific constitutional symptoms (eg, fatigue and low-grade fever).

SLE is considered primarily a disease of women of childbearing age, although males or females of any age can be affected. The typical age at diagnosis is between 15 and 45 years. The female to male ratio for the development of SLE is 9:1, although it is interesting that lung involvement is proportionally more common in men. African Americans and Hispanic Americans have a threefold increased incidence of SLE, develop SLE at an earlier age, and have increased morbidity and mortality compared with Caucasians.[2,3]

Although SLE has the potential to affect any organ, the lungs are commonly involved later in the course of the disease in the setting of other organ involvement. The most common pulmonary manifestation attributable to SLE is pleuritis, but other pleural involvement can be seen, as well as parenchymal disease, pulmonary vascular disease, diaphragmatic dysfunction, and upper airway dysfunction (**Table 1**).[4] Finding the true prevalence of lung involvement with SLE is complicated by the high rates of pulmonary infections. Lung involvement occurring in 80% of SLE patients at autopsy and chart review from past reports is now thought to be largely a result of infection and not directly SLE-induced.[4] A more recent autopsy study of 90 patients with SLE found pleuropulmonary involvement in 97.8%, the most common being pleuritis (77.8%), bacterial infections (57.8%), primary and secondary alveolar hemorrhages (25.6%), followed by distal airway alterations (21.1%), opportunistic infections (14.4%), and pulmonary thromboembolism (7.8%).[5] In a series of 216 consecutive patients with SLE followed in the United Kingdom, 25% had evidence of lung involvement diagnosed clinically and/or by imaging.[6]

EPIDEMIOLOGY AND RISK FACTORS

Susceptibility to SLE has a genetic component, and familial clustering of cases is seen. From 5% to 12% of first-degree relatives of SLE patients will themselves develop the disease during their

Financial disclosures: None.

[a] Division of Rheumatology and Immunology, Medical University of South Carolina, 96 Jonathan Lucas Street, Suite 912, Charleston, SC 29425, USA

[b] Division of Pulmonary and Critical Care Medicine, Medical University of South Carolina, Charleston, SC, USA

* Corresponding author.

E-mail address: kamend@musc.edu

Table 1
Most common pulmonary manifestations of SLE

Pleural disease	Pleural effusion Pleurisy
Parenchymal disease	Acute lupus pneumonitis Acute respiratory distress syndrome Diffuse alveolar hemorrhage Chronic interstitial pneumonitis Diaphragmatic dysfunction/Shrinking lung syndrome
Vascular involvement	Acute reversible hypoxemia Pulmonary embolism/Thromboembolic disease Pulmonary arterial hypertension
Airway disease	Obstructive lung disease Upper airway disease

Data from Pego-Reigosa JM, Medeiros DA, Isenberg DA. Respiratory manifestations of systemic lupus erythematosus: old and new concepts. Best Pract Res Clin Rheumatol 2009;23:469–80; and Strange C, Highland KB. Interstitial lung disease in the patient who has connective tissue disease. Clin Chest Med 2004;25:549–59, vii.

lifetime. Several susceptibility loci as well as specific gene polymorphisms have been identified, although the relationships are complex and vary by ethnicity.[7] Not all studies of SLE-related genetic markers have looked separately at lung involvement; but among those that have, both protective haplotypes and risk haplotypes have been identified.[8] Identified genetic factors do not fully explain why some patients have lung involvement. Therefore, multiple environmental factors have been implicated as potential triggers to explain why SLE has a variable pulmonary presentation.

Tissue chimerism, the presence of cells from one individual in another individual, may also play a role in lung disease in SLE. In an autopsy series of 7 women with SLE, the lungs (67%) were second only to the kidneys (86%) in the prevalence of chimerism in organs of women with SLE, compared with very little chimerism (17%) seen in the lungs of 34 controls.[9] These data support the idea that tissue chimerism is the result of the repair process rather than the etiology of the organ involvement.[9]

CLINICAL FEATURES
Pleural Disease

More so than in any other connective tissue disease, the pleura is often involved in patients with SLE. Approximately 30% to 50% of patients with SLE will develop symptomatic pleural inflammation over the course of their disease, and a larger number if asymptomatic effusions are included.[10,11] In 5% to 10% of patients, pleuritis is an initial manifestation of their SLE.[12] The typical presentation of pleural involvement in SLE is sharp chest pain with a deep breath (pleurisy). Nonpleuritic musculoskeletal chest wall pain is also common, and can usually be distinguished from pleural disease if the symptoms are reproducible on palpation of the painful areas.

Pleural effusions in SLE tend to be bilateral but small, and may not be evident on radiographic imaging.[13] A friction rub may be present on examination; however, these can be transient. The pleural fluid in SLE is exudative with a predominance of either lymphocytes or polymorphonuclear cells, low glucose concentration (but not as low as in rheumatoid arthritis effusions), and low complement levels.[14] Serologic testing of the pleural fluid shows low complement levels and positive antinuclear antibody; however, these tests are not sufficiently sensitive to assist in making a diagnosis.[15] Lupus erythematosus cells occasionally can be found on cytologic examination of pleural fluid, but this test is rarely performed due to the prolonged preparation time of this assay.[13] On rare occasions pleural fibrosis and a trapped lung can occur as a long-term complication of pleural inflammation.

Pleural disease in SLE typically responds well to nonsteroidal anti-inflammatory drugs or low-dose corticosteroids. Small asymptomatic effusions usually resolve spontaneously without therapy.[12] Occasionally, moderate to high dose corticosteroids are needed for resolution of the pleural inflammation and only rarely are other immunosuppressants required to control refractory or recurrent pleuritis. Tetracycline or talc pleurodesis has been used successfully for recurrent large effusions.[16–18]

Parenchymal Lung Disease

Acute lupus pneumonitis

Albeit rare, occurring in 1% to 12% of patients, acute lupus pneumonitis is one of the most dreaded complications of SLE.[19,20] Patients usually present with fever, cough, pleurisy, dyspnea with hypoxia, and sometimes hemoptysis. Most patients with lupus pneumonitis will be anti-dsDNA antibody positive. Examination usually finds basilar rales. Chest radiography shows pleural effusions and alveolar pulmonary infiltrates, particularly in the lower lung fields. Bronchoalveolar lavage in lupus pneumonitis reveals increased cellularity with activated polymorphonuclear leukocytes.[21] Noninvasive clues of active disease include increased gallium-67 uptake, late inspiratory crackles, and an abnormal interstitial pattern (either ground-glass or honeycomb appearance) on chest computed tomography (CT).[21] It can be difficult to distinguish acute lupus pneumonitis from diffuse alveolar hemorrhage (discussed later).

Older studies suggest that the prognosis is poor for patients with acute lupus pneumonitis, with a short-term mortality of 50%. The outcome is reported to be worse for postpartum lupus pneumonitis.[22,23] However, in the modern era with advanced critical care support, frequent use of plasmapheresis, and an improved ventilatory armamentarium, the true mortality of this condition remains unknown. Long-term morbidity includes persistent pulmonary function abnormalities and restrictive lung disease. Bronchoalveolar lavage (BAL) fluid analysis can be helpful, with eosinophilic or neutrophilic lavage fluid predicting a worse prognosis compared with lymphocytic fluid.[21]

The most immediate concern for patients with suspected lupus pneumonitis is to exclude the presence of a pulmonary infection, because these 2 diseases have similar presentations but very different treatments. Empiric antibiotics are often started early, then discontinued as cultures return negative for infections. The mainstay of acute lupus pneumonitis treatment is systemic corticosteroids (prednisone 1–1.5 mg/kg/d in divided doses), although the mortality of lupus pneumonitis remains high despite corticosteroids.[24] If the response to oral corticosteroids is not adequate within 72 hours or the patient has marked tachypnea, hypoxemia, or suspected diffuse alveolar hemorrhage, treatment should include intravenous pulse corticosteroids (ie, 1 g methylprednisolone per day for 3 days). In addition, immunosuppressants such as cyclophosphamide should be considered.[22] One case has been reported of clinical improvement with addition of rituximab to a background of immunosuppression with mycophenolate mofetil and corticosteroids in a patient with refractory lupus pneumonitis.[25]

Chronic interstitial lung disease

Chronic interstitial lung disease (ILD), also called fibrotic lupus pneumonitis, is seen in 3% to 13% of patients with SLE, primarily in patients with long-standing disease.[26,27] There is an association with anti-SSA antibodies, and in one series anti-SSA antibodies were found in 81% of patients with lupus pneumonitis, compared with 38% for all patients with SLE.[28] Because ILD can occur in primary Sjögren syndrome or with other lupus overlap syndromes, controversy remains concerning the prevalence of chronic interstitial lung disease in SLE. ILD often develops insidiously, with gradually worsening nonproductive cough, dyspnea on exertion, and recurrent pleurisy, but can also appear following an episode of acute lupus pneumonitis.[22] Similar to idiopathic pulmonary fibrosis, examination reveals bibasilar inspiratory pulmonary crackles. Lung function tests show a restrictive pattern with reduced lung volumes and reduced diffusing capacity for carbon monoxide (DLCO).

Chest radiographs may be normal or reveal bibasilar irregular linear opacities early in the course. More diffuse infiltrates, pleural disease, or honeycombing appear later in the course. High-resolution computed tomography (HRCT) is helpful to evaluate for the ground-glass appearance associated with cellular infiltration or fibrosis and for the reticular pattern associated with fibrotic disease (**Fig. 1**). Although HRCT findings are predictive of the pathologic pattern of ILD seen on lung biopsy, a biopsy is occasionally used to exclude other causes, including infections. The histopathologic findings of chronic ILD in SLE include alveolar septal thickening, interstitial fibrosis, lymphocytic infiltrates, alveolar septal immune deposits, and type II pneumocyte hyperplasia. The most common pathologic patterns include nonspecific interstitial pneumonia , usual interstitial pneumonia and, less often, lymphocytic interstitial pneumonia.[29]

Similar to acute lupus pneumonitis, there have been no controlled treatment trials for chronic ILD in SLE. Oral corticosteroids are a reasonable first-line therapy for symptomatic patients. An open-label trial of prednisone (60 mg/d for at least 4 weeks) in 14 patients with SLE-related ILD found that respiratory symptoms in all of the patients improved. At a mean follow-up of 7.3 years, 3 of the patients had died, 2 of lung fibrosis and 1 of bacterial pneumonia, but the DLCO was improved in the majority of the survivors.[26] Beyond

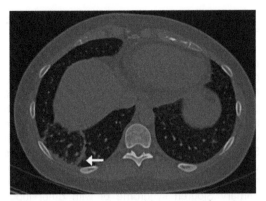

Fig. 1. Chest CT in a 33 year-old woman with a 13-year history of SLE, showing a focal area of traction bronchiectasis with mucoid impaction (*arrow*) surrounded by ground-glass opacities in the right lower lobe, felt to be postinflammatory in nature. She also has interstitial markings in the lung bases, which have remained unchanged for 7 years.

corticosteroids, the authors' guidance on the choice of immunosuppressant treatments is borrowed from the scleroderma ILD experience, supported by a similar histopathologic appearance between the 2 diseases. The optimal choice for SLE-related ILD is uncertain, but cyclophosphamide, azathioprine, and mycophenolate have all been tried in situations of inadequate response to corticosteroids.

Shrinking lung syndrome

The shrinking or "vanishing" lung syndrome (SLS) has been reported in patients with SLE who have unexplained dyspnea, elevation of the diaphragm (usually bilateral), and reduced lung volumes without evidence of ILD.[30,31] Lung function tests show a restrictive defect, and DLCO is usually normal when corrected for lung volume. To date there have been 77 patients with SLS reported in the literature, with a prevalence of 0.6% to 0.9%.[6,32] A review of these SLS cases found that episodes of pleuritic chest pain are common (65% at the time of evaluation).[32]

The underlying etiology of SLS is debated. One possibility is that diaphragmatic weakness results from an inflammatory myopathy or phrenic neuropathy, resulting in elevation of the diaphragms and reduced lung volumes.[33,34] Other reports, however, have found normal diaphragmatic muscle strength among patients with SLS on testing.[35,36]

The prognosis of SLS is overall good with treatment.[37] Based on case reports in the literature, corticosteroids and immunosuppressive therapy may be effective therapeutic options for symptomatic patients with SLS.[38,39] Immunosuppressants

reported in the literature as having potential benefit include azathioprine, methotrexate, cyclophosphamide, and rituximab.[30,32,40] In addition, theophylline has been used in SLS to improve diaphragmatic strength.[30,41] There are some patients with residual diaphragmatic weakness that may respond to surgical diaphragmatic plication.

Diffuse alveolar hemorrhage

Diffuse alveolar hemorrhage (DAH) is a rare and potentially fatal complication of SLE.[42–44] The exact prevalence is not known, but in one study of hospitalized patients with SLE, DAH occurred in 19 of 510 patients over 10 years.[43]

Patients with DAH present acutely ill, often with dyspnea, cough, hemoptysis, and sometimes fever. DAH typically presents in patients with established SLE, often in the setting of active lupus nephritis or other active organ involvement. The hematocrit of a patient with active DAH will usually drop quickly. If lung function tests have been done, a significantly elevated DLCO may be suggestive of pulmonary hemorrhage. Chest radiography shows bilateral alveolar infiltrates and chest magnetic resonance image may show evidence of hemorrhage, because the paramagnetic effects of iron in the hemorrhagic blood result in preferential T2 shortening.[45]

BAL is useful in excluding infection. The presence of persistently bloody fluid with hemosiderin-laden macrophages helps confirm DAH.[43] It is also important to look for other forms of pulmonary vasculitis, such as antineutrophil cytoplasmic antibody–associated vasculitis, and screen for coagulopathies and thrombotic thrombocytopenic purpura as part of the evaluation.[46]

On lung biopsy, 1 of 2 histologic patterns can be seen: (1) capillaritis with immune complex deposition (14% of DAH cases) and, more commonly, (2) bland hemorrhage (72% of DAH cases).[43,47,48]

Improved treatment options are needed for patients with DAH. High-dose corticosteroids used alone have historically been associated with a high mortality. One study of 12 patients with DAH reported no survivors.[49] Concomitant cyclophosphamide given with the high-dose corticosteroids improves the prognosis greatly.[48] DAH is also one of the few indications for plasmapheresis in SLE and has been shown to improve survival. Treatment with plasmapheresis in 11 patients who failed high-dose corticosteroids and cyclophosphamide treatment resulted in the survival of 7, or 64%, of the patients.[50]

Acute respiratory distress syndrome

Acute respiratory distress syndrome (ARDS), as defined by international consensus, can occur from acute lupus pneumonitis, DAH, or pulmonary infection.[51,52] Patients with ARDS associated with SLE are younger and have more rapid ARDS progression than non-SLE patients.[51] ARDS has been most often described in patients with SLE in association with bacteremia or sepsis with gram-negative bacilli. In a series of 19 patients with SLE and ARDS, recent treatment with corticosteroids was a risk factor and the overall prognosis was very poor, with a 68% mortality.[51]

Vascular Lung Disease

Pulmonary hypertension

Symptomatic pulmonary hypertension (PH) is considered a rare complication of SLE, and is more often seen with SLE overlaps with other connective tissue diseases, particularly scleroderma or mixed connective tissue disease. The prevalence of PH in patients with SLE (SLE-PH) is estimated at between 0.5% and 43%, depending on the cohort studied and the method of diagnosis used.[53–56] A large multiethnic community-based cohort from the United Kingdom found the prevalence of SLE-PH to be only 4.2% out of 288 patients.[57] Even without documented PH, however, patients with SLE are more likely to have abnormal exercise hemodynamics, with higher PA pressures at rest and at each stage of exercise compared with controls.[58] The duration of SLE and the extrapulmonary activity of SLE do not correlate with the development of PH, and PH can be a presenting manifestation of SLE.[59–62] Symptoms of SLE-PH most commonly include dyspnea, chest pain, nonproductive cough, and fatigue. Patients may also develop peripheral edema and other findings consistent with PH, including jugular venous distension, fixed S2 splitting, murmurs of tricuspid regurgitation or pulmonic insufficiency, and hepatomegaly with ascites.

The first-line of diagnostic testing for patients with suspected SLE-PH involves obtaining a Doppler echocardiogram to look for elevations in estimated pulmonary artery pressure and resistance and/or tricuspid valve insufficiency.[53] Finding an isolated diffusion defect on lung function testing may be an early predictor of SLE-PH.[63] Right heart catheterization (RHC) is required to confirm the diagnosis and gauge the severity of PH. There is less of a clear consensus on the role of vasoreactivity testing.[64,65] Exercise during the echocardiogram or RHC increases the diagnostic yield.[66] The majority of SLE-PH patients will be positive for antiribonuclear protein antibodies and/or rheumatoid factor.[56,62,67]

Other studies to consider as part of the evaluation for secondary causes of PH, even in a patient with known SLE, include polysomnography to evaluate for disordered breathing during sleep, and testing for human immunodeficiency virus. To evaluate for recurrent thromboemboli underlying SLE-PH, testing should be done for antiphospholipid antibodies and consideration made for a ventilation-perfusion lung scan.

Although the pathogenesis of SLE-PH is unknown, the high prevalence of lupus anticoagulant and/or antiphospholipid antibodies suggests that thrombosis may play an important role,[57] and the increased prevalence of Raynaud phenomenon among SLE-PH patients suggests that pulmonary arterial vasospasm may be involved.[62,68] The histopathology behind PH in SLE includes plexiform angiomatous lesions, thickening of the muscular wall of the pulmonary arteries, and intimal fibrosis, virtually identical to what is seen in idiopathic pulmonary arterial hypertension (IPAH). In addition, there is immunoglobulin and complement deposition in the arterial walls.[56]

There is no uniformly successful treatment for SLE-PH. Management is similar to that of patients with IPAH, although in SLE-PH calcium channel blockers have not shown efficacy.[61] Potential therapies include oxygen, anticoagulation, vasodilators, selective and nonselective endothelial antagonists, phosphodiesterase-5 inhibitors, and the prostanoids. There is usually not an acute measurable drop in mean pulmonary artery pressure (PAP) from nitric oxide or epoprostenol. However, in one case series, long-term therapy with epoprostenol in patients with severe SLE-PH improved PAP and pulmonary vascular resistance.[61] All 6 patients improved from New York Heart Association class III or IV to class I or II symptoms.[61]

A controlled trial of the nonselective endothelin-1 antagonist, bosentan, in patients with primary and connective tissue disease–related pulmonary arterial hypertension showed a dose-related improvement in function assessed by 6-minute walk distance with bosentan compared with placebo.[69] Sixteen of the 213 patients had SLE; however, subgroup analysis of the patients with SLE is not available.[69]

Treatment of the underlying SLE with immunosuppressants may provide added benefit when combined with PAH-specific therapy, based on studies of cyclophosphamide therapy in patients with SLE-PH.[70,71] One study of 23 patients with either SLE-PH (n = 13) or PAH with mixed connective tissue disease (n = 10) compared first-line immunosuppressive therapy alone (monthly intravenous cyclophosphamide, 600 mg/m^2 plus prednisone, 0.5–1.0 mg/kg/d for 4 weeks then tapered) to immunosuppressive therapy with vasodilators to conventional therapy.[71] Approximately half of the patients had improved functional class, 6-minute walking distance, and mean PAP. Although the number of patients was small, it would seem that mild SLE-PH can benefit from immunosuppression alone, whereas more severe SLE-PH requires PAH-specific therapy in combination with immunosuppression.[71] When available, lung or heart-lung transplantation may be an option for some people with SLE-PH.[72,73]

SLE-PH tends to have a worse prognosis than IPAH. This tendency was particularly noted in a retrospective Korean study showing a 5-year survival of 16.8% in SLE-PH patients compared with 68.2% in the IPAH patients.[74] Because of the high maternal mortality of 66% among patients with SLE-PH, experts suggest PH screening for all women with SLE who are planning to conceive.[75,76]

Thromboembolic disease

The presence of antiphospholipid IgG and IgM antibodies increases the risk of thromboembolic events from approximately 9% to between 35% and 42%. These antibodies may be associated with a wide array of clinical presentations including pulmonary embolism, pulmonary infarction, PH, pulmonary arterial thrombosis, pulmonary microthrombosis, ARDS, intra-alveolar pulmonary hemorrhage, and postpartum hemolytic-uremic syndrome.

Immunosuppressive therapy alone is rarely effective, and most patients are given chronic anticoagulation. Prophylactic treatment with daily aspirin is often used in SLE patients with antiphospholipid antibodies but no history of a thrombotic event, although definitive evidence to support this practice is lacking. Patients with a known thrombotic event history should be treated with anticoagulation with heparin in the short term and coumadin in the long term, with a target international normalized ratio of at least 2.0 to 3.0.

Acute reversible hypoxemia

Unexplained hypoxemia by arterial blood gas without obvious parenchymal lung disease has been described among hospitalized patients with SLE.[77,78] In one series of 22 hospitalized patients, 6 had 9 episodes of hypoxemia and/or hypocapnia. Gas exchange improved within 72 hours of initiating corticosteroid therapy.[77] Although traditional workup was unrevealing regarding etiology of the reversible hypoxemia, plasma C3a levels were markedly elevated, suggesting pulmonary leukoaggregation and complement activation within pulmonary capillaries.[77] Upregulation of adhesion molecules E-selectin, VCAM-1, and ICAM-1 has also been reported.[79]

The majority of published cases report good responses to corticosteroids, either alone or in combination with aspirin.[78]

Airway Disease

SLE can involve the upper airways in up to 30% of patients, ranging from laryngeal mucosal inflammation, mucosal ulcerations, cricoarytenoiditis, vocal cord paralysis and edema, to life-threatening necrotizing vasculitis with airway obstruction.[80,81] Presenting symptoms can also range from hoarseness, dyspnea and, much more rarely, airway obstruction from edema requiring mechanical ventilation. Corticosteroids are the first-line therapy and symptoms typically respond well.

Symptomatic bronchiolar disorders in SLE are rare, but bronchial wall thickening and/or bronchiectasis was seen in 21% of 34 patients with SLE in a prospective study using HRCT.[82] In a different series, features consistent with small airway dysfunction were found in 24% of 70 nonsmoking patients with SLE.[83]

Secondary Causes of Lung Disease in SLE

Infectious complications

When a patient with SLE presents with lung involvement, infection must always be considered. Symptoms of lupus pneumonitis can be indistinguishable from infection. Patients with SLE presenting with diffuse lung disease require bronchoscopy to evaluate for infection or alveolar hemorrhage.[46] Many of the patients are immunosuppressed, and opportunistic infections can be seen (**Fig. 2**). In one study, 43 pneumonia events in patients with SLE were caused by bacterial infections in 75%, mycobacteria in 12%, fungal infections in 7%, and viruses in 5% of patients.[84] Imaging can be helpful; however, the definitive diagnosis requires waiting for culture results.

Initial antibiotic coverage should be broad-spectrum until specificities and sensitivities are obtained and therapy can become more targeted. To help with prevention, it is important for patients to stay up to date with influenza and pneumococcal vaccinations.

Drug-induced pulmonary disease

Several immunosuppressants used for SLE can cause or contribute to pulmonary disease as an adverse effect. The most notorious of the agents is methotrexate, which can cause pulmonary toxicity that is acute, subacute, or chronic in presentation. Subacute pneumonitis, presenting with dyspnea, dry cough, fever, crackles, and hypoxemia, is the most common. Patients usually

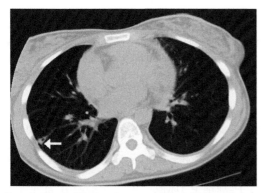

Fig. 2. Chest CT showing a small right lower lobe peripheral cavitary lesion (*arrow*) in a 22-year-old woman with active SLE, complicated by pericarditis and lupus nephritis. She was receiving immunosuppression with cyclophosphamide and corticosteroids. Initial cultures were negative; however, biopsy later revealed *Nocardia* infection involving her lungs, heart, brain, and retina.

recover following discontinuation of methotrexate and administration of corticosteroids; however, 10% may progress to pulmonary fibrosis and a mortality rate of 1% has been reported.[85]

Drug-induced lupus can include a full spectrum of pulmonary manifestations, most commonly pleurisy and pleural effusions.[24,86] Symptoms of drug-induced lupus typically resolve following the discontinuation of the offending drug.

SUMMARY

Pulmonary disease may complicate SLE and is an important cause of morbidity and mortality. Early detection of pulmonary disease in a patient with SLE is of importance because therapy ranges from aggressive immunosuppression for lupus pneumonitis, to anticoagulation for antiphospholipid antibody syndrome, to lowering immunosuppression while starting antimicrobial therapy in settings where infection is the culprit. Treatment strategies for pulmonary disease in SLE are based on limited data (primarily small, uncontrolled series and case reports) and the experience from other connective tissue disorders. Continued investigations into the pathogenesis and treatment of SLE-related lung involvement are needed to improve morbidity and mortality outcomes for patients with SLE.

REFERENCES

1. Pisetsky DS, Gilkeson G, St Clair EW. Systemic lupus erythematosus. Diagnosis and treatment. Med Clin North Am 1997;81:113–28.

2. Alarcon GS, Friedman AW, Straaton KV, et al. Systemic lupus erythematosus in three ethnic groups: III. A comparison of characteristics early in the natural history of the LUMINA cohort. LUpus in MInority populations: NAture vs. Nurture. Lupus 1999;8:197–209.

3. Bernatsky S, Boivin JF, Joseph L, et al. Mortality in systemic lupus erythematosus. Arthritis Rheum 2006;54:2550–7.

4. Orens JB, Martinez FJ, Lynch JP 3rd. Pleuropulmonary manifestations of systemic lupus erythematosus. Rheum Dis Clin North Am 1994;20: 159–93.

5. Quadrelli SA, Alvarez C, Arce SC, et al. Pulmonary involvement of systemic lupus erythematosus: analysis of 90 necropsies. Lupus 2009;18:1053–60.

6. Pego-Reigosa JM, Medeiros DA, Isenberg DA. Respiratory manifestations of systemic lupus erythematosus: old and new concepts. Best Pract Res Clin Rheumatol 2009;23:469–80.

7. Tsao BP. Update on human systemic lupus erythematosus genetics. Curr Opin Rheumatol 2004;16: 513–21.

8. Pullmann R Jr, Bonilla E, Phillips PE, et al. Haplotypes of the HRES-1 endogenous retrovirus are associated with development and disease manifestations of systemic lupus erythematosus. Arthritis Rheum 2008;58:532–40.

9. Kremer Hovinga IC, Koopmans M, Baelde HJ, et al. Tissue chimerism in systemic lupus erythematosus is related to injury. Ann Rheum Dis 2007;66:1568–73.

10. Good JT Jr, King TE, Antony VB, et al. Lupus pleuritis. Clinical features and pleural fluid characteristics with special reference to pleural fluid antinuclear antibodies. Chest 1983;84:714–8.

11. Pines A, Kaplinsky N, Olchovsky D, et al. Pleuropulmonary manifestations of systemic lupus erythematosus: clinical features of its subgroups. Prognostic and therapeutic implications. Chest 1985;88:129–35.

12. Winslow WA, Ploss LN, Loitman B. Pleuritis in systemic lupus erythematosus: its importance as an early manifestation in diagnosis. Ann Intern Med 1958;49:70–88.

13. Bouros D, Pneumatikos I, Tzouvelekis A. Pleural involvement in systemic autoimmune disorders. Respiration 2008;75:361–71.

14. Hunder GG, McDuffie FC, Hepper NG. Pleural fluid complement in systemic lupus erythematosus and rheumatoid arthritis. Ann Intern Med 1972;76:357–63.

15. Small P, Frank H, Kreisman H, et al. An immunological evaluation of pleural effusions in systemic lupus erythematosus. Ann Allergy 1982;49:101–3.

16. Gilleece MH, Evans CC, Bucknall RC. Steroid resistant pleural effusion in systemic lupus erythematosus

treated with tetracycline pleurodesis. Ann Rheum Dis 1988;47:1031–2.

17. McKnight KM, Adair NE, Agudelo CA. Successful use of tetracycline pleurodesis to treat massive pleural effusion secondary to systemic lupus erythematosus. Arthritis Rheum 1991;34:1483–4.

18. Kaine JL. Refractory massive pleural effusion in systemic lupus erythematosus treated with talc poudrage. Ann Rheum Dis 1985;44:61–4.

19. Wiedemann HP, Matthay RA. Pulmonary manifestations of systemic lupus erythematosus. J Thorac Imaging 1992;7:1–18.

20. Cheema GS, Quismorio FP Jr. Interstitial lung disease in systemic lupus erythematosus. Curr Opin Pulm Med 2000;6:424–9.

21. Witt C, Dorner T, Hiepe F, et al. Diagnosis of alveolitis in interstitial lung manifestation in connective tissue diseases: importance of late inspiratory crackles, 67 gallium scan and bronchoalveolar lavage. Lupus 1996;5:606–12.

22. Matthay RA, Schwarz MI, Petty TL, et al. Pulmonary manifestations of systemic lupus erythematosus: review of twelve cases of acute lupus pneumonitis. Medicine (Baltimore) 1975;54:397–409.

23. Leikin JB, Arof HM, Pearlman LM. Acute lupus pneumonitis in the postpartum period: a case history and review of the literature. Obstet Gynecol 1986;68: 29S–31S.

24. Wiedemann HP, Matthay RA. Pulmonary manifestations of the collagen vascular diseases. Clin Chest Med 1989;10:677–722.

25. Lim SW, Gillis D, Smith W, et al. Rituximab use in systemic lupus erythematosus pneumonitis and a review of current reports. Intern Med J 2006;36:260–2.

26. Weinrib L, Sharma OP, Quismorio FP Jr. A long-term study of interstitial lung disease in systemic lupus erythematosus. Semin Arthritis Rheum 1990;20:48–56.

27. Haupt HM, Moore GW, Hutchins GM. The lung in systemic lupus erythematosus. Analysis of the pathologic changes in 120 patients. Am J Med 1981;71: 791–8.

28. Boulware DW, Hedgpeth MT. Lupus pneumonitis and anti-SSA(Ro) antibodies. J Rheumatol 1989;16: 479–81.

29. Tansey D, Wells AU, Colby TV, et al. Variations in histological patterns of interstitial pneumonia between connective tissue disorders and their relationship to prognosis. Histopathology 2004;44:585–96.

30. Karim MY, Miranda LC, Tench CM, et al. Presentation and prognosis of the shrinking lung syndrome in systemic lupus erythematosus. Semin Arthritis Rheum 2002;31:289–98.

31. Warrington KJ, Moder KG, Brutinel WM. The shrinking lungs syndrome in systemic lupus erythematosus. Mayo Clin Proc 2000;75:467–72.

32. Toya SP, Tzelepis GE. Association of the shrinking lung syndrome in systemic lupus erythematosus with pleurisy: a systematic review. Semin Arthritis Rheum 2009;39:30–7.

33. Rubin LA, Urowitz MB. Shrinking lung syndrome in SLE—a clinical pathologic study. J Rheumatol 1983;10:973–6.

34. Hardy K, Herry I, Attali V, et al. Bilateral phrenic paralysis in a patient with systemic lupus erythematosus. Chest 2001;119:1274–7.

35. Laroche CM, Mulvey DA, Hawkins PN, et al. Diaphragm strength in the shrinking lung syndrome of systemic lupus erythematosus. Q J Med 1989;71: 429–39.

36. Hawkins P, Davison AG, Dasgupta B, et al. Diaphragm strength in acute systemic lupus erythematosus in a patient with paradoxical abdominal motion and reduced lung volumes. Thorax 2001;56:329–30.

37. Martens J, Demedts M, Vanmeenen MT, et al. Respiratory muscle dysfunction in systemic lupus erythematosus. Chest 1983;84:170–5.

38. Walz-Leblanc BA, Urowitz MB, Gladman DD, et al. The "shrinking lungs syndrome" in systemic lupus erythematosus—improvement with corticosteroid therapy. J Rheumatol 1992;19:1970–2.

39. Soubrier M, Dubost JJ, Piette JC, et al. Shrinking lung syndrome in systemic lupus erythematosus. A report of three cases. Rev Rhum Engl Ed 1995;62: 395–8.

40. Benham H, Garske L, Vecchio P, et al. Successful treatment of shrinking lung syndrome with rituximab in a patient with systemic lupus erythematosus. J Clin Rheumatol 2010;16:68–70.

41. Van Veen S, Peeters AJ, Sterk PJ, et al. The "shrinking lung syndrome" in SLE, treatment with theophylline. Clin Rheumatol 1993;12:462–5.

42. Eagen JW, Memoli VA, Roberts JL, et al. Pulmonary hemorrhage in systemic lupus erythematosus. Medicine (Baltimore) 1978;57:545–60.

43. Zamora MR, Warner ML, Tuder R, et al. Diffuse alveolar hemorrhage and systemic lupus erythematosus. Clinical presentation, histology, survival, and outcome. Medicine (Baltimore) 1997;76:192–202.

44. Badsha H, Teh CL, Kong KO, et al. Pulmonary hemorrhage in systemic lupus erythematosus. Semin Arthritis Rheum 2004;33:414–21.

45. Hsu BY, Edwards DK 3rd, Trambert MA. Pulmonary hemorrhage complicating systemic lupus erythematosus: role of MR imaging in diagnosis. AJR Am J Roentgenol 1992;158:519–20.

46. Strange C, Highland KB. Interstitial lung disease in the patient who has connective tissue disease. Clin Chest Med 2004;25:549–59, vii.

47. Myers JL, Katzenstein AA. Microangiitis in lupus-induced pulmonary hemorrhage. Am J Clin Pathol 1986;85:552–6.

48. Schwab EP, Schumacher HR Jr, Freundlich B, et al. Pulmonary alveolar hemorrhage in systemic lupus erythematosus. Semin Arthritis Rheum 1993;23:8–15.

49. Abud-Mendoza C, Diaz-Jouanen E, Alarcon-Segovia D. Fatal pulmonary hemorrhage in systemic lupus erythematosus. Occurrence without hemoptysis. J Rheumatol 1985;12:558–61.

50. Erickson RW, Franklin WA, Emlen W. Treatment of hemorrhagic lupus pneumonitis with plasmapheresis. Semin Arthritis Rheum 1994;24:114–23.

51. Kim WU, Kim SI, Yoo WH, et al. Adult respiratory distress syndrome in systemic lupus erythematosus: causes and prognostic factors: a single center, retrospective study. Lupus 1999;8:552–7.

52. Andonopoulos AP. Adult respiratory distress syndrome: an unrecognized premortem event in systemic lupus erythematosus. Br J Rheumatol 1991;30:346–8.

53. Winslow TM, Ossipov MA, Fazio GP, et al. Five-year follow-up study of the prevalence and progression of pulmonary hypertension in systemic lupus erythematosus. Am Heart J 1995;129:510–5.

54. Simonson JS, Schiller NB, Petri M, et al. Pulmonary hypertension in systemic lupus erythematosus. J Rheumatol 1989;16:918–25.

55. Johnson SR, Gladman DD, Urowitz MB, et al. Pulmonary hypertension in systemic lupus. Lupus 2004; 13:506–9.

56. Quismorio FP Jr, Sharma O, Koss M, et al. Immunopathologic and clinical studies in pulmonary hypertension associated with systemic lupus erythematosus. Semin Arthritis Rheum 1984;13:349–59.

57. Prabu A, Patel K, Yee CS, et al. Prevalence and risk factors for pulmonary arterial hypertension in patients with lupus. Rheumatology (Oxford) 2009; 48:1506–11.

58. Winslow TM, Ossipov M, Redberg RF, et al. Exercise capacity and hemodynamics in systemic lupus erythematosus: a Doppler echocardiographic exercise study. Am Heart J 1993;126:410–4.

59. Asherson RA, Mackworth-Young CG, Boey ML, et al. Pulmonary hypertension in systemic lupus erythematosus. Br Med J (Clin Res Ed) 1983;287: 1024–5.

60. Boumpas DT, Austin HA 3rd, Fessler BJ, et al. Systemic lupus erythematosus: emerging concepts. Part 1: renal, neuropsychiatric, cardiovascular, pulmonary, and hematologic disease. Ann Intern Med 1995;122:940–50.

61. Robbins IM, Gaine SP, Schilz R, et al. Epoprostenol for treatment of pulmonary hypertension in patients with systemic lupus erythematosus. Chest 2000; 117:14–8.

62. Asherson RA, Higenbottam TW, Dinh Xuan AT, et al. Pulmonary hypertension in a lupus clinic: experience with twenty-four patients. J Rheumatol 1990; 17:1292–8.

63. Hodson P, Klemp P, Meyers OL. Pulmonary hypertension in systemic lupus erythematosus: a report of four cases. Clin Exp Rheumatol 1983;1:241–5.

64. Pope J. An update in pulmonary hypertension in systemic lupus erythematosus—do we need to know about it? Lupus 2008;17:274–7.

65. Minai O. An update in pulmonary hypertension in systemic lupus erythematosus—do we need to know about it? Lupus 2009;18:92.

66. Steen V, Chou M, Shanmugam V, et al. Exercise-induced pulmonary arterial hypertension in patients with systemic sclerosis. Chest 2008;134:146–51.

67. Asherson RA, Oakley CM. Pulmonary hypertension and systemic lupus erythematosus. J Rheumatol 1986;13:1–5.

68. Kasparian A, Floros A, Gialafos E, et al. Raynaud's phenomenon is correlated with elevated systolic pulmonary arterial pressure in patients with systemic lupus erythematosus. Lupus 2007;16: 505–8.

69. Rubin LJ, Badesch DB, Barst RJ, et al. Bosentan therapy for pulmonary arterial hypertension. N Engl J Med 2002;346:896–903.

70. Gonzalez-Lopez L, Cardona-Munoz EG, Celis A, et al. Therapy with intermittent pulse cyclophosphamide for pulmonary hypertension associated with systemic lupus erythematosus. Lupus 2004; 13:105–12.

71. Jais X, Launay D, Yaici A, et al. Immunosuppressive therapy in lupus- and mixed connective tissue disease-associated pulmonary arterial hypertension: a retrospective analysis of twenty-three cases. Arthritis Rheum 2008;58:521–31.

72. Levy RD, Guerraty AJ, Yacoub MH, et al. Prolonged survival after heart-lung transplantation in systemic lupus erythematosus. Chest 1993;104:1903–5.

73. Hutter JA, Despins P, Higenbottam T, et al. Heart-lung transplantation: better use of resources. Am J Med 1988;85:4–11.

74. Chung SM, Lee CK, Lee EY, et al. Clinical aspects of pulmonary hypertension in patients with systemic lupus erythematosus and in patients with idiopathic pulmonary arterial hypertension. Clin Rheumatol 2006;25:866–72.

75. Greenstone MA. Delayed diagnosis of systemic lupus erythematosus associated pulmonary hypertension. Br J Rheumatol 1991;30:391.

76. Ray J, Sermer M. Systemic lupus erythematosus and pulmonary hypertension during pregnancy: report of a case fatality. Can J Cardiol 1996;12: 753–6.

77. Abramson SB, Dobro J, Eberle MA, et al. Acute reversible hypoxemia in systemic lupus erythematosus. Ann Intern Med 1991;114:941–7.

78. Martinez-Taboada VM, Blanco R, Armona J, et al. Acute reversible hypoxemia in systemic lupus erythematosus: a new syndrome or an index of disease activity? Lupus 1995;4:259–62.

79. Belmont HM, Buyon J, Giorno R, et al. Up-regulation of endothelial cell adhesion molecules characterizes

disease activity in systemic lupus erythematosus. The Shwartzman phenomenon revisited. Arthritis Rheum 1994;37:376–83.

80. Teitel AD, MacKenzie CR, Stern R, et al. Laryngeal involvement in systemic lupus erythematosus. Semin Arthritis Rheum 1992;22:203–14.

81. Langford CA, Van Waes C. Upper airway obstruction in the rheumatic diseases. Rheum Dis Clin North Am 1997;23:345–63.

82. Fenlon HM, Doran M, Sant SM, et al. High-resolution chest CT in systemic lupus erythematosus. AJR Am J Roentgenol 1996;166:301–7.

83. Keane MP, Lynch JP 3rd. Pleuropulmonary manifestations of systemic lupus erythematosus. Thorax 2000;55:159–66.

84. Kinder BW, Freemer MM, King TE Jr, et al. Clinical and genetic risk factors for pneumonia in systemic lupus erythematosus. Arthritis Rheum 2007;56: 2679–86.

85. Lateef O, Shakoor N, Balk RA. Methotrexate pulmonary toxicity. Expert Opin Drug Saf 2005;4:723–30.

86. Abunasser J, Forouhar FA, Metersky ML. Etanercept-induced lupus erythematosus presenting as a unilateral pleural effusion. Chest 2008;134:850–3.

Pulmonary Involvement in Sjögren Syndrome

Maria Kokosi, MD[a], Ellen C. Riemer, MD, JD[b],
Kristin B. Highland, MD, MSCR[c],*

KEYWORDS

- Sjögren syndrome • Interstitial lung disease
- Airway disease • Lymphocytic interstitial pneumonitis
- Lymphoma

Sjögren syndrome (SS) is a chronic inflammatory autoimmune disease characterized by lymphocytic infiltration of exocrine glands and other numerous extraglandular sites. The disease can present in isolation (primary Sjögren syndrome, pSS) or in association with other connective tissue diseases, most commonly rheumatoid arthritis (secondary Sjögren syndrome, sSS). pSS is one of the 3 most common autoimmune disorders, with a population prevalence of 0.04% to 0.6%.[1] It affects predominantly women in the fourth and fifth decades of life, with a female/male ratio of 9:1.[2]

The clinical manifestations of the disease vary from exocrinopathy to systemic benign extraglandular disease and, in some cases, B-cell lymphoid malignancy. Its predilection for the lacrimal and salivary glands leads to the typical sicca symptoms (xerophthalmia/keratoconjunctivitis sicca, xerostomia), whereas decreased glandular secretions in other sites manifest as dryness of the nose, airways, and skin; atrophic gastritis; and subclinical pancreatitis. The extraglandular manifestations of the disease are present in 40% to 50% of Sjögren patients and are a result of lymphocytic infiltration of epithelial tissues. Extraglandular manifestations commonly occur in the lungs, but may also involve the thyroid, kidney (interstitial nephritis), and hepatobiliary tract. Vasculitis, secondary to immunocomplex deposition, may result in leukocytoclastic skin rash, glomerulonephritis, peripheral neuropathy, and low C4 levels. In less than 5% of patients, this lymphoproliferation may undergo malignant transformation. The most frequent malignancy is non-Hodgkin lymphoma, although cases of Waldenström macroglobulinemia have also been described.[3] The presence of the immunocomplex form of the disease increases the risk of development of lymphoma.[4]

The pathogenesis of SS may include several genetic, environmental, and hormonal factors. pSS has been linked to a higher frequency of HLA-DR2 and HLA-DR3 subtypes and a decreased frequency of HLA-DR4, whereas sSS has a frequency of HLA-DR2, HLA-DR3, and HLA-DR4 similar to that of the general population. Some investigators have suggested that the association of SS with various HLA markers is present only in patients with positive Ro (SSA) or La (SSB) autoantibodies.[5] An association of these autoantibodies (especially Ro) with extraglandular manifestations, immunocomplex disease, and

Funding: none.
[a] 3rd Pulmonary Department, Sismanoglio General Hospital, 1 Sismanogliou Street, Marousi 15126, Athens, Greece
[b] Department of Pathology and Laboratory Medicine, Medical University of South Carolina, 171 Ashley Avenue, MSC 908, Charleston, SC 29425, USA
[c] Divisions of Pulmonary, Critical Care, Allergy and Sleep Medicine and Rheumatology and Immunology, Medical University of South Carolina, 96 Johnathan Lucas Street, Suite 812 CSB, Charleston, SC 29425, USA
* Corresponding author.
E-mail address: highlakb@musc.edu

Clin Chest Med 31 (2010) 489–500
doi:10.1016/j.ccm.2010.05.007
0272-5231/10/$ – see front matter © 2010 Elsevier Inc. All rights reserved.

hematologic disorders has also been described.[6] The possibility that estrogen increases the risk of developing sicca symptoms is suggested by the predominance of women with pSS and by the increased prevalence of ocular dryness in postmenopausal women receiving hormone replacement therapy.[7] It is believed that an environmental trigger incites the development of SS in genetically predisposed individuals. For example, viral infections (eg, Epstein-Barr and cytomegalovirus) have been shown to stimulate the epithelial glandular cells to produce chemokines, resulting in the consequent migration and accumulation of T (mainly CD4) and B lymphocytes. The destruction of the glandular tissues is caused by this infiltration of lymphocytes and the production of cytokines (eg, interferon-γ and interleukin [IL]-2), metalloproteinases, and numerous circulating autoantibodies, such as those against the ribonucleoproteins Ro and La or against muscarinic receptors.[8,9] Similar pathogenetic events have been described in parenchymal organs such as the liver, thyroid, lungs, and kidneys. The epithelial cell has a major role in the pathogenesis of SS; therefore, the term autoimmune epithelitis has been suggested by researchers.[10]

DIAGNOSTIC CRITERIA

The diagnosis of SS is based on 6 criteria proposed by the American-European consensus group[11]: (1) ocular symptoms of dryness, (2) oral symptoms of dryness or persistently swollen salivary glands, (3) objective evidence of ocular involvement (positive results on Schirmer test or Rose Bengal), (4) lymphocytic sialoadenitis on minor salivary gland biopsy, (5) objective evidence of salivary gland involvement (abnormal salivary flow, parotid salography, or salivary scintigraphy), and (6) antibodies to Ro (SSA) and/or La (SSB) antigens. pSS can be established when 4 of these 6 criteria are present, one of which must be either lymphocytic sialadenitis or positive anti-Ro or anti-La antibodies. Alternatively, SS may also be established by the presence of 3 of the following: objective evidence of ocular involvement, supportive histopathologic findings, objective evidence of salivary gland involvement, or presence of autoantibodies.

The diagnosis of sSS in a patient with a potentially associated rheumatologic disease requires ocular or oral symptoms in combination with any 2 criteria including positive minor salivary gland biopsy, objective evidence of salivary gland involvement, or objective evidence of ocular involvement. Common rheumatic diseases associated with SS include systemic sclerosis, rheumatoid arthritis, systemic lupus erythematosus, mixed connective tissue disease, idiopathic inflammatory muscle disease, autoimmune liver disease, and autoimmune thyroid disease.

Factors mitigating against a diagnosis of SS include sarcoidosis, preexisting lymphoma, hepatitis C infection, acquired immunodeficiency syndrome, graft-versus-host disease, and previous head and neck radiation. Avoidance of drugs with anticholinergic properties is also necessary during the evaluation of sicca symptoms.

PREVALENCE OF PULMONARY INVOLVEMENT

A plethora of pulmonary manifestations is found in pSS (**Box 1**). The most frequent are interstitial lung disease (ILD), airway disease (xerotrachea and small airway obstruction), and lymphoproliferative disorders. The diagnosis of lung disease in SS is based on clinical evaluation, radiographic findings, pulmonary functional testing, bronchoalveolar lavage (BAL), and histopathology. The prevalence of pulmonary involvement in pSS has been reported

---

Box 1
Pulmonary manifestations in pSS

- Interstitial lung disease
    Nonspecific interstitial pneumonia
    Lymphocytic interstitial pneumonia
    Usual interstitial pneumonitis
    Organizing pneumonia
- Airway disease
    Rhinitis sicca
    Xerostomia
    Xerotrachea
    Lymphocytic bronchitis/bronchiolitis
    Atelectasis
    Bronchiectasis
    Follicular bronchiolitis
- Lymphoma
- Pseudolymphoma
- Amyloidosis
- Pleural involvement
    Pleural effusion
    Pleural thickening
- Vascular disease
    Pulmonary vasculitis
    Pulmonary hypertension

to be between 9% and 75%.[12,13] Lung abnormalities seen in sSS may be attributed to the underlying primary rheumatic disease, making it difficult to evaluate the relationship between sSS and pulmonary disease. Therefore, the subject of this article is the pulmonary involvement in *primary* SS.

A recent study by Yazisiz and colleagues[14] reported an 11.4% prevalence of lung involvement in pSS based on radiological findings and suggested several factors that could possibly play an important role in predicting lung disease in pSS, including hypergammaglobulinemia, lymphopenia, positivity for rheumatoid factor (RF), presence of anti-Ro and anti-La antibodies, decreased forced vital capacity (FVC), and forced expiratory volume in 1 second (FEV_1). The study suggests that a history of smoking, male gender, and higher age appear to be risk factors for development of lung disease in pSS. This is supported by a longitudinal study of 19 patients with pSS who had pulmonary function testing (PFT) during a median follow-up of 10 years.[15] In the latter study, a restrictive ventilatory defect developed more often in the patients with baseline laboratory signs of immunologic activity such as increased levels of serum protein, IgG, erythrocyte sedimentation rate, and β_2-microglobulin. These laboratory findings were also associated with mild interstitial changes on high-resolution computed tomography (HRCT). These 2 studies are consistent with a large retrospective study of 343 patients with both pSS and sSS, which demonstrated pulmonary involvement in 31 patients (9%). Histology was used to confirm pulmonary involvement in approximately 50% of the patients. In the other 50%, chest roentgenogram, symptoms, and PFT were used. In contrast, Constantopoulos and colleagues[13] reported a prevalence of 75% of pulmonary involvement in pSS, based either on clinical symptoms or on functional or histologic data. Similarly, Ufmann and colleagues[16] reported the prevalence of pulmonary manifestations in 65% of patients with pSS, based solely on HRCT findings. However, abnormal radiographic findings were mostly subtle and may not necessarily be attributable to pSS. The difference in the methods used to detect pulmonary involvement is one of the reasons for the wide variability in its reported prevalence. The value of chest roentgenogram in the diagnosis of ILD is low, and histologic evaluation, which is more specific, is not always available. The characteristics and the size of the population in each study (patients with both pSS and sSS vs patients with just pSS), the enrolling criteria, and the criteria used for the diagnosis of SS also contribute to the huge difference in the reported prevalence of lung involvement.

CLINICAL MANIFESTATIONS

Although many patients remain asymptomatic, the main clinical manifestations of pulmonary involvement in pSS are cough and exertional dyspnea. These symptoms are associated with ILD and airway involvement, and their frequency depends on the dominating feature of lung disease. Dry cough is associated with xerotrachea and airway disease, which may remain undiagnosed when cough is the only sign or symptom of lung disease. Constantopoulos and colleagues[13] reported dry cough as the primary symptom in patients with pSS. Papiris and colleagues[17] evaluated 61 patients with pSS and found dry cough to be the only symptom in 41%, whereas dyspnea was present in a mere 9%. Only 14% of the patients in this series had findings detectable on auscultation (bibasilar crackles). In a series of 18 patients with pSS and histologically proven ILD, dyspnea was present in 94%, cough in 67%, chest pain in 22%, and wheeze in 17%. The most frequent physical finding in the same study was inspiratory crackles found in 67%, whereas in 28% the lung examination findings were normal.[18]

PULMONARY FUNCTION

In patients with pSS and ILD, PFT commonly reveals a restrictive pattern with a low diffusing capacity.[19,20] In one study of 100 patients with pSS, significant reductions in FEV_1, FVC, and diffusing capacity of lung for carbon monoxide (D_{LCO}) were present in 14, 12, and 10 patients, respectively.[20] The presence of small airway dysfunction is common in nonsmoking patients with pSS and is often asymptomatic.[16,17] The correlations between radiological findings and PFT vary among different case series. In a study of 37 patients by Uffmann and colleagues,[16] there was no correlation found between HRCT and PFT. This is in contrast to a study by Taouli and colleagues,[21] in which patients with radiologically large or small airway abnormalities predominantly had an obstructive pattern on PFT, and a significant correlation was found between the scores for air trapping and FEV_1. Likewise, a restrictive pattern was found in patients with evidence of ILD on HRCT, and there was a correlation between total lung capacity (TLC), D_{LCO}, and ground glass attenuation.

BRONCHOALVEOLAR LAVAGE

The role of BAL in the evaluation of SS-related lung disease is not clear. Dalavanga and colleagues[22] studied BAL in patients with pSS and found alveolitis in 52% of patients, characterized by an increase in the total cell count and a predominance of lymphocytes on the differential count. The CD4/CD8 ratio was reduced in the patients with pSS and a lymphocytic alveolitis compared with patients with pSS without alveolitis and healthy nonsmoking controls. The patients with a lymphocytic alveolitis more frequently had dyspnea and cough, restrictive physiology on PFT, and radiographic findings consistent with ILD. In a series of 18 patients with pSS but no symptoms or radiographic findings of pulmonary involvement, Salaffi and colleagues[23] found that 88% had a lymphocytic alveolitis, whereas 22% had mixed lymphocytic and neutrophilic alveolitis. BAL was repeated after 2 years, and almost 50% of the patients with a prior lymphocytic alveolitis had a normal BAL cell count, whereas the rest of the patients remained unchanged. Patients with a lymphocytic alveolitis had a smaller decrease in their diffusion capacity than patients with the mixed pattern. BAL lymphocytic alveolitis tended to predict a better prognosis even if other findings of lung disease were present. In contrast, patients with a neutrophilic BAL tended to have a less favorable clinical outcome.

RADIOGRAPHIC FINDINGS

The chest radiograph may be normal or show bilateral alveolar, reticular, or nodular markings or a combination thereof, mainly localized in the middle and lower lung zones. The chest radiograph, however, has a low diagnostic value in the detection of pulmonary involvement in SS, especially in the early stages of lung disease. In a series of 37 asymptomatic patients with pSS, all chest radiographs were normal, whereas abnormal computed tomographic (CT) findings were detected in 24.[16] These results highlight the role of HRCT in the detection of lung disease, especially in its subclinical forms.

The main HRCT findings in pSS are those of airway involvement and ILD. Large airway disorders manifest with bronchial wall thickening and bronchiectasis. Small airway disease presents with bronchiolectasis, centrilobular nodules, mosaic attenuation, and air trapping. Interstitial lung disease presents radiographically with a reticular or reticulonodular pattern, ground glass opacities, honeycombing, traction bronchiectasis, and thin-walled cysts.

Ground glass attenuation is a very common finding in patients with SS-related lung disease and has been reported to be present in 40% to 92% of patients with SS screened by HRCT.[14,21,24,25] Findings of ground glass are suggestive of an underlying histopathologic diagnosis of airway disease as well as early stages of nonspecific interstitial pneumonia (NSIP), lymphocytic interstitial pneumonia (LIP), and organizing pneumonia (OP). Other frequent findings on HRCT series include linear opacities (septal and nonseptal thickening) (75%–55%),[25] nodules (subpleural and centrilobular) (78%–23%),[25] honeycombing (24%–43%),[14,24] cysts (7%–13%),[14,16] and findings associated with airway disease, including bronchiectasis (37%–50%),[14,21] bronchial or bronchiolar wall thickening (14%–60%), and air trapping (9%).[21] Lower zone predominance is a common finding in all of the studies. Expiratory images on HRCT may be particularly useful in the detection of early airway disease and may be seen before abnormal physiology on PFT.[26]

AIRWAY MANIFESTATIONS

Upper airway involvement is a common phenomenon in SS. Dryness of nasal and oral mucosa due to diminished glandular function can be the cause of smell and taste disorders, bleeding, sinusitis, and septal perforation. Freeman and colleagues[27] reported that in 111 patients with pSS, 50% complained of nasal symptoms, although only 20% had abnormal rhinoscopy. Similarly, 60% complained of throat symptoms, but only 20% had pathologic findings on indirect laryngoscopy.

Involvement of the trachea and large airway manifests as dryness of the mucosa of the trachea (xerotrachea) and large airways (xerobronchitis) and presents almost exclusively as a nonproductive cough. In the largest series in which desiccation of the tracheobronchial tree was documented by bronchoscopy, xerotrachea was present in 17% of patients with pSS.[13] Xerotrachea was first described by Henrik Sjögren in 1933 when he reported histopathologic changes in the bronchial glands similar to those in salivary exocrine glands. Papiris and colleagues[28] studied lobar bronchial biopsies of patients with SS and found an increased number of $CD4^+$ T lymphocytes in the bronchial mucosa of the large airways (lymphocytic bronchitis).

Small airway involvement has been described in several studies and represents a common finding in pSS but rarely causes severe clinical problems. Common symptoms include cough, dyspnea, and wheezing, similar to those symptoms that are usually present in xerotrachea. Decreased maximum expiratory flow (MEF) values and hyperinflation are the earliest signs of small airway involvement. In one study, approximately 50% of 61 patients with pSS had a decline in MEF_{25} or

MEF_{50}, whereas only 10% had a low FEV_1.[17] A second study revealed hyperinflation in 53% of patients with pSS as measured by static lung volumes.[29] Bronchial hyperresponsiveness is also an early finding of small airway involvement. In a series of 21 patients with pSS, 60% had mild to severe bronchial hyperresponsiveness; only half of these patients had small airway obstruction on PFT.[30] As the disease progresses, air trapping, mosaic attenuation, and bronchiectasis may be present on CT.

Small airway disease is a result of inflammatory infiltration of bronchial submucosa characterized by the presence of large numbers of neutrophils, mast cells, and lymphocytes, resulting in bronchial epithelial and subepithelial damage.[31] An elevated level of serum β_2-microglobulin is believed to be a marker of lymphoproliferation and has been shown to be associated with those patients with pSS with significantly lower maximal expiratory flows.[29]

FOLLICULAR BRONCHIOLITIS

Follicular bronchiolitis is a type of lymphoproliferative disorder of the lung and usually coexists with lymphocytic bronchitis, bronchiolitis, or LIP in patients with pSS. Histologically, follicular bronchiolitis is characterized by nodules of lymphocytic infiltrates with reactive germinal centers surrounding the terminal and respiratory bronchioles (bronchi-associated lymphoid tissue hyperplasia). Clinically it presents with cough and dyspnea. A reticular or reticulonodular pattern is seen radiographically, and pulmonary function tests may be normal or have features of restriction and/or obstruction. Follicular bronchiolitis associated with pSS usually responds well to corticosteroids.[32]

INTERSTITIAL LUNG DISEASE

Diffuse ILD is the most common form of lung involvement in pSS and includes LIP, NSIP, usual interstitial pneumonia (UIP), and OP.

Nonspecific Interstitial Pneumonia

Several studies determined NSIP as the most common ILD disorder in patients with pSS. Parambil and colleagues[18] performed biopsies in 18 patients (14 surgical biopsies and 9 bronchoscopic biopsies) and found a prevalence of NSIP in 28%. This prevalence is similar to that found in the study by Yamadori and colleagues,[33] who reported that biopsy-proven NSIP was present in one-third of patients with SS and radiographically evident lung disease. In contrast, Ito and colleagues[19] retrospectively examined 33 biopsies and found that NSIP was the most common histopathologic pattern, with a prevalence of 61%. Clinical manifestations of NSIP include cough and dyspnea, with fever in approximately 30%.[34] NSIP is usually a restrictive ventilatory defect with decreased D_{LCO} on PFT. The most frequent HRCT findings are increased reticular markings, traction bronchiectasis, lobar volume loss, and ground glass opacities.[35] As the disease progresses, honeycombing may develop. Histopathologically, NSIP is characterized by alveolar wall interstitial inflammation and/or fibrosis in a temporally homogeneous pattern. Based on the relative degree of inflammation to fibrosis, it is classified into 3 groups: cellular type with interstitial inflammation, fibrotic type with primarily fibrosis, and mixed type with a combination of inflammation and fibrosis.[36]

Lymphocytic Interstitial Pneumonia

Lymphocytic interstitial pneumonitis is a pattern of benign lymphoproliferative disease. Its prevalence in patients with SS is 0.9%, whereas 25% of adults with LIP suffer from SS. SS-associated LIP has a female predominance.[37] The most frequent clinical manifestations are cough and dyspnea, while other systemic symptoms such as fever, sweats, and weight loss are less common. A radiographic pattern of ground glass opacities with some thin-walled cysts is seen in approximately 50% of patients (**Fig. 1**). Centrilobular nodules, interlobular septal thickening, and bronchovascular bundle thickening are also frequent findings. Pleural effusions are rare.[38] A restrictive defect with a decreased D_{LCO} is seen on PFT. About 80% of patients with LIP have polyclonal hypergammaglobulinemia of unknown cause. A definitive diagnosis is made only by a surgical lung biopsy. Histopathologically, LIP is characterized by an infiltrate of B and T lymphocytes, plasma cells, and histiocytes localized in the interstitial septa often filling the alveolar spaces (**Fig. 2**). The interstitial lymphoid cells are mainly T cells, whereas B cells are mostly located in peribronchial germinal centers. Interstitial fibrosis and honeycombing can be present in the late stages of the disease. Often, LIP coexists with follicular bronchiolitis. These 2 entities can both progress to lymphoma. LIP may respond well to corticosteroids or immunosuppressive therapy.[39]

Usual Interstitial Pneumonia

Usual interstitial pneumonitis is a rare feature in patients with pSS. Kadota and colleagues[40] reported the first documented case of UIP in

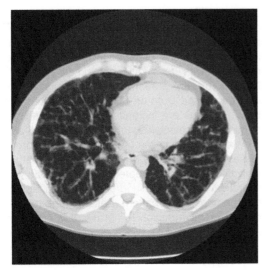

Fig. 1. HRCT scan of a patient with lymphocytic interstitial pneumonia. Diffuse central and peripheral interstitial disease is present with associated fibrosis. There is irregular septal thickening, associated thick-walled bronchi, and mild peripheral honeycombing. Mild centrilobular bronchiectasis is also present diffusely.

pSS. Clinical manifestations do not differ from those in other ILDs. PFT shows restriction, and CT findings are consistent, with fibrosis, honeycombing, and traction bronchiectasis predominantly at the lower lobes. Histologically it is characterized by a variety of changes ranging from normal alveolar walls to architectural effacement with characteristic interstitial fibroblastic foci. Parampil and colleagues[18] reported 17% of their patients having UIP documented by biopsy.

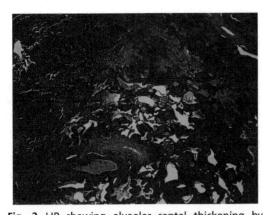

Fig. 2. LIP showing alveolar septal thickening by a dense cellular infiltrate, with some architectural distortion. A proteinaceous exudate is present in alveolar spaces. (Hematoxylin & eosin, original magnification ×40.)

Organizing Pneumonia

pSS is not usually associated with OP, and only a few cases documented by surgical lung biopsy have been reported in the literature. Matteson and Ike[41] described the first case of pSS-associated OP in 1990. A few years later, Usui and colleagues,[42] Lambert and colleagues,[43] and Ioannou and colleagues[44] described 3 more patients with pSS and histologically proven OP. In most published reports, the diagnosis of OP was made concurrently with the diagnosis of pSS. This is in contrast to the series by Parambil and colleagues[18] in which 4 of 18 patients (22%) were diagnosed with OP; however, in 3 patients the diagnosis was established by transbronchial biopsy, not surgical lung biopsy.

LYMPHOMA

The evolution from the benign lymphocytic infiltration characteristic of SS to lymphoma is a multistep process. Epithelial infiltration consists of polyclonal B and T lymphocytes, whereas lymphoma represents monoclonal B-cell proliferation. The risk of lymphoma in patients with SS is 44 times higher than the incidence in a healthy population.[45] It has been estimated by several studies that 4% to 8% of patients with SS will develop lymphoma in the course of their disease.[46,47] The most common type is non-Hodgkin lymphoma. Multiple histologic types of non-Hodgkin lymphoma have been described in patients with pSS, such as follicular, lymphoplasmacytoid, and diffuse large B-cell lymphoma, with mucosa-associated lymphoid tissue (MALT) lymphoma, a subtype of marginal zone B-cell lymphoma, being the most frequent. Voulgarelis and colleagues[48] reported that the presence of severe involvement of the exocrine glands, vasculitis, hypocomplementemia, and cryoglobulinemia at diagnosis increases the risk of developing lymphoma among patients with pSS.

The prevalence of primary pulmonary lymphoma is estimated to be 1% to 2% in patients with SS. Franquet and colleagues[24] described 1 case of pulmonary lymphoma among 50 patients with pSS. Similarly, Strimlan and colleagues[12] found 3 patients with pulmonary lymphoma in a series of 343 patients with pSS and sSS. Primary pulmonary lymphoma accounts for approximately 20% of all lymphoma in patients with SS. Hansen and colleagues[49] reported 10 patients with pulmonary lymphoma in a series of 50 patients with SS-related malignancy. Primary pulmonary lymphoma in these patients is usually a low-grade extranodal marginal B-cell lymphoma of the MALT type

(**Fig. 3**) and clinically manifests with cough, dyspnea, weight loss, sweats, and fatigue. Radiographically, it can present as solitary or multifocal nodules, bilateral alveolar infiltrates, or interstitial markings randomly distributed with a mild predilection for the lower lobes (**Fig. 4**). Mediastinal lymphadenopathy and pleural effusions may accompany the parenchymal abnormalities. MALT lymphomas can occasionally progress to high-grade lymphomas.

Thymic MALToma is a rare entity described in SS, which appears radiographically as an anterior mediastinal mass with multiple cystic formations. It is difficult to distinguish thymic MALToma from other types of mediastinal lymphomas and thymomas based exclusively on imaging techniques (CT and magnetic resonance imaging). Biopsy is considered necessary for a definitive diagnosis.[50]

PSEUDOLYMPHOMA

Pseudolymphoma or pulmonary nodular lymphoid hyperplasia is considered a benign lesion characterized pathologically by infiltration of

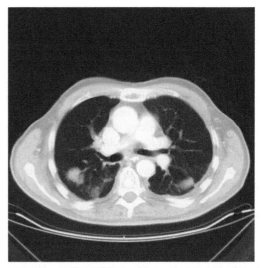

Fig. 4. CT demonstrates a 2.4 × 2.1-cm parenchymal opacity in the posterior segment of the right upper lobe.

mature polyclonal lymphocytes and plasma cells. Strimlan and colleagues[12] reported 1 case of pseudolymphoma in a large series of patients with pSS and sSS. There are some controversial data on whether pseudolymphoma is different from extranodal marginal zone B-cell lymphoma. Differentiation of pseudolymphoma from other lymphoproliferative disorders can be based only on immunohistochemical and molecular studies.[50] Pseudolymphoma is more often seen in patients with lone sicca syndrome. Patients are usually asymptomatic but can also present with cough and dyspnea. The typical CT finding is a solitary nodule or mass. Pseudolymphoma can also present as parenchymal consolidation with air bronchograms or even as multiple nodules with vascular involvement. If pleural effusions or mediastinal lymph nodes are found, a diagnosis of lymphoma should be considered. Pseudolymphoma usually regresses after treatment with corticosteroids or immunosuppressive therapy; rarely it can progress to frank lymphoma.[51]

AMYLOIDOSIS

Amyloidosis is caused by the extracellular deposition of an abnormal fibrillar protein. The secondary form of the disease has been occasionally described in SS and is often associated with lymphoproliferative disorders. In the study of 343 patients with pSS and sSS by Strimlan and colleagues,[12] 2 patients were diagnosed with pulmonary amyloidosis. Jeong and colleagues[52] studied CT scans in 5 women with pSS with pulmonary amyloidosis and lymphoproliferative

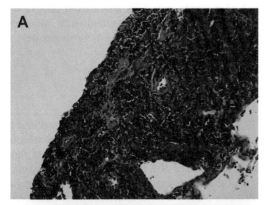

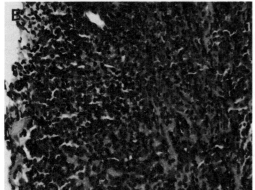

Fig. 3. (*A*, *B*) Pulmonary lymphoma of MALT type with infiltration and marked distortion of alveolar architecture by a diffuse infiltrate of small monoclonal lymphoid cells of B-cell phenotype. (*A*, hematoxylin & eosin, original magnification ×40; *B*, hematoxylin & eosin, original magnification ×400.)

disorders and described multiple thin-walled cysts and nodules, parenchymal opacities, and bronchiectasis (**Fig. 5**). In the series of Parambil and colleagues,[18] 1 of 18 patients with pSS was diagnosed with pulmonary amyloidosis.

Pulmonary amyloidosis may involve the larynx, tracheobronchial tree, pulmonary interstitium, and/or mediastinum and usually presents as bilateral micronodular lesions, predominantly peripheral subpleural and lower lobe in location. These nodules may calcify or cavitate. Histopathologic evaluation with positive staining for amyloid is necessary for the diagnosis.[53]

PULMONARY ARTERIAL HYPERTENSION

Pulmonary arterial hypertension (PAH) is associated with several connective tissue disorders, most commonly with scleroderma. Although pulmonary involvement in SS is relatively frequent, the prevalence of pulmonary hypertension is rare.[54,55] Pulmonary hypertension is one of the more severe pulmonary complications of SS, with survival rates of 73% at 1 year and 66% at 3 years.[56]

The pathogenesis of pulmonary hypertension in pSS is not clear, but it is believed that it results from vasculitis with prolonged vasospasm followed by structural vessel remodeling, eventually leading to irreversible thrombotic obstruction of the pulmonary arterioles. Raynaud phenomenon often accompanies SS-associated pulmonary hypertension and either precedes or appears concurrently with pulmonary vasculitis. There are about 41 known cases of pSS-pulmonary hypertension of which only 28 are well documented. Launay and colleagues[56] studied 9 new patients with pSS and pulmonary hypertension diagnosed by catheterization of the right side of the heart and reviewed the data on an additional 19 already reported cases. Patients with pSS-related pulmonary hypertension were more likely to have Raynaud phenomenon, skin vasculitis, and ILD. They were also more likely to have anti-Ro and antiribonucleoprotein autoantibodies as well as a positive RF and hypergammaglobulinemia. These data suggest that vasculopathy, B-cell activation, and autoimmunity contribute to the pathogenesis of pulmonary hypertension in pSS.

The best treatment strategy is unknown. Standard PAH therapy has been shown to be effective in some patients; however, failures with these therapies have also been documented. There are case reports of patients with pSS-associated pulmonary hypertension also treated with immunosuppression as monotherapy with initial improvement. Generally, it is believed that all patients with pSS-associated pulmonary hypertension should be treated with standard PAH therapy with or without an immunosuppressive regimen.[56]

OTHER MANIFESTATIONS

Pleural effusions in SS are more often associated with sSS in rheumatoid arthritis or systemic lupus erythematosus. Pleural effusions in pSS are rare. So far, 9 cases of pSS complicated by pleural effusions have been reported in the literature. Pleural effusions are more often bilateral but can be unilateral. The pleural fluid is exudative with predominant lymphocytic cell counts, normal glucose levels and pH, and low adenosine deaminase levels. In 2 of the reported cases, pleural effusions have regressed with corticosteroid therapy or improved spontaneously.[57] Pleural thickening in patients with pSS has been associated with recurrent pneumonias and atelectasis.

There is one reported case of pulmonary gangrene associated with pSS. A pulmonary vasculitis in combination with small airway involvement seemed to be involved in the pathogenesis. The vasculitis, with local activation of the coagulation cascade, could explain the presence of thrombosis and associated infarction.[58]

Cysts or bullae have been described in patients with pSS and are often associated with lymphoproliferative disorders including LIP. The mechanism of cyst formation includes peribronchial

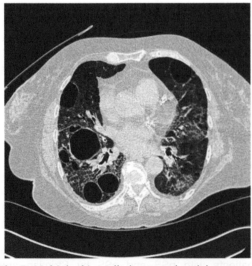

Fig. 5. Multiple thin-walled cysts and nodules, parenchymal opacities, interlobular thickening, and bronchiectasis are seen on high-resolution chest CT in a patient with pSS, pulmonary amyloidosis, and lymphocytic interstitial pneumonia.

lymphocytic infiltration, bronchiolar obstruction, and hyperinflation of the terminal lobules.[59]

TREATMENT AND PROGNOSIS

pSS usually is a slowly progressing disease; if extraglandular involvement or lymphoma is present, the progression is faster. The most common pSS symptoms (sicca) are not treated with corticosteroids or other immunosuppressive drugs because of lack of efficacy. Topical treatment is recommended for symptom amelioration, such as lubricants for the mouth and eyes, nonsteroid antiinflammatory for joint pains, and normal saline nebulizers for xerotrachea. Systemic therapies are reserved for severe extraglandular manifestations. Corticosteroids are commonly used for the treatment of LIP, OP, and follicular bronchiolitis. UIP and NSIP related to pSS have been treated with corticosteroids alone or in combination with other immunosuppressives such as azathioprine.

Of the new biologic therapies, rituximab (anti-CD20) appears to be well suited for the treatment of pSS by targeting B cells, although it has no effect on sicca symptoms. Systemic manifestations, such as fatigue; synovitis; arthralgia; cryoglobulinemia-related vasculitis; and neurologic, renal, and pulmonary involvement, may improve.[60] Seror and colleagues,[61] in their series of 18 patients with pSS and various systemic presentations, studied 2 patients with pulmonary involvement. One patient with pulmonary infiltrates and pleural effusion, recalcitrant to traditional immunosuppressive therapy, had complete remission with 4 infusions of rituximab. The other patient, with diagnosed LIP, was free of symptoms (cough and dyspnea) after 4 infusions of rituximab. The effect on pSS-related non-Hodgkin lymphoma is also impressive. In a review of 5 studies on the efficacy of rituximab on systemic manifestations of pSS, 7 of 12 patients with pSS-associated lymphoma had full remission of the disease after treatment with rituximab alone.[60] Voulgarelis and colleagues[62] described good results combining rituximab with cyclophosphamide, hydroxydaunorubicin (doxorubicin), vincristine (Oncovin), and prednisone (CHOP) in the treatment of pSS-aggressive B-cell lymphoma. One report describes a case of MALT lymphoma that had complete remission after monotherapy with rituximab.[63]

Unlike rituximab, anti–tumor necrosis factor therapies have no efficacy in the treatment of pSS. Infliximab was studied in a double-blind, placebo-controlled trial that included 103 patients and was shown to be no more effective than placebo in local and systemic symptoms; this study provides no information about its efficacy on pulmonary manifestations.[64,65] Etanercept has also shown negative results in the treatment of the disease.[66] New targets among cytokines, such as IL-16, IL-17, and IL-12 and/or IL-23, may be effective on pSS.[67]

In general, pSS has a rather slow and temperate course, taking 6 to 10 years to fully develop. Periepithelial lymphocytic infiltration of glandular organs results in sicca symptoms. Lymphocytic infiltration of extraglandular organs has mild, often subclinical manifestations, such as interstitial nephritis or lymphocytic bronchiolitis. The manifestations of immunocomplex disease (eg, skin vasculitis, glomerulonephritis) carry the worst prognosis. Factors such as severe exocrinopathy, decreased levels of C4 complement, presence of purpura, and mixed monoclonal cryoglobulinemia at the time of diagnosis are each identified as negative prognostic factors, as these are often associated with glomerulonephritis and lymphoma, the latter being the main cause of death.[48] Based on this fact, Ioannidis and colleagues[68] suggested a predictive model that divides patients with pSS into 2 groups. Patients with low C4 levels and palpable purpura are classified as high risk for development of lymphoma and death and those without hypocomplimentemia are classified as low risk. In conclusion, of all the pulmonary manifestations of pSS, development of lymphoma, although rare, has the highest effect on overall mortality. The discovery of factors that identify high-risk patients even at the time of diagnosis may suggest closer follow-up and more aggressive therapeutic regimens.

REFERENCES

1. Gabriel SE, Michaud K. Epidemiological studies in incidence, prevalence, mortality, and comorbidity of the rheumatic diseases. Arthritis Res Ther 2009; 11:229.

2. Mavragani CP, Moutsopoulos HM. The geoepidemiology of Sjogren's syndrome. Autoimmun Rev 2010; 9:A305–10.

3. Ferreiro JE, Pasarin G, Quesada R, et al. Benign hypergammaglobulinemic purpura of Waldenstrom associated with Sjogren's syndrome. Case report and review of immunologic aspects. Am J Med 1986;81:734–40.

4. Tzioufas AG, Voulgarelis M. Update on Sjogren's syndrome autoimmune epithelitis: from classification to increased neoplasias. Best Pract Res Clin Rheumatol 2007;21:989–1010.

5. Bolstad AI, Wassmuth R, Haga HJ, et al. HLA markers and clinical characteristics in Caucasians

with primary Sjogren's syndrome. J Rheumatol 2001; 28:1554–62.

6. Alexander EL, Arnett FC, Provost TT, et al. Sjogren's syndrome: association of anti-Ro (SS-A) antibodies with vasculitis, hematologic abnormalities, and serologic hyperreactivity. Ann Intern Med 1983;98:155–9.

7. Schaumberg DA, Buring JE, Sullivan DA, et al. Hormone replacement therapy and dry eye syndrome. JAMA 2001;286:2114–9.

8. Fox RI. Sjogren's syndrome. Lancet 2005;366:321–31.

9. Dawson L, Tobin A, Smith P, et al. Antimuscarinic antibodies in Sjogren's syndrome: where are we, and where are we going? Arthritis Rheum 2005;52:2984–95.

10. Mitsias DI, Kapsogeorgou EK, Moutsopoulos HM. The role of epithelial cells in the initiation and perpetuation of autoimmune lesions: lessons from Sjogren's syndrome (autoimmune epithelitis). Lupus 2006;15:255–61.

11. Vitali C, Bombardieri S, Jonsson R, et al. Classification criteria for Sjogren's syndrome: a revised version of the European criteria proposed by the American-European Consensus Group. Ann Rheum Dis 2002;61:554–8.

12. Strimlan CV, Rosenow EC 3rd, Divertie MB, et al. Pulmonary manifestations of Sjogren's syndrome. Chest 1976;70:354–61.

13. Constantopoulos SH, Papadimitriou CS, Moutsopoulos HM. Respiratory manifestations in primary Sjogren's syndrome. A clinical, functional, and histologic study. Chest 1985;88:226–9.

14. Yazisiz V, Arslan G, Ozbudak IH, et al. Lung involvement in patients with primary Sjogren's syndrome: what are the predictors? Ann Rheum Dis 2002; 61(6):554–8.

15. Pertovaara M, Korpela M, Saarelainen S, et al. Long-term follow-up study of pulmonary findings in patients with primary Sjogren's syndrome. Scand J Rheumatol 2004;33:343–8.

16. Uffmann M, Kiener HP, Bankier AA, et al. Lung manifestation in asymptomatic patients with primary Sjogren syndrome: assessment with high resolution CT and pulmonary function tests. J Thorac Imaging 2001;16:282–9.

17. Papiris SA, Maniati M, Constantopoulos SH, et al. Lung involvement in primary Sjogren's syndrome is mainly related to the small airway disease. Ann Rheum Dis 1999;58:61–4.

18. Parambil JG, Myers JL, Lindell RM, et al. Interstitial lung disease in primary Sjogren syndrome. Chest 2006;130:1489–95.

19. Ito I, Nagai S, Kitaichi M, et al. Pulmonary manifestations of primary Sjogren's syndrome: a clinical, radiologic, and pathologic study. Am J Respir Crit Care Med 2005;171:632–8.

20. Kelly C, Gardiner P, Pal B, et al. Lung function in primary Sjogren's syndrome: a cross sectional and longitudinal study. Thorax 1991;46:180–3.

21. Taouli B, Brauner MW, Mourey I, et al. Thin-section chest CT findings of primary Sjogren's syndrome: correlation with pulmonary function. Eur Radiol 2002;12:1504–11.

22. Dalavanga YA, Constantopoulos SH, Galanopoulou V, et al. Alveolitis correlates with clinical pulmonary involvement in primary Sjogren's syndrome. Chest 1991;99:1394–7.

23. Salaffi F, Manganelli P, Carotti M, et al. A longitudinal study of pulmonary involvement in primary Sjogren's syndrome: relationship between alveolitis and subsequent lung changes on high-resolution computed tomography. Br J Rheumatol 1998;37:263–9.

24. Franquet T, Gimenez A, Monill JM, et al. Primary Sjogren's syndrome and associated lung disease: CT findings in 50 patients. AJR Am J Roentgenol 1997;169:655–8.

25. Koyama M, Johkoh T, Honda O, et al. Pulmonary involvement in primary Sjogren's syndrome: spectrum of pulmonary abnormalities and computed tomography findings in 60 patients. J Thorac Imaging 2001;16:290–6.

26. Franquet T, Diaz C, Domingo P, et al. Air trapping in primary Sjogren syndrome: correlation of expiratory CT with pulmonary function tests. J Comput Assist Tomogr 1999;23:169–73.

27. Freeman SR, Sheehan PZ, Thorpe MA, et al. Ear, nose, and throat manifestations of Sjogren's syndrome: retrospective review of a multidisciplinary clinic. J Otolaryngol 2005;34:20–4.

28. Papiris SA, Saetta M, Turato G, et al. CD4-positive T-lymphocytes infiltrate the bronchial mucosa of patients with Sjogren's syndrome. Am J Respir Crit Care Med 1997;156:637–41.

29. Lahdensuo A, Korpela M. Pulmonary findings in patients with primary Sjogren's syndrome. Chest 1995;108:316–9.

30. Gudbjornsson B, Hedenstrom H, Stalenheim G, et al. Bronchial hyperresponsiveness to methacholine in patients with primary Sjogren's syndrome. Ann Rheum Dis 1991;50:36–40.

31. Amin K, Ludviksdottir D, Janson C, et al. Inflammation and structural changes in the airways of patients with primary Sjogren's syndrome. Respir Med 2001; 95:904–10.

32. Wells AU, du Bois RM. Bronchiolitis in association with connective tissue disorders. Clin Chest Med 1993;14:655–66.

33. Yamadori I, Fujita J, Bandoh S, et al. Nonspecific interstitial pneumonia as pulmonary involvement of primary Sjogren's syndrome. Rheumatol Int 2002; 22:89–92.

34. Fujita J, Yamadori I, Suemitsu I, et al. Clinical features of non-specific interstitial pneumonia. Respir Med 1999;93:113–8.

35. Travis WD, Hunninghake G, King TE Jr, et al. Idiopathic nonspecific interstitial pneumonia: report of

an American Thoracic Society project. Am J Respir Crit Care Med 2008;177:1338–47.

36. Katzenstein AL, Fiorelli RF. Nonspecific interstitial pneumonia/fibrosis. Histologic features and clinical significance. Am J Surg Pathol 1994;18:136–47.

37. Cha SI, Fessler MB, Cool CD, et al. Lymphoid interstitial pneumonia: clinical features, associations and prognosis. Eur Respir J 2006;28:364–9.

38. Johkoh T, Muller NL, Pickford HA, et al. Lymphocytic interstitial pneumonia: thin-section CT findings in 22 patients. Radiology 1999;212:567–72.

39. Dalvi V, Gonzalez EB, Lovett L. Lymphocytic interstitial pneumonitis (LIP) in Sjogren's syndrome: a case report and a review of the literature. Clin Rheumatol 2007;26:1339–43.

40. Kadota J, Kusano S, Kawakami K, et al. Usual interstitial pneumonia associated with primary Sjogren's syndrome. Chest 1995;108:1756–8.

41. Matteson EL, Ike RW. Bronchiolitis obliterans organizing pneumonia and Sjogren's syndrome. J Rheumatol 1990;17:676–9.

42. Usui Y, Kimula Y, Miura H, et al. A case of bronchiolitis obliterans organizing pneumonia associated with primary Sjogren's syndrome who died of superimposed diffuse alveolar damage. Respiration 1992; 59:122–4.

43. Lambert M, Hebbar M, Viget N, et al. [Bronchiolitis obliterans with organized pneumonia: a rare complication of primary Gougerot-Sjogren syndrome]. Rev Med Interne 2000;21:74–7 [in French].

44. Ioannou S, Toya SP, Tomos P, et al. Cryptogenic organizing pneumonia associated with primary Sjogren's syndrome. Rheumatol Int 2008;28:1053–5.

45. Kassan SS, Thomas TL, Moutsopoulos HM, et al. Increased risk of lymphoma in sicca syndrome. Ann Intern Med 1978;89:888–92.

46. Voulgarelis M, Dafni UG, Isenberg DA, et al. Malignant lymphoma in primary Sjogren's syndrome: a multicenter, retrospective, clinical study by the European Concerted Action on Sjogren's syndrome. Arthritis Rheum 1999;42:1765–72.

47. Tonami H, Matoba M, Kuginuki Y, et al. Clinical and imaging findings of lymphoma in patients with Sjogren syndrome. J Comput Assist Tomogr 2003;27: 517–24.

48. Voulgarelis M, Tzioufas AG, Moutsopoulos HM. Mortality in Sjogren's syndrome. Clin Exp Rheumatol 2008;26:S66–71.

49. Hansen LA, Prakash UB, Colby TV. Pulmonary lymphoma in Sjogren's syndrome. Mayo Clin Proc 1989;64:920–31.

50. Sunada K, Hasegawa Y, Kodama T, et al. Thymic and pulmonary mucosa-associated lymphoid tissue lymphomas in a patient with Sjogren's syndrome and literature review. Respirology 2007;12:144–7.

51. Song MK, Seol YM, Park YE, et al. Pulmonary nodular lymphoid hyperplasia associated with Sjogren's syndrome. Korean J Intern Med 2007;22: 192–6.

52. Jeong YJ, Lee KS, Chung MP, et al. Amyloidosis and lymphoproliferative disease in Sjogren syndrome: thin-section computed tomography findings and histopathologic comparisons. J Comput Assist Tomogr 2004;28:776–81.

53. Adzic TN, Stojsic JM, Radosavljevic-Asic GD, et al. Multinodular pulmonary amyloidosis in primary Sjogren's syndrome. Eur J Intern Med 2008;19: e97–8.

54. Bertoni M, Niccoli L, Porciello G, et al. Pulmonary hypertension in primary Sjogren's syndrome: report of a case and review of the literature. Clin Rheumatol 2005;24:431–4.

55. Hedgpeth MT, Boulware DW. Pulmonary hypertension in primary Sjogren's syndrome. Ann Rheum Dis 1988;47:251–3.

56. Launay D, Hachulla E, Hatron PY, et al. Pulmonary arterial hypertension: a rare complication of primary Sjogren syndrome: report of 9 new cases and review of the literature. Medicine (Baltimore) 2007;86: 299–315.

57. Bouros D, Pneumatikos I, Tzouvelekis A. Pleural involvement in systemic autoimmune disorders. Respiration 2008;75:361–71.

58. Perez-Castrillon JL, Gonzalez-Castaneda C, Del Campo F, et al. Cavitary lung lesion in a patient with Sjogren's syndrome. Postgrad Med J 1999;75: 765–6.

59. Hubscher O, Re R, Iotti R. Cystic lung disease in Sjogren's syndrome. J Rheumatol 2002;29:2235–6.

60. Isaksen K, Jonsson R, Omdal R. Anti-CD20 treatment in primary Sjogren's syndrome. Scand J Immunol 2008;68:554–64.

61. Seror R, Sordet C, Guillevin L, et al. Tolerance and efficacy of rituximab and changes in serum B cell biomarkers in patients with systemic complications of primary Sjogren's syndrome. Ann Rheum Dis 2007;66:351–7.

62. Voulgarelis M, Giannouli S, Tzioufas AG, et al. Long term remission of Sjogren's syndrome associated aggressive B cell non-Hodgkin's lymphomas following combined B cell depletion therapy and CHOP (cyclophosphamide, doxorubicin, vincristine, prednisone). Ann Rheum Dis 2006;65:1033–7.

63. Pijpe J, van Imhoff GW, Vissink A, et al. Changes in salivary gland immunohistology and function after rituximab monotherapy in a patient with Sjogren's syndrome and associated MALT lymphoma. Ann Rheum Dis 2005;64:958–60.

64. Mariette X, Ravaud P, Steinfeld S, et al. Inefficacy of infliximab in primary Sjogren's syndrome: results of the randomized, controlled Trial of Remicade in Primary Sjogren's Syndrome (TRIPSS). Arthritis Rheum 2004;50:1270–6.

65. Steinfeld SD, Demols P, Salmon I, et al. Infliximab in patients with primary Sjogren's syndrome: a pilot study. Arthritis Rheum 2001;44:2371–5.

66. Sankar V, Brennan MT, Kok MR, et al. Etanercept in Sjogren's syndrome: a twelve-week randomized, double-blind, placebo-controlled pilot clinical trial. Arthritis Rheum 2004;50:2240–5.

67. Roescher N, Tak PP, Illei GG. Cytokines in Sjogren's syndrome: potential therapeutic targets. Ann Rheum Dis 2010;69:945–8.

68. Ioannidis JP, Vassiliou VA, Moutsopoulos HM. Long-term risk of mortality and lymphoproliferative disease and predictive classification of primary Sjogren's syndrome. Arthritis Rheum 2002;46:741–7.

Pulmonary Manifestations of the Idiopathic Inflammatory Myopathies

Meena Kalluri, MD[a],*, Chester V. Oddis, MD[b]

KEYWORDS

- Myositis • Pulmonary complications
- Interstitial lung disease

The idiopathic inflammatory myopathies (IIMs) are chronic, acquired, autoimmune disorders causing muscle weakness due to skeletal muscle inflammation. Based on clinical, histopathologic, and immunologic features, IIMs have been classified into 3 general subtypes including polymyositis (PM), adult and juvenile dermatomyositis (DM), and inclusion body myositis (IBM). However, overlap syndromes of myositis with other connective tissue diseases (CTD) and malignancy-associated myositis also occur under the rubric of IIM. These subsets of IIM are characterized by proximal muscle weakness, elevation of serum muscle enzymes (most commonly creatine kinase [CK]), electromyographic features of myopathy, and inflammatory cell infiltrates in muscle tissue. Patients manifesting any of several characteristic rashes are classified as having DM (**Fig. 1**); and various organs may be involved in PM or DM including the lungs, heart, gastrointestinal tract and joints. Many investigators include amyopathic dermatomyositis (ADM) with the IIM as a potentially distinct category; these patients have skin findings consistent with DM but no muscle involvement. This review focuses on the pulmonary manifestations seen in the inflammatory myopathies, and here the term myositis or PM-DM is used interchangeably with IIM.

CLASSIFICATION AND EPIDEMIOLOGY

Many classification systems have been suggested in IIM. Bohan and Peter[1,2] proposed the 5 criteria already mentioned for the diagnosis of PM and DM, which are still used today; Dalakas and Hohlfeld[3] suggested new criteria based on immunohistochemical and pathologic features. The subsequent discovery of autoantibodies associated with the myositis syndromes led to a different classification scheme incorporating serologic features.[4] The Bohan and Peter criteria have come under considerable scrutiny,[1,2] and myositis investigators are currently pursuing efforts to update IIM classification criteria.[5] **Table 1** compares the 2 classification systems, the original Bohan and Peter classification and the later proposal relying on immunohistochemistry.

IIM is a rare disease, with an overall incidence ranging from 2 to 10 new cases per million persons at risk per year in various populations.[6–10] The prevalence and incidence may be increasing as a result of better physician awareness and the availability of laboratory tests. Although inflammatory myopathy can occur at any age, there are childhood and adult peaks with a 3:1 to 4:1 Afro-American to Caucasian ratio of incidence.

[a] Division of Pulmonary Medicine, University of Alberta, Edmonton, Canada
[b] Division of Rheumatology and Clinical Immunology, University of Pittsburgh, PA, USA
* Corresponding author. 2-25 D, College Plaza, 8215-112th Street, Edmonton, Alberta T6G2C8, Canada.
E-mail address: meenakalluri@med.ualberta.ca

Clin Chest Med 31 (2010) 501–512
doi:10.1016/j.ccm.2010.05.008

chestmed.theclinics.com

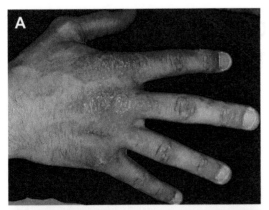

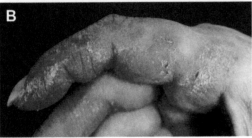

Fig. 1. (A) DM-associated rashes. Extensor erythema over the knuckles and interphalangeal joints of a patient with DM consistent with Gottron papules. (B) DM-associated cutaneous features. "Mechanic's hands" in a patient with the anti–Jo-1 autoantibody. Erythema, hyperkeratosis, and cracking of the lateral aspects of the fingers is noted.

IMMUNOPATHOGENESIS OF THE MYOSITIS SYNDROMES

The pathogenesis of myositis is incompletely understood. The presence of T cells and B cells in muscle tissue, the finding of serum autoantibodies in many patients, and the coexistence of myositis with other autoimmune diseases certainly support an immune-mediated cause. The spectrum of myositis is thought to be triggered by environmental (eg, infectious agents such as viruses) factors in individuals with a genetic predisposition to autoimmunity. Many recent reports strongly support this genetic component in the immunopathogenesis of myositis, as there are significant correlations of HLA class II haplotypes with clinical and serologic profiles in large cohorts of primarily Caucasian patients with myositis.[11–13] Histopathologic changes in muscle provide strong evidence for autoimmunity in PM and DM. In PM, the myofiber appears to be the target of immunologic attack because non-necrotic fibers are surrounded and invaded by mononuclear CD8+ T cells (Fig. 2). These fibers demonstrate major histocompatibility complex (MHC) class I expression suggesting that the pathology of PM is mediated by the recognition of a surface antigen on the muscle fiber by antigen-specific T cells (Fig. 3). On the contrary, DM is thought to be more humorally mediated, with the blood vessel being the

Table 1
Diagnosis of PM-DM

Criteria	Features	Diagnosis
Bohan and Peter (1975)[1,2]	1. Symmetric proximal muscle weakness 2. Elevated serum muscle enzymes 3. EMG consistent with myopathy 4. Muscle biopsy with characteristic features 5. Typical rash	1–4 criteria present: definite PM Any 3 of 1–4 present: probable PM Any 2 of 1–4 present: possible PM Rash + any 3 of 1–4: definite DM
Dalakas and Hohlfeld[3]: emphasis on histology and immunopathology	1. Subacute proximal muscle weakness 2. Elevated serum muscle enzymes 3. Muscle biopsy 4. Typical rash	Criteria 1,2 with muscle biopsy showing inflammation with CD8/MHC-I complex and no vacuoles: definite PM Criteria 1 and 2 with muscle biopsy showing MHC-I expression without T cells or vacuoles: probable PM Rash + muscle biopsy: definite DM No rash + typical biopsy: probable DM Rash without muscle weakness: ADM

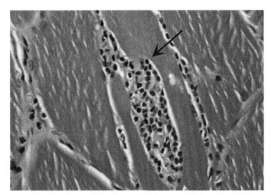

Fig. 2. Muscle biopsy (H&E stain) in PM. Invasion of a non-necrotic muscle fiber by lymphocytes in a patient with PM.

immunologic target. CD4$^+$ T cells and B cells are more common with complement activation, leading to C5-9 membrane attack complex deposition in muscle capillaries. Antinuclear or anticytoplasmic autoantibodies are found in up to 90% of patients with PM or DM and are useful in defining clinically homogeneous subsets of patients.[14] Myositis-specific autoantibodies (MSAs) have been previously reported to occur exclusively in IIM but have been detected in patients without evidence of myositis (**Table 2**).[15] A negative antinuclear antibody test does not exclude an MSA because the antigens targeted by these autoantibodies may be cytoplasmic in location. Autoantibodies seen in other CTD may also be found in patients with myositis and are termed myositis-associated autoantibodies (MAA). Of relevance to the pulmonary problems seen with myositis is anti–Jo-1, which is directed against histidyl-tRNA synthetase, one of a group of antiaminoacyl-tRNA synthetases. The clinical associations of the various antisynthetase antibodies are similar

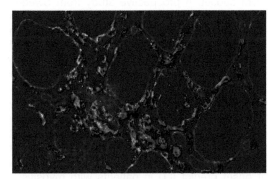

Fig. 3. MHC-I/CD8 complexes in PM. MHC-I is up-regulated on all muscle fibers (*green*). CD8$^+$ T cells that also express MHC-I invade muscle fibers. (*From* Dalakas MC, Hohlfeld R. Seminars: polymyositis and dermatomyositis. Lancet 2003;362:974; with permission.)

and comprise the "antisynthetase syndrome" that includes myositis, fever, Raynaud phenomenon, "mechanic's hands" (cracking and hyperkeratosis of the lateral surfaces of the fingers), polyarthritis, and interstitial lung disease (ILD).[4]

LUNG AND MYOSITIS

The lung is the most common extramuscular organ involved in PM-DM. Pulmonary complications occur in more than 40% of patients, causing significant morbidity and mortality.[16] Complications include ILD, aspiration, pneumonia, drug-induced lung diseases, and nonparenchymal problems such as ventilatory (diaphragmatic and intercostal) muscle weakness. However, ventilatory muscle weakness leading to respiratory failure or significant dyspnea is uncommon, occurring in less than 5% of patients.[4,17] Pulmonary disease may be observed in patients without overt muscle involvement.[18] Beyond these issues, parenchymal lung involvement may include pulmonary arterial hypertension and diffuse alveolar hemorrhage with pulmonary capillaritis, the latter being uncommon but frequently fatal.[19] On the other hand, pneumomediastinum and pneumothorax are being increasingly reported, and may be associated with rapidly progressive ILD even in the setting of ADM (see **Table 2**).[20,21]

NONPULMONARY CAUSES OF DYSPNEA
Muscle Weakness

Respiratory failure due to respiratory muscle weakness is a rare complication in adult PM, the prevalence of which is unknown.[22,23] Chronic respiratory failure has been described in patients with advanced myositis and a history of dysphagia. Only 4 cases with acute respiratory failure due to respiratory muscle weakness have been reported.[22] Patients without obvious parenchymal lung involvement or respiratory complaints may show a higher than expected proportion of diaphragmatic abnormalities. The standard pulmonary function tests (PFTs) may be unremarkable, with only reduced inspiratory or expiratory pressures.[24] With progressive disease restrictive physiology is seen, showing low total lung capacity and vital capacity, and low maximal inspiratory pressure (MIP) and maximal expiratory pressure (MEP),[25] with normal forced expiratory volume in 1 second (FEV$_1$) and forced vital capacity (FVC), diffusion, and alveolar-arterial oxygen tension difference. Supine respiratory function tests are useful for clinical diagnosis and respiratory risk stratification. The critical predictive parameters include respiratory muscle strength

Table 2
Lung in myositis

Lung Disease in Myositis	Diagnosis	Prevalence (40–65%)
Parenchymal disease	Aspiration pneumonia	17%
	Infectious pneumonia	
	ILD	5%–65%
	Drug-induced ILD	
	PAH	
	Diffuse alveolar hemorrhage	
	Pneumomediastinum	
	Pneumothorax	
Nonparenchymal disease	Ventilatory failure	<5%

(MIP and MEP) less than 30% of predicted and vital capacity less than 55% predicted.[26] In one study, the most severe degree of diaphragmatic dysfunction was found in DM.[24] The presence of diaphragmatic weakness may also be an independent risk factor for sleep-disordered breathing and for respiratory failure.

Cardiac Causes

Serious cardiac involvement in IIM is unusual, but dyspnea is a common symptom from any of the several cardiac issues. Congestive heart failure,[27] left ventricular diastolic dysfunction, coronary artery disease, and arrhythmias may contribute to dyspnea. Pulmonary edema due to myocarditis and/or cardiomyopathy usually occurs together with active muscle disease; subclinical cardiac manifestations of myositis include various conduction blocks and occasionally atrial or ventricular arrhythmias.[28]

PULMONARY CAUSES OF DYSPNEA
Infections Including Aspiration Pneumonia

Infectious complications have been reported in up to 26% of patients resulting in an increased mortality rate.[29] Immunosuppressive medications have been implicated, with most patients developing lung infections in the first year following diagnosis. In a study of 156 patients with PM-DM, 33% of the cohort developed infectious complications led by aspiration pneumonia (17%), opportunistic infections (11.5%), septicemia, and pneumonia (2% each). *Pneumocystis jiroveci* and *Candida albicans* were responsible for 50% of all infections while *Pseudomonas* and *Staphylococcus* were common organisms in patients with pneumonia. Predisposing factors include dysphagia, lymphopenia, low serum total protein, thoracic muscle myopathy,[30] and concurrent immunosuppressive therapy.[29]

Interstitial Lung Diseases

ILD is a common manifestation in IIM with a prevalence of 5% to 65%, varying depending on the means of detection.[31] In an enriched population of 90 Jo-1 antibody positive patients with clinical, radiographic, and pulmonary function data, 77 (86%) met criteria for ILD.[32] ILD is an important prognostic factor and may cause life-threatening complications. Myositis-associated ILD (MA-ILD) can precede, occur concomitantly with, or present after the diagnosis of IIM.[31] The clinical presentation is variable because patients may be asymptomatic, present acutely, develop rapidly progressive respiratory failure, or follow a subacute or chronic course.

In a study of 36 patients with ILD, most (58%) had a chronic course, 25% were asymptomatic at diagnosis, and 17% presented with acute respiratory failure. ILD was diagnosed concomitantly with skin and muscle disease in 42% of the patients and preceded IIM in 19% of the patients.[33] The most common symptom was dyspnea, followed by cough. Acute ILD is more frequently seen in DM, particularly the ADM subset. A prospective study from Sweden identified 11 of 17 (65%) new PM and DM patients over a 2.5-year period with lung disease, 18% of whom had subclinical ILD.[34] Of note, DM-associated ILD (DM-ILD) may be more commonly associated with diffuse alveolar damage (DAD) and be more resistant to treatment and progressive,[35] reflecting pulmonary histologic differences and high-resolution computed tomography (HRCT) findings that may further distinguish PM from DM.[36,37] Joint symptoms, anti–Jo-1 positivity, and older age at onset predict ILD in patients with myositis.[38] In a retrospective Korean study of 72 patients with myositis, a Hamman-rich like presentation, features of ADM, and an initial FVC less than or equal to 60% were predictive of poor prognosis.[39] In addition, the concomitant finding of anti-Ro/SSA autoantibodies in patients with an antisynthetase antibody may be associated with more severe and progressive ILD.[40,41] Another study demonstrated that poor survival rate corresponds to an initial bronchoalveolar lavage (BAL) showing neutrophilic alveolitis.[42]

The most common histologic subtype reported in myositis is nonspecific interstitial pneumonia (NSIP).[42,43] Other histologic subtypes in MA-ILD include usual interstitial pneumonia (UIP), DAD, and organizing pneumonia (OP)[31,33,44] (**Fig. 4**). Lymphocytic interstitial pneumonitis is uncommon,[43,45] and only 1 of 17 biopsies was positive for this histology.[43] A new histologic pattern, acute fibrinous and organizing pneumonia, has been described in 17 reported cases, of which one had PM. This subgroup should also be taken into consideration.[46]

Pulmonary Hypertension

Pulmonary hypertension (PH) is poorly defined and is limited to case reports in IIM.[45,47] Patients typically present with exertional dyspnea, restriction on PFTs, or an isolated reduction in the diffusion capacity. PH seems to be predominant in the female population, and in one autopsy series, 4 of 20 patients with myositis had medial hypertrophy in the pulmonary artery.[48] Progressive pulmonary fibrosis may lead to severe PH that is poorly responsive to vasodilator therapy. Mortality is high despite treatment with immunosuppressive agents and vasodilators. Although a decreased diffusion on PFTs warrants an echocardiogram, the diagnosis should be confirmed by documentation of elevated pulmonary pressures by cardiac catheterization. Early referral for lung transplantation should be considered, given the grim prognosis.

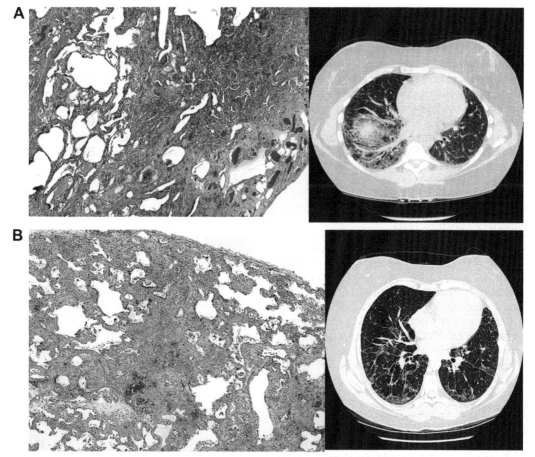

Fig. 4. Lung biopsy and CT images of MA-ILD. (*A*) H&E stained open lung biopsy (*left*) shows features of usual interstitial pneumonia (fibroblastic foci, mild inflammatory infiltrate, fibrosis and cystic changes); chest CT shows basal, peripheral honeycombing along with septal thickening. (*B*) H&E stained open lung biopsy (*left*) shows features of diffuse alveolar damage (edema, protein exudate, and inflammatory cell infiltrate in the alveolar spaces and interstitium). Chest CT shows patchy, peripheral ground-glass opacities in the lower lobes.

Pneumomediastinum and Pneumothorax

Considered rare in other CTDs, pneumomediastinum and pneumothorax may occur early in myositis (including ADM) resulting from rupture of alveoli or pericardiac blebs. In one report, the investigators identified 62 patients with CTD-associated pneumomediastinum, of whom 80% had DM and nearly half had ADM.[21] Thus, ADM should be considered in the setting of ILD and pneumothorax/pneumomediastinum. Pneumomediastinum was treated symptomatically in all cases, but pneumothorax, seen in 4 patients, was treated with thoracic drainage followed by pleurectomy. Although 3 patients died, 7 patients had a favorable outcome with relatively mild impairment of their PFTs. Lung histology varied and the overall mortality was 34%, with a cumulative estimated survival of 55% at 2 years.

Drug-Induced Lung Diseases

Several immunosuppressive agents used to treat myositis have specific pulmonary toxicities. Cyclophosphamide can cause an early, acute interstitial pneumonitis that is generally reversible with discontinuation.[49] Chronic, low-dose therapy can cause irreversible fibrosis that presents after years of therapy.[49] Methotrexate-induced pneumonitis, accompanied by dyspnea, cough, and constitutional symptoms, has been reported in 2% to 7% of rheumatoid patients and is idiosyncratic, and often occurs within the first year of treatment.[50] The reported mortality rate is 17% with a recurrence rate of 50%.[51]

DIAGNOSIS OF LUNG DISEASE IN MYOSITIS
Pulmonary Function Tests

PFTs are necessary for diagnosis, long-term follow-up, and monitoring the response to therapy. Restrictive impairment is characterized by a decrease in total lung capacity (TLC), functional residual capacity (FRC), FVC, FEV_1, diffusion lung capacity for carbon monoxide (DLCO) and a normal or increased FEV_1/FVC. Respiratory muscle weakness can also cause a reduction in TLC and FVC, but measurement of the MIP and MEP distinguishes it from restriction due to ILD.

Radiography

HRCT scanning correlates well with the open lung biopsy findings.[31] The most common HRCT pattern in PM or DM involves reticular and/or ground-glass opacities with or without consolidation and without honeycombing, correlating best with underlying NSIP histology.[17] The ground-glass opacities are potentially treatment-

responsive inflammatory conditions with a more favorable prognosis.[52] With treatment, serial computed tomography (CT) scans show improvement in opacities and limited fibrotic progression.[53] "Honeycombing," which corresponds to fibrosis, is less amenable to anti-inflammatory or immunosuppressive therapy.[52] Of the 32 retrospectively studied anti-Jo-1 positive patients who had HRCT, 15 (47%) presented acutely with respiratory insufficiency, whereas 17 (53%) had a more gradual onset of ILD symptoms.[54] Fever and HRCT findings of diffuse ground-glass opacities were common in the acute-onset group, contrasting with the gradual-onset patients in whom neutrophil-predominant BAL fluid and non–Jo-1 autoantibodies were characteristic along with traction bronchiectasis and honeycombing on CT. Although patients in the acute-onset group had a better initial treatment response at 3 months, they ultimately had more long-term ILD progression requiring combined therapy. Chest radiographs are less sensitive than HRCT; **Fig. 5** shows basal predominant alveolar infiltrate in a Jo-1–positive patient with acute dyspnea.

However, outcomes may not always correlate with the varied HRCT patterns that may be seen in PM and DM, as evidenced by a retrospective study showing a fatal outcome in DM-associated ILD characterized by ground-glass attenuation and reticular opacities without significant fibrosis.[36] When changes on HRCT are seen in the setting of normal PFTs, their clinical significance and outcome is not known.

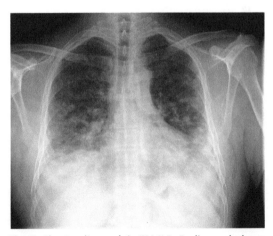

Fig. 5. Chest radiograph in IIM-ILD. Radiograph shows bilateral, basal, predominant alveolar opacities in a Jo-1–positive PM patient with acute-onset dyspnea and subsequent ARDS. (*Courtesy of* Chester V. Oddis, MD, Pittsburgh, PA.)

Bronchoalveolar Lavage

BAL, mostly done to rule out infection in the setting of MA-ILD, primarily reveals CD8$^+$ T cells and a minor B-cell component.[17] One report notes increased CD8$^+$ and CD 25$^+$ T cells in a corticosteroid-resistant group, while the CD4/CD8 ratio was not significantly different between steroid-sensitive and steroid-resistant patients.[55] Protein expression in BAL fluid was significantly different in the 3 subgroups of 11 patients with myositis and overlap syndrome, suggesting that a proteomic approach may provide pathogenic clues to MA-ILD.[56]

Lung Biopsy

Tissue biopsy may not be necessary if there are classic findings on HRCT.[57] When performed, surgical lung biopsies are preferred to transbronchial specimens because of the patchy nature of the disease. The histopathology was discussed earlier,[38,42,44] but different patterns may coexist, as reported retrospectively in a review of 13 patients.[44]

Biomarkers for ILD

The strongest predictor of ILD is the presence of anti–Jo-1, directed against histidyl-tRNA synthetase, one of a group of antiaminoacyl tRNA synthetases (**Table 3**). The prevalence of ILD in this group approximates 70% in synthetase-positive patients.[4,34] The clinical associations of the various antisynthetase antibodies are similar and have been described as comprising the "antisynthetase syndrome," but the reason for such patients having such a high frequency of lung involvement is poorly understood. One thought-provoking observation is that a proteolytically sensitive conformation of histidyl-tRNA synthetase exists in the lung, suggesting that an immune response to this antigen may be initiated and propagated in this tissue.[58] Similarly, the occurrence of shared T-cell receptor gene segment usage in the muscle and lungs of a small group of IIM patients (some with the Jo-1 autoantibody) could indicate a common target antigen in these organs.[59] Multiplex enzyme-linked immunosorbent assays (ELISAs) have demonstrated disease-specific associations between anti–Jo-1 antibody positive ILD and serum levels of interferon-γ–inducible chemokines.[32]

Other peripheral blood markers indicating lung involvement include antiendothelial antibodies, found in 20 of 56 patients with myositis and 10 of 15 with ILD.[60] The concentration of KL-6, a mucinous glycoprotein expressed on type II pneumocytes and bronchiolar epithelial cells, decreases with treatment in adults with myositis and children with JDM.[61] Cytokeratin 19 fragment, a cytoskeletal structural protein of bronchial epithelial cells, was significantly increased in the serum of patients with myositis who have ILD; it correlated with DAD and fluctuated with ILD progression or improvement.[62] Serum surfactant protein D, a phospholipid and protein moiety that

Table 3
Clinical profile of myositis-specific antibodies

Antisynthetase	Antigen	Clinical Profile	Prevalence
Anti–Jo-1	Histidyl-tRNA synthetase	Antisynthetase syndrome (AS)	20%
Anti–PL 7	Threonyl-tRNA synthetase	AS; milder myositis	5%–10%
Anti–PL-12	Alanyl-tRNA synthetase	AS; ILD > myositis	1%–5%
Anti–EJ	Glycyl-tRNA synthetase	AS: ILD > myositis	<5%
Anti–OJ	Isoleucyl-tRNA synthetase	AS; ILD > myositis	1%–5%
Anti–KS	Asparaginyl-tRNA synthetase	AS; ILD > myositis	1%–5%
Anti–YRS	Tyrosyl-tRNA synthetase	AS	<1%
Anti–Zo	Phenylalanyl-tRNA synthetase	AS; relapsing ILD	1%
Other MSA Anti-SRP Anti–Mi-2	SRP–intracytoplasmic protein translocation Helicase protein	Acute necrotizing myositis; cardiomyopathy DM with hallmark cutaneous features, mild muscle disease, low risk of ILD, good response to treatment	<1% <10%
Anti–CADM-140		Associated with cancer	Unknown

Data from Kalluri M, Sahn SA, Oddis CV, et al. Clinical profile of anti-PL-12 autoantibody: cohort study and review of the literature. Chest 2009;135(6):1550–6; and Gunawardena H, Betteridge ZE, McHugh NJ. Myositis-specific autoantibodies: their clinical and pathogenic significance in disease expression. Rheumatology (Oxford) 2009;48(6):607–12.

covers the alveolar surface, was found to be a useful marker for ILD when assayed in patients with PM and DM.[63]

The antisynthetase antibodies, in particular anti–Jo-1 anti–PL-12, have been strongly associated with ILD. Two recently published studies on anti–PL-12 confirmed this association, as the presence of anti–PL-12 was associated with ILD more than myositis.[64,65] In a Japanese study of 64 PM-DM and 28 IPF patients, the prevalence of antisynthetase autoantibodies was 51%, and 96% of antibody-positive patients had ILD, again suggesting that presence of antibody is a stronger marker of ILD than myositis in PM-DM.[66] In addition, the antibody-positive subset required immunosuppressive agents in addition to prednisone.

TREATMENT

The optimal treatment for MA-ILD remains to be determined. There are no controlled trials of any agents for ILD, but the standard therapeutic approach includes corticosteroids to which 50% of patients may respond favorably.[67] Patients with DM and normal CK levels tend to be resistant to corticosteroid therapy and have a poor survival compared with MA-ILD patients with an elevated CK.[68] Other immunosuppressive or immunomodulatory agents used to treat ILD include cyclophosphamide,[69–71] azathioprine,[72,73] methotrexate,[42] cyclosporine,[68,74] intravenous immune globulin (IVIg), and plasma exchange (Table 4).[75,76] IVIg was used in a small number of patients with refractory ILD and an acute presentation.[76] Calcineurin inhibitors have also demonstrated consistent efficacy. Cyclosporine inhibits interleukin-2 production and T-cell proliferation, and may be an appropriate choice for early, slowly progressive, nondiffuse ILD. Tacrolimus, which is 100 fold more potent than cyclosporine in inhibiting T-cell activation,

was efficacious in several case series of patients, including those refractory to cyclosporine and in patients with ILD associated with antisynthetase autoantibodies.[35,77,78] Tacrolimus may have a more favorable safety profile than cyclosporine. Mycophenolate mofetil (MMF), an antimetabolite, not only disrupts T-cell activation via inactivation of inosine monophosphate dehydrogenase but also interferes with fibroblast activity, proliferation, and release of profibrotic cytokines such as transforming growth factor-β.[79,80] MMF has potential efficacy in reversing progression or stabilization of disease activity in CTD-ILD including MA-ILD.[80,81]

Early administration of aggressive therapy may be beneficial in a select subgroup of patients. There is increasing evidence that cyclosporine may induce a response and prolong survival, but most of these studies are retrospective case series or open-label trials.[68] Combination therapy is often used. One study of chronic ILD compared 23% of the patients treated with prednisone with 77% of the patients who were given combination immunosuppressive therapy; after 6 months, the improvement in FVC in the latter group was statistically better and was maintained for up to 3 years.[82]

PROGNOSIS

In a study by Marie and colleagues,[33] the survival of IIM-associated ILD was reported to be 94%, 90%, and 87% at 1, 3, and 5 years, respectively. This rate is similar to that reported for idiopathic NSIP. The presence or absence of anti-Jo-1 did not influence survival in this group of 36 patients with PM or DM-ILD. The predictors of poor outcome include: acute presentations; neutrophilic alveolitis[33]; initial DLCO lesser than 45%; FVC lesser than or equal to 60%[39]; DM, microangiopathy and digital infarcts in DM, ADM[39,83]; and histologic UIP.[31,33]

Table 4
Treatment of IIM-ILD

Drug/Dose	Outcome
Methotrexate (15–25 mg/wk by mouth or by injection)	Generally favorable results with myositis; rarely used for ILD
Azathioprine (2–3 mg/kg/d)	Used for myositis and ILD
Cyclosporine (2–5 mg/kg/d)	Efficacy reported in ILD
Tacrolimus—dose depends on trough level	Check drug levels; effective in refractory Jo-1 patients with ILD
Mycophenolate mofetil (1g twice a day)	Used for refractory DM rash; ILD
Cyclophosphamide (1–2 mg/kg/d by mouth or monthly intravenous pulse	Conflicting results; effective in ILD

In a study of 17 patients with biopsy-proven ILD and a median follow-up of 3.4 years, 5 died, 1 received lung transplant, and the survival rate at 5 years was 50%. The cause of death was progressive respiratory failure in all cases. The remaining 11 patients improved with combination immunosuppressive therapy. NSIP was seen in 65% of the cases.[35] Histopathology of ILD has prognostic value. NSIP and organizing pneumonia tend to have the best prognosis and respond to therapy, whereas UIP has intermediate prognosis and the worst outcomes are seen in DAD.[33,84]

SUMMARY

ILD is common in myositis and may precede the onset of CTD-related symptoms, so an early or occult rheumatologic disease should be considered in this setting. The relatively low incidence and prevalence of many forms of ILD has hampered attempts at performing adequately powered and soundly designed clinical trials to evaluate pharmacologic treatments for these disorders. More insight into the etiopathogenesis from ongoing clinical trials is likely, and additional well-designed prospective studies are necessary to answer the questions of optimal treatment strategies for all forms of autoimmune ILD.

REFERENCES

1. Bohan A, Peter JB. Polymyositis and dermatomyositis (first of two parts). N Engl J Med 1975;292(7): 344–7.
2. Bohan A, Peter JB. Polymyositis and dermatomyositis (second of two parts). N Engl J Med 1975;292(8): 403–7.
3. Dalakas MC, Hohlfeld R. Polymyositis and dermatomyositis. Lancet 2003;362(9388):971–82.
4. Love LA, Leff RL, Fraser DD, et al. A new approach to the classification of idiopathic inflammatory myopathy: myositis-specific autoantibodies define useful homogeneous patient groups. Medicine 1991; 70(6):360–74.
5. Amato AA, Griggs RC. Unicorns, dragons, polymyositis, and other mythological beasts. Neurology 2003;61(3):288–9.
6. Benbassat J, Geffel D, Zlotnick A. Epidemiology of polymyositis-dermatomyositis in Israel, 1960-76. Isr J Med Sci 1980;16(3):197–200.
7. Koh ET, Seow A, Ong B, et al. Adult onset polymyositis/dermatomyositis: clinical and laboratory features and treatment response in 75 patients. Ann Rheum Dis 1993;52(12):857–61.
8. Kaipiainen-Seppanen O, Aho K. Incidence of rare systemic rheumatic and connective tissue diseases in Finland. J Intern Med 1996;240(2):81–4.
9. Oddis CV, Conte CG, Steen VD, et al. Incidence of polymyositis-dermatomyositis: a 20-year study of hospital diagnosed cases in Allegheny County, PA 1963-1982. J Rheumatol 1990;17(10): 1329–34.
10. Weitoft T. Occurrence of polymyositis in the county of Gavleborg, Sweden. Scand J Rheumatol 1997; 26(2):104–6.
11. Chinoy H, Salway F, Fertig N, et al. In adult onset myositis, the presence of interstitial lung disease and myositis specific/associated antibodies are governed by HLA class II haplotype, rather than by myositis subtype. Arthritis Res Ther 2006;8(1): R13.
12. O'Hanlon TP, Carrick DM, Arnett FC, et al. Immunogenetic risk and protective factors for the idiopathic inflammatory myopathies: distinct HLA-A, -B, -Cw, -DRB1 and -DQA1 allelic profiles and motifs define clinicopathologic groups in Caucasians. Medicine (Baltimore) 2005;84(6):338–49.
13. O'Hanlon TP, Carrick DM, Targoff IN, et al. Immunogenetic risk and protective factors for the idiopathic inflammatory myopathies: distinct HLA-A, -B, -Cw, -DRB1, and -DQA1 allelic profiles distinguish European American patients with different myositis autoantibodies. Medicine (Baltimore) 2006;85(2):111–27.
14. Targoff IN. Laboratory testing in the diagnosis and management of idiopathic inflammatory myopathies. Rheum Dis Clin North Am 2002;28(4):859 90, viii.
15. Brouwer R, Hengstman GJ, Vree Egberts W, et al. Autoantibody profiles in the sera of European patients with myositis. Ann Rheum Dis 2001;60(2): 116–23.
16. Torres C, Belmonte R, Carmona L, et al. Survival, mortality and causes of death in inflammatory myopathies. Autoimmunity 2006;39(3):205–15.
17. Schnabel A, Hellmich B, Gross WL. Interstitial lung disease in polymyositis and dermatomyositis. Curr Rheumatol Rep 2005;7(2):99–105.
18. Friedman AW, Targoff IN, Arnett FC. Interstitial lung disease with autoantibodies against aminoacyl-tRNA synthetases in the absence of clinically apparent myositis. Semin Arthritis Rheum 1996; 26(1):459–67.
19. Schwarz MI, Sutarik JM, Nick JA, et al. Pulmonary capillaritis and diffuse alveolar hemorrhage. A primary manifestation of polymyositis. Am J Respir Crit Care Med 1995;151(6):2037–40.
20. Korkmaz C, Ozkan R, Akay M, et al. Pneumomediastinum and subcutaneous emphysema associated with dermatomyositis. Rheumatology (Oxford) 2001;40(4):476–8.
21. Goff BL, Cherin P, Cantagrel A, et al. Pneumomediastinum in interstitial lung disease associated with dermatomyositis and polymyositis. Arthritis Rheum 2009;61(1):108–18.

22. Sano M, Suzuki M, Sato M, et al. Fatal respiratory failure due to polymyositis. Intern Med 1994;33(3):185–7.

23. Selva-O'Callaghan A, Sanchez-Sitjes L, Munoz-Gall X, et al. Respiratory failure due to muscle weakness in inflammatory myopathies: maintenance therapy with home mechanical ventilation. Rheumatology (Oxford) 2000;39(8):914–6.

24. Teixeira A, Cherin P, Demoule A, et al. Diaphragmatic dysfunction in patients with idiopathic inflammatory myopathies. Neuromuscul Disord 2005; 15(1):32–9.

25. Martin L, Chalmers IM, Dhingra S, et al. Measurements of maximum respiratory pressures in polymyositis and dermatomyositis. J Rheumatol 1985; 12(1):104–7.

26. Braun NM, Arora NS, Rochester DF. Respiratory muscle and pulmonary function in polymyositis and other proximal myopathies. Thorax 1983;38(8):616–23.

27. Lundberg IE. The heart in dermatomyositis and polymyositis. Rheumatology (Oxford) 2006;45(Suppl 4): iv18–21.

28. Stern R, Godbold JH, Chess Q, et al. ECG abnormalities in polymyositis. Arch Intern Med 1984; 144(11):2185–9.

29. Marie I, Hachulla E, Cherin P, et al. Opportunistic infections in polymyositis and dermatomyositis. Arthritis Rheum 2005;53(2):155–65.

30. Hepper NG, Ferguson RH, Howard FM Jr. Three types of pulmonary involvement in polymyositis. Med Clin North Am 1964;48:1031–42.

31. Fathi M, Lundberg IE. Interstitial lung disease in polymyositis and dermatomyositis. Curr Opin Rheumatol 2005;17(6):701–6.

32. Richards TJ, Eggebeen A, Gibson K, et al. Characterization and peripheral blood biomarker assessment of anti-Jo-1 antibody-positive interstitial lung disease. Arthritis Rheum 2009;60(7):2183–92.

33. Marie I, Hachulla E, Cherin P, et al. Interstitial lung disease in polymyositis and dermatomyositis. Arthritis Rheum 2002;47(6):614–22.

34. Fathi M, Dastmalchi M, Rasmussen E, et al. Interstitial lung disease, a common manifestation of newly diagnosed polymyositis and dermatomyositis. Ann Rheum Dis 2004;63(3):297–301.

35. Takada K, Nagasaka K, Miyasaka N. Polymyositis/dermatomyositis and interstitial lung disease: a new therapeutic approach with T-cell-specific immunosuppressants. Autoimmunity 2005;38(5): 383–92.

36. Hayashi S, Tanaka M, Kobayashi H, et al. High-resolution computed tomography characterization of interstitial lung diseases in polymyositis/dermatomyositis. J Rheumatol 2008;35(2):260–9.

37. Fujisawa T, Suda T, Nakamura Y, et al. Differences in clinical features and prognosis of interstitial lung diseases between polymyositis and dermatomyositis. J Rheumatol 2005;32(1):58–64.

38. Chen IJ, Jan Wu YJ, Lin CW, et al. Interstitial lung disease in polymyositis and dermatomyositis. Clin Rheumatol 2009;28(6):639–46.

39. Kang EH, Lee EB, Shin KC, et al. Interstitial lung disease in patients with polymyositis, dermatomyositis and amyopathic dermatomyositis. Rheumatology (Oxford) 2005;44(10):1282–6.

40. Vancsa A, Csipo I, Nemeth J, et al. Characteristics of interstitial lung disease in SS-A positive/Jo-1 positive inflammatory myopathy patients. Rheumatol Int 2009;29(9):989–94.

41. La Corte R, Lo Mo Naco A, Locaputo A, et al. In patients with antisynthetase syndrome the occurrence of anti-Ro/SSA antibodies causes a more severe interstitial lung disease. Autoimmunity 2006; 39(3):249–53.

42. Douglas WW, Tazelaar HD, Hartman TE, et al. Polymyositis-dermatomyositis-associated interstitial lung disease. Am J Respir Crit Care Med 2001; 164(7):1182–5.

43. Cottin V, Thivolet-Bejui F, Reynaud-Gaubert M, et al. Interstitial lung disease in amyopathic dermatomyositis, dermatomyositis and polymyositis. Eur Respir J 2003;22(2):245–50.

44. Tansey D, Wells AU, Colby TV, et al. Variations in histological patterns of interstitial pneumonia between connective tissue disorders and their relationship to prognosis. Histopathology 2004;44(6): 585–96.

45. Minai OA. Pulmonary hypertension in polymyositis-dermatomyositis: clinical and hemodynamic characteristics and response to vasoactive therapy. Lupus 2009;18(11):1006–10.

46. Beasley MB, Franks TJ, Galvin JR, et al. Acute fibrinous and organizing pneumonia: a histological pattern of lung injury and possible variant of diffuse alveolar damage. Arch Pathol Lab Med 2002;126(9): 1064–70.

47. Yaqub S, Moder KG, Lacy MQ. Severe, reversible pulmonary hypertension in a patient with monoclonal gammopathy and features of dermatomyositis. Mayo Clin Proc 2004;79(5):687–9.

48. Denbow CE, Lie JT, Tancredi RG, et al. Cardiac involvement in polymyositis: a clinicopathologic study of 20 autopsied patients. Arthritis Rheum 1979;22(10):1088–92.

49. Malik SW, Myers JL, DeRemee RA, et al. Lung toxicity associated with cyclophosphamide use. Two distinct patterns. Am J Respir Crit Care Med 1996;154(6 Pt 1):1851–6.

50. Cannon GW, Ward JR, Clegg DO, et al. Acute lung disease associated with low-dose pulse methotrexate therapy in patients with rheumatoid arthritis. Arthritis Rheum 1983;26(10):1269–74.

51. Marder W, McCune WJ. Advances in immunosuppressive therapy. Semin Respir Crit Care Med 2007;28(4):398–417.

52. Bonnefoy O, Ferretti G, Calaque O, et al. Serial chest CT findings in interstitial lung disease associated with polymyositis-dermatomyositis. Eur J Radiol 2004;49(3):235–44.

53. Arakawa H, Yamada H, Kurihara Y, et al. Nonspecific interstitial pneumonia associated with polymyositis and dermatomyositis: serial high-resolution CT findings and functional correlation. Chest 2003;123(4): 1096–103.

54. Tillie-Leblond I, Wislez M, Valeyre D, et al. Interstitial lung disease and anti-Jo-1 antibodies: difference between acute and gradual onset. Thorax 2008; 63(1):53–9.

55. Kurasawa K, Nawata Y, Takabayashi K, et al. Activation of pulmonary T cells in corticosteroid-resistant and -sensitive interstitial pneumonitis in dermatomyositis/polymyositis. Clin Exp Immunol 2002; 129(3):541–8.

56. Passadore I, Iadarola P, Di Poto C, et al. 2-DE and LC-MS/MS for a comparative proteomic analysis of BALf from subjects with different subsets of inflammatory myopathies. J Proteome Res 2009;8(5): 2331–40.

57. Wells AU, Hansell DM, Corrin B, et al. High resolution computed tomography as a predictor of lung histology in systemic sclerosis. Thorax 1992;47(9):738–42.

58. Levine SM, Raben N, Xie D, et al. Novel conformation of histidyl-transfer RNA synthetase in the lung: the target tissue in Jo-1 autoantibody-associated myositis. Arthritis Rheum 2007;56(8):2729–39.

59. Englund P, Wahlstrom J, Fathi M, et al. Restricted T cell receptor BV gene usage in the lungs and muscles of patients with idiopathic inflammatory myopathies. Arthritis Rheum 2007;56(1):372–83.

60. D'Cruz D, Keser G, Khamashta MA, et al. Antiendothelial cell antibodies in inflammatory myopathies: distribution among clinical and serologic groups and association with interstitial lung disease. J Rheumatol 2000;27(1):161–4.

61. Bandoh S, Fujita J, Ohtsuki Y, et al. Sequential changes of KL-6 in sera of patients with interstitial pneumonia associated with polymyositis/dermatomyositis. Ann Rheum Dis 2000;59(4):257–62.

62. Fujita J, Dobashi N, Tokuda M, et al. Elevation of cytokeratin 19 fragment in patients with interstitial pneumonia associated with polymyositis/dermatomyositis. J Rheumatol 1999;26(11):2377–82.

63. Ihn H, Asano Y, Kubo M, et al. Clinical significance of serum surfactant protein D (SP-D) in patients with polymyositis/dermatomyositis: correlation with interstitial lung disease. Rheumatology (Oxford) 2002; 41(11):1268–72.

64. Hervier B, Wallaert B, Hachulla E, et al. Clinical manifestations of anti-synthetase syndrome positive for anti-alanyl-tRNA synthetase (anti-PL12) antibodies: a retrospective study of 17 cases. Rheumatology (Oxford) 2010;49(5):972–6.

65. Kalluri M, Sahn SA, Oddis CV, et al. Clinical profile of anti-PL-12 autoantibody: cohort study and review of the literature. Chest 2009;135(6):1550–6.

66. Matsushita T, Hasegawa M, Fujimoto M, et al. Clinical evaluation of anti-aminoacyl tRNA synthetase antibodies in Japanese patients with dermatomyositis. J Rheumatol 2007;34(5):1012–8.

67. Schwarz MI, Matthay RA, Sahn SA, et al. Interstitial lung disease in polymyositis and dermatomyositis: analysis of six cases and review of the literature. Medicine (Baltimore) 1976;55(1):89–104.

68. Nawata Y, Kurasawa K, Takabayashi K, et al. Corticosteroid resistant interstitial pneumonitis in dermatomyositis/polymyositis: prediction and treatment with cyclosporine. J Rheumatol 1999; 26(7):1527–33.

69. Maccioni FJ, Colebatch HJ. Management of fibrosing alveolitis with polymyositis dermatomyositis. Aust N Z J Med 1990;20(6):806–10.

70. al-Janadi M, Smith CD, Karsh J. Cyclophosphamide treatment of interstitial pulmonary fibrosis in polymyositis/dermatomyositis. J Rheumatol 1989; 16(12):1592–6.

71. Yoshida T, Koga H, Saitoh F, et al. Pulse intravenous cyclophosphamide treatment for steroid-resistant interstitial pneumonitis associated with polymyositis. Intern Med 1999;38(9):733–8.

72. Marie I, Hatron PY, Hachulla E, et al. Pulmonary involvement in polymyositis and in dermatomyositis. J Rheumatol 1998;25(7):1336–43.

73. Rowen AJ, Reichel J. Dermatomyositis with lung involvement, successfully treated with azathioprine. Respiration 1983;44(2):143–6.

74. Gruhn WB, Diaz-Buxo JA. Cyclosporine treatment of steroid resistant interstitial pneumonitis associated with dermatomyositis/polymyositis. J Rheumatol 1987;14(5):1045–7.

75. Ideura G, Hanaoka M, Koizumi T, et al. Interstitial lung disease associated with amyopathic dermatomyositis: review of 18 cases. Respir Med 2007; 101(7):1406–11.

76. Suzuki Y, Hayakawa H, Miwa S, et al. Intravenous immunoglobulin therapy for refractory interstitial lung disease associated with polymyositis/dermatomyositis. Lung 2009;187(3):201–6.

77. Bongartz T, Ryu JH, Matteson EL. Is tacrolimus effective for treating antisynthetase-associated interstitial lung disease? Nat Clin Pract Rheumatol 2005; 1(2):80–1.

78. Wilkes MR, Sereika SM, Fertig N, et al. Treatment of antisynthetase-associated interstitial lung disease with tacrolimus. Arthritis Rheum 2005;52(8): 2439–46.

79. Roos N, Poulalhon N, Farge D, et al. In vitro evidence for a direct antifibrotic role of the immunosuppressive drug mycophenolate mofetil. J Pharmacol Exp Ther 2007;321(2):583–9.

80. Hervier B, Masseau A, Mussini JM, et al. Long-term efficacy of mycophenolate mofetil in a case of refractory antisynthetase syndrome. Joint Bone Spine 2009;76(5):575–6.

81. Swigris JJ, Olson AL, Fischer A, et al. Mycopheno-late mofetil is safe, well tolerated, and preserves lung function in patients with connective tissue disease-related interstitial lung disease. Chest 2006;130(1):30–6.

82. Won Huh J, Soon Kim D, Keun Lee C, et al. Two distinct clinical types of interstitial lung disease associated with polymyositis-dermatomyositis. Respir Med 2007;101(8):1761–9.

83. Ye S, Chen XX, Lu XY, et al. Adult clinically amyo-pathic dermatomyositis with rapid progressive inter-stitial lung disease: a retrospective cohort study. Clin Rheumatol 2007;26(10):1647–54.

84. Tazelaar HD, Viggiano RW, Pickersgill J, et al. Inter-stitial lung disease in polymyositis and dermatomyo-sitis. Clinical features and prognosis as correlated with histologic findings. Am Rev Respir Dis 1990; 141(3):727–33.

Pulmonary Manifestations of Relapsing Polychondritis

Samaan Rafeq, MD[a], David Trentham, MD[b],
Armin Ernst, MD[a,c,*]

KEYWORDS

- Relapsing polychondritis • Pulmonary manifestations

Relapsing polychondritis (RP) is a chronic multi-systemic disease characterized by recurrent episodes of cartilage inflammation throughout the body with the ears, nose, and airways being the most frequently affected areas.[1] The lower respiratory tract is involved in 20% to 50% of patients,[2–4] and specific diagnoses include sub-glottic stenosis, tracheal stenosis, tracheal wall thickening and calcification with sparing of the posterior membranous wall, and tracheobroncho-malacia (TBM). Medical therapies and airway inter-ventions are available and effective when used in experienced centers; however, no single treat-ment is curative, and the prognosis of RP with airway disease remains overall guarded.

This article reviews particular aspects of the clinical features, pathology, treatment, and prog-nosis of the pulmonary manifestations of RP.

EPIDEMIOLOGY

RP has been reported in almost all age groups, ranging from childhood to geriatric patients.

There is a female predominance with a ratio of 2:1 to 3:1,[2–4] and an association with other autoim-mune and rheumatic diseases has been described.[3,4]

CLINICAL FEATURES

McAdam and colleagues[4] have defined the diag-nosis of RP as the presence of any three out of the following six clinical features: (1) bilateral auric-ular chondritis, (2) nonerosive seronegative inflam-matory arthritis, (3) nasal chondritis, (4) ocular inflammation, (5) respiratory tract chondritis, or (6) audiovestibular damage.

Twenty percent to 50% of RP patients will develop airway symptoms, which maybe the pre-senting symptoms in up to 50% of those patients.[2–4] Symptoms including dyspnea, cough, chest discomfort, hoarseness, and stridor can be signs of serious airway involvement, and in the past, they were thought to indicate a poor prog-nosis, potentially leading to sudden unexpected death.[5,6] In the present time, however, the combi-nation of medical treatments with airway interven-tions that are available in specialized centers has led to better symptom control, airway patency, and improved survival.[2]

There are different mechanisms thought to be responsible for the airway obstruction depending on the stage of disease: inflammatory airway edema in the active stage, followed by dynamic collapse of the airway secondary to progressive

a Division of Interventional Pulmonary, Beth Israel Deaconess Medical Center, One Deaconess Road, Deaconess Building-201, Boston, MA 02215, USA
b Division of Rheumatology, Beth Israel Deaconess Medical Center, 330 Brookline Avenue, Boston, MA 02215, USA
c Department of Medicine and Surgery, Harvard Medical School, Boston, MA, USA
* Corresponding author. Division of Interventional Pulmonary, Beth Israel Deaconess Medical Center, One Deaconess Road, Deaconess Building-201, Boston, MA 02215.
E-mail address: aernst@bidmc.harvard.edu

Clin Chest Med 31 (2010) 513–518
doi:10.1016/j.ccm.2010.04.004

cartilage destruction, followed by fibrous tissue formation leading to contraction[7] and subsequent airway stenosis.

Radiologically, the most common and pathognomonic finding on dynamic airway imaging is anterior airway wall thickening with or without calcification with sparing of the posterior membranous wall (**Fig. 1**), followed by airway stenosis that may be focal or more extensive, involving larger segments or multiple segments of the tracheobronchial tree. The third finding is tracheobronchomalacia.[8]

There is no known involvement of the lung interstitium or the pulmonary vasculature in RP.

PATHOGENESIS

Patients with RP have been found to have an immunologic reaction to type 2 collagen, forming both autoantibodies and cellular response.[9,10]

Autoantibodies against the minor cartilage collagens, type 9 and type 11 also have been reported in a case report in a patient with fatal RP.[11]

LABORATORY TESTS

There are no specific markers for diagnosis or progression; however, anemia, leukocytosis, thrombocytosis, elevated C-reactive protein level, and sedimentation rate may be associated with disease activity.[3] Other markers such as rheumatoid factor (RF), antinuclear antibodies (ANA), and antineutrophil cytoplasmic antibodies (ANCA) may be positive in RP cases associated with other systemic vasculitis processes.[12] There are no clearly recognized markers or laboratory values that either indicate presence of airway involvement or are correlated with severity of progression. In

a prior survey, the presence of a saddle nose deformity correlated with pulmonary involvement.[3]

PULMONARY FUNCTION TESTS

Pulmonary function tests (PFTs), including spirometry, flow volume loop, and resistance measurements may reveal early findings of airway involvement in asymptomatic patients. An abnormal contour to the flow volume loop may be seen in patients with suspected central airway obstruction before any abnormal findings on spirometry.[13]

Clinically, pulmonary involvement of RP manifests with airway obstruction and significant reduction in exercise capacity, (**Fig. 2**) all well demonstrated with standard testing. There is no involvement of the pulmonary vasculature, however. Ventilation and perfusion remain well matched, and diffusion capacity, gas exchange, alveolar–arterial oxygen tension difference, calculated physiologic shunt, and dead space are usually normal.[14]

The elastic recoil forces are also generally normal. Therefore, the flow limitation is usually a result of pure airway obstruction, which is related to different mechanisms based on the stage of disease. In the early stages, inflammatory edema causes airway narrowing, which then progresses to destruction of the airway cartilage causing dynamic collapse followed by the formation of fibrosing contraction in the late stages.

There are three patterns of airway obstruction in RP patients with airway involvement: (1) fixed

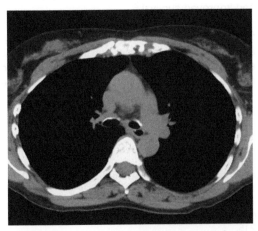

Fig. 1. Noncontrast chest computed tomography scan representing anterior tracheal wall calcification in a 46-year-old patient with relapsing polychondritis.

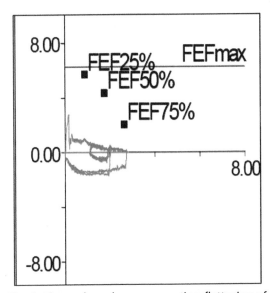

Fig. 2. Flow volume loop representing flattening of the expiratory and inspiratory limbs in a 40-year-old patient with early stages of relapsing polychondritis and no respiratory symptoms.

obstruction, (2) dynamic or variable extrathoracic obstruction, and (3) dynamic or variable intrathoracic obstruction.[15] Staats and colleagues[16] reported that the fixed obstruction pattern is the most commonly seen type in RP.

Reduction in maximal ventilatory ventilation (MVV) is seen in RP and is related mainly to a reduction in maximal expiratory flow. If severe enough, this may lead to a compromise in ventilation and eventual hypercapnia. Hypoxemia is less affected during the course of disease as described by Gibson and Davis,[14] where blood gases checked at baseline were normal and only revealed a nonsignificant reduction of PaO_2 with exercise as opposed to a significant rise of $PaCO_2$ indicating alveolar hypoventilation.

RADIOLOGY

Computed tomography (CT) abnormalities including malacia and air trapping during dynamic expiration are found in most RP patients with airway disease and may represent the only findings identified.

In a retrospective review by Lee and colleagues[8] to assess the prevalence of CT airway abnormalities, 8 of 18 patients (44%) had morphologic abnormalities seen on inspiratory CT, including airway wall thickening sparing the posterior membranous wall, airway wall calcification sparing the posterior membranous wall (see **Fig. 1**), and airway stenosis.

On dynamic expiratory CT scans, 17 of 18 patients had abnormalities including air trapping and airway malacia. The eight patients with CT abnormalities on inspiration were all found to have expiratory CT abnormalities also. The authors concluded that most patients with relapsing polychondritis with suspected airway involvement, have evidence of expiratory CT abnormalities, whereas abnormalities may be seen less than with inspiratory CT. Dynamic CT imaging should be a routine standard of evaluation of RP patients who have suspected airway involvement given that many patients will have normal findings on CT during inspiration. The identification of early airway involvement will allow for early treatment and hopefully improved outcomes in this subset of RP patients with a generally poor prognosis.

Newer imaging protocols such as three-dimensional rendering will allow improved detection and description of areas of stenosis and narrowing (**Fig. 3**). Other imaging modalities have been described in the past including magnetic resonance imaging (MRI), positron emission tomography (PET) scan, and gallium scintigraphy. All have been in the setting of case reports and

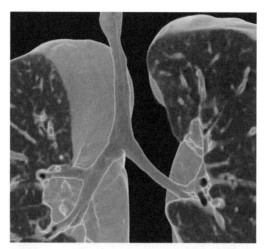

Fig. 3. Noncontrast chest computed tomography scan representing a focal tracheal stenosis in a 39-year-old patient with relapsing polychondritis.

have not been widely used for the work-up or follow-up of the disease.

BRONCHOSCOPY

Bronchoscopy is performed in RP patients who experience respiratory symptoms to assess for mucosal inflammation as a sign of active disease, define the severity of airway involvement, and allow for dynamic assessment of potential airway collapse. It should be performed cautiously because of the possibility of increased morbidity and mortality from anesthesia as well as the morbidity and mortality of the actual procedure itself including acute flare of disease leading to supraglottic or airway edema, bronchospasm, bleeding, respiratory failure, or death.[13] Trained personnel with emergent airway management skills should be available to perform intubation or emergency tracheotomy if needed.[17]

The most common finding is TBM (**Fig. 4**), followed by subglottic stenosis (**Fig. 5**), followed by focal stenosis in the tracheobronchial tree as reported by Ernst and colleagues.[2] In this study, 31 patients with airway involvement from RP were reviewed; 14 patients had TBM. Eight patients had subglottic stenosis, and three had focal stenosis. Special attention also should be paid to vocal cord function and signs of mucosal airway inflammation (**Fig. 6**), which can be localized or more commonly appears generalized throughout the central airways.

PATHOLOGY

Biopsies should be considered during bronchoscopy if the cause of airway process is otherwise unclear,

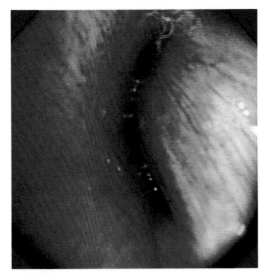

Fig. 4. Bronchoscopy image representing severe tracheobronchomalacia at the level of distal trachea in a 52-year-old patient with relapsing polychondritis who has been experiencing progressive dyspnea on exertion.

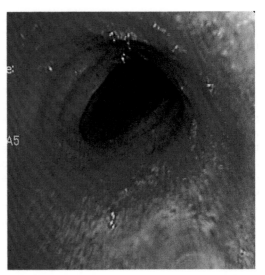

Fig. 6. Bronchoscopy image representing airway inflammation in a 43-year-old patient with relapsing polychondritis who has been experiencing cough and progressive dyspnea for months.

and when performed, they should include deep biopsies of the anterior cartilaginous tracheal wall.

There are no specific pathognomonic findings in specimens obtained from the airways or other parts of the lung for RP. Samples of the cartilage may reveal signs of inflammation. The main reason to perform biopsies is the exclusion of alternative diagnoses, and they only should be performed if necessary, because biopsies of the tracheobronchial tree may also contribute to anatomic damage in the biopsied area.

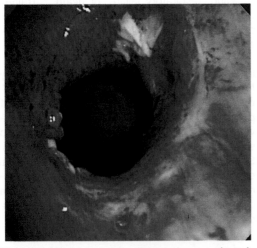

Fig. 5. Bronchoscopy image representing complex subglottic stenosis in a 39-year-old patient with relapsing polychondritis who has been experiencing progressive dyspnea on exertion, wheezing, and stridor.

TREATMENT OF AIRWAY DISEASE

Treatment of RP requires a multidisciplinary approach by rheumatologists, pulmonologists, and occasionally thoracic surgeons experienced in the management of RP and central airway obstruction, which is usually only available at specialized centers. Most of the treatments are based on case reports and series with no reported randomized controlled trials available due to the rarity of this disease. The main goal of treatment is to achieve symptom control and maintain airway stability and patency.

MEDICAL TREATMENT

Medications used for the treatment of airway manifestations are the same used for any other manifestation of the disease, and treatment usually is individualized based on the manifestations and severity of disease. In the authors' experience, corticosteroids alone are inferior in the control of airway symptoms when compared with combination therapy or antitumor necrosis factor (anti-TNF) drugs. However, there have not been any randomized controlled trials to determine what the best regimen is. Corticosteroids remain an important part of treatment, with doses up to 1 mg/kg/d depending on the severity of the disease. High-dose intravenous pulse methylprednisolone may be needed if oral therapy is not effective or the patient has acute airway obstruction.[18] Corticosteroids help resolve the acute chondritis episodes and decrease the severity, duration, and frequency of attacks including airway symptoms. Most patients will require long-term therapy up to months or even years.

Many steroid-sparing agents have been used including azathioprine, cyclophosphamide, methotrexate, dapsone, and cyclosporine. There are no data to compare these agents with each other to determine which has a greater benefit. Methotrexate, however, has been reported in one case series by Trentham and Le[1] to reduce the daily dose of prednisone by almost fourfold in patients with an average weekly methotrexate dose of 17.5 mg.

These medications have been administered individually as well as in combination for varying periods of time, and it may take few weeks for effects to be noticed.

ENDOSCOPIC INTERVENTIONS

There are a variety of interventions that are available for the symptomatic RP patient with airway disease including endobronchial laser therapy, argon plasma coagulation (APC), balloon dilation, airway stenting, and tracheotomy.

These interventions are usually reserved for:

Patients with significant findings on bronchoscopy that are associated with a higher risk for morbidity and mortality such as central airway obstruction, severe diffuse or focal stenosis

Patients who have failed medical therapy

Patients requiring a bridging intervention while awaiting for medical therapy to take its effects.

The decision for single intervention versus combination of interventions or therapies should be based on expert opinion on what works best for an individual patient, the availability of these treatments and interventions, and the ability to manage any complications that might arise from such treatments.

From the authors' experience, patients who benefit the most from early intervention are the ones with severe focal stenosis or diffuse TBM. Re-establishing airway patency is evidenced by clinical improvement and improvement in PFTs, shape of the flow volume loop, and appearance on bronchoscopy.

Patients, referring physicians, and interventionalists should be aware of the possible complications associated with each intervention such as acute flare of disease, life-threatening airway obstruction or perforation during or after the procedure, stent occlusion or migration, increased mucus secretions, bronchospasm, and worsening cough.

Metallic stents have been placed in the past,[19,20] until that practice changed following the US Food and Drug Administration's (FDA) warning regarding the use of metallic stents in benign diseases.[21] Stents may cause worsening of airway inflammation and erosion. They can migrate or fracture, causing acute airway obstruction.

Silicone stents are the gold standard for nonmalignant airway stenosis and are also considered when tracheobronchomalacia is the predominant feature. Stenting is considered especially in patients who are limited due to dyspnea and are found on dynamic bronchoscopy and CT to have a severe degree of TBM (**Fig. 7**). In most cases, they are placed as a trial to assess for symptomatic improvement and select patients who might benefit from more extensive surgical procedures such as tracheobronchoplasty, which involves supporting the posterior membranous wall with mesh. This surgery has been performed in a subset of RP patient with diffuse TBM at very few specialized centers, but no long- term outcome data are available at this time.

Other endobronchial therapies such as laser therapy or APC are considered in patients who have focal symptomatic stenosis as soon as the diagnosis is made to ensure airway patency.

Tracheotomy may be necessary in cases of severe subglottic stenosis given the critical nature of this finding and the high likelihood of loosing the airway and death.[19]

Noninvasive mechanical ventilation via a continuous positive airway pressure or bi-level positive airway pressure mask or directly through

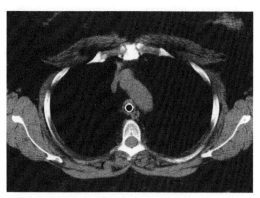

Fig. 7. Noncontrast chest computed tomography scan representing a silicone stent seen with its tracheal limb maintaining patency of the airway in a 43-year-old patient with relapsing polychondritis and severe tracheobronchomalacia.

a tracheotomy tube has been applied in a subset of RP patients with tracheal collapse.

PROGNOSIS

Availability of new interventional treatment modalities has led to the improvement of morbidity and mortality, although RP in general and airway manifestations of the disease in particular, continue to carry a substantial morbidity and mortality. RP patients treated with immunosuppressive agents are also at high risk of infections and sepsis, which might lead to death. Survival rates for 10 years are close to 55% in one series,[3] but these numbers vary considerably in different series and are likely due to the level of disease extent based on different institutions. In one of the largest case series reported so far,[2] which included 31 patients, there was only one death reported over the 4-year period of data analysis.

SUMMARY

Knowledge about the pulmonary manifestations of RP and its management continues to evolve. Further studies and long-term follow-up are required to assess the best medical and interventional treatment options and outcomes of these patients.

REFERENCES

1. Trentham DE, Le CH. Relapsing polychondritis. Ann Intern Med 1998;129(2):114–22.
2. Ernst A, Rafeq S, Boiselle P, et al. Relapsing polychondritis and airway involvement. Chest 2009; 135:1024–30.
3. Michet CJ, McKenna CH, Luthra HS, et al. Relapsing polychondritis: survival and predictive role of early disease manifestations. Ann Intern Med 1986;104:74–8.
4. McAdam LP, O'Hanlan MA, Bluestone R, et al. Relapsing polychondritis: prospective study of 23 patients and a review of the literature. Medicine 1976;55:193–215.
5. Thould AK, Stansfeld AG, Wykeham Balme H. Chronic atrophic perichondritis. Ann Rheum Dis 1965;24(6):563–8.
6. Dolan DL, Lemmon GB Jr, Teitelbaum SL. Relapsing polychondritis, analytical literature review and studies on pathogenesis. Am J Med 1966;41(2):285–99.
7. Mohsenifar Z, Tashkin DP, Carson SA, et al. Pulmonary function in patients with relapsing polychondritis. Chest 1982;81:711–7.
8. Lee KS, Ernst A, Trentham D, et al. Prevalence of functional airway abnormalities in relapsing polychondritis. Radiology 2006;240:565–73.
9. Foidart JM, Abe S, Martin GR, et al. Antibodies to type II collagen in relapsing polychondritis. N Engl J Med 1978;929:1203–7.
10. Giroux L, Paquin F, Guerard-Desjardins MJ, et al. Relapsing polychondritis: an autoimmune disease. Semin Arthritis Rheum 1983;13:182–7.
11. Alsalemeh S, Mollenhauer J, Scheuplein F, et al. Preferential cellular and humoral immune reactivities to native and denatured collagen types IX and XI in a patient with fatal relapsing polychondritis. J Rheumatol 1993;20:1419–24.
12. Handrock K, Gross WL. Relapsing polychondritis as a secondary phenomenon of primary systemic vasculitis [letter; comment]. Ann Rheum Dis 1993; 52(12):895–7.
13. Ernst A, Feller-Kopman D, Becker H, et al. Central airway obstruction. Am J Respir Crit Care Med 2004;169:1278–97.
14. Gibson GJ, Davis P. Respiratory complications of relapsing polychondritis. Thorax 1974;29:726–31.
15. Miller RD, Hyatt RE. Evaluation of obstructing lesions of the trachea and larynx by flow volume loops. Am Rev Respir Dis 1986;133:1120–3.
16. Staats B, Utz J, Michet C. Relapsing Polychondritis. Semin Respir Crit Care Med 2002;23(2):145–54.
17. Self J, Hammarsten JF, Lyne B, et al. Relapsing Polychondritis. Arch Intern Med 1967;120:109–12.
18. Lipnick RN, Fink CW. Acute airway obstruction in relapsing polychondritis: treatment with pulse methylprednisolone. J Rheumatol 1991;18:98–9.
19. Sarodia BD, Dasguta A, Mehta AC. Management of airway complications of relapsing polychondritis. Case reports and review of the literature. Chest 1999;116:1669–75.
20. Faul JL, Kee AT, Rizk NW. Endobronchial stenting for severe airway obstruction in relapsing polychondritis. Chest 1999;116:825–7.
21. US Food and Drug Administration. FDA public health notification: complications from metallic tracheal stents in patients with benign airway disorders. Washington, DC: US Food and Drug Administration; 2005.

The Pulmonary Vasculitides

Stephen K. Frankel, MD[a,b,*], David Jayne, MBBchir, MD[c]

KEYWORDS

- Pulmonary vasculitides • Wegener granulomatosis
- Microscopic polyangitiis • Churg-Strauss vasculitis

The vasculitides are a group of disorders characterized by cellular infiltration, inflammation, and necrosis of the walls of blood vessels, or the histopathologic finding of vasculitis. These disorders occur as primary, presumed autoimmune, syndromes or occur secondary to another process such as infection, malignancy, drug reaction, or connective tissue disease (**Table 1**). Primary vasculitides are subgrouped according to the predominant involvement of small, medium, or large vessels, and the small or microscopic group is further divided into those syndromes associated with antineutrophil cytoplasmic antibody (ANCA) and those associated with immune-complex deposition (see **Table 1**). The ANCA-associated vasculitides (AAV) of Wegener granulomatosis (WG), microscopic polyangitiis (MPA), and CSV (CSV) are known to preferentially attack the lungs and they are the main focus of this review. However, secondary vasculitis associated with systemic lupus erythematosus and immune-complex vasculitides, such as Goodpasture syndrome, also known as antiglomerular basement membrane (GBM) disease, also have a predilection for the lungs. In addition, the large-vessel vasculitides can affect the respiratory system, although these disorders primarily affect the pulmonary vasculature and large branches of the aorta rather than the pulmonary parenchyma itself.

EPIDEMIOLOGY

The cause of primary systemic vasculitis is not understood but there is evidence for a genetic contribution from the increased frequency in relatives of affected individuals and from candidate gene associations with HLA and other immune response genes. Although environmental factors are likely to be important, only silica exposure has been convincingly shown to increase the frequency of vasculitis. The incidence of AAV is 15 to 20/million/y with prevalence rates ranging from 90 to more than 300/million. Both WG and CSV are more common in northern latitudes in the Northern Hemisphere and southern latitudes in the Southern Hemisphere, which has been associated with ultraviolet light exposure.[1] The average age of onset of WG is 55 to 65 years; MPA increases in frequency in older age groups. Both syndromes occur but are rare in children. The frequency of MPA is unaffected by latitude. Japanese and Chinese ethnic populations have a different distribution of vasculitis with MPA, associated with myeloperoxidase (MPO)-ANCA, being much more common than the other ANCA vasculitides.[2]

DIAGNOSIS

The diagnosis of vasculitis challenges even the most experienced of clinicians. This is because

[a] Interstitial Lung Disease Program, Critical Care & Hospital Medicine, National Jewish Health, 1400 Jackson Street, G-012, Denver, CO 80206, USA
[b] Division of Pulmonary Sciences & Critical Care Medicine, Anschutz Medical Campus, University of Colorado School of Medicine, 1645 Ursula Street, Aurora, CO 80045, USA
[c] Vasculitis and Lupus Clinic, Addenbrooke's Hospital, Cambridge University Hospitals, NHS Foundation Trust, Hills Road, Cambridge CB2 0QQ, UK
* Corresponding author. Interstitial Lung Disease Program, Critical Care & Hospital Medicine, National Jewish Health, 1400 Jackson Street, G-012, Denver, CO 80206.
E-mail address: frankels@NJHealth.org

Clin Chest Med 31 (2010) 519–536
doi:10.1016/j.ccm.2010.04.005

Table 1 The vasculitides	
Primary vasculitis	Small-vessel vasculitis Wegener granulomatosis Microscopic polyangiitis Churg-Strauss vasculitis Medium-vessel vasculitis Polyarteritis nodosa Kawasaki disease Larger-vessel vasculitis Takayasu arteritis Giant cell arteritis
Immune complex– mediated vasculitis	Goodpasture syndrome Henoch-Schönlein purpura
Secondary vasculitis	Infection Malignancy (paraneoplastic) Drug-induced vasculitis Connective tissue diseases Antiphospholipid antibody syndrome Inflammatory bowel disease Essential cryoglobulinemia

Data from Frankel SK, Cosgrove GP, Brown KK. Small vessel vasculitis of the lung. Chron Respir Dis 2005;2:75; Frankel SK, Cosgrove GP, Fischer A, et al. Update in the diagnosis and management of pulmonary vasculitis. Chest 2006;129:452; Jennette JC, Falk, RJ. Small-vessel vasculitis. N Engl J Med 1997;337:1512; Jennette JC, Falk R, Andrassay K, et al. Nomenclature of systemic vasculitides. Arthritis Rheum 1990;37:187.

of (1) the rarity of the vasculitides (AAV incidence 20/million/y)[3–5] relative to competing diagnostic considerations such as infection, malignancy, thromboembolic disease, and primary rheumatologic disorders/connective tissue diseases; (2) the multitude of manifestations that an individual entity may present with; and (3) the absence of a single diagnostic test or criterion by which to make the diagnosis.

Within the accepted nomenclature systems for vasculitis, the 1990 American College of Rheumatology (ACR) classification criteria[6–8] and the 1994 Chapel Hill consensus definitions[9] were developed to assist in the classification of these conditions (**Table 2**). However, these criteria were never intended to be used as diagnostic criteria, and perform poorly when used as such.[10] The diagnosis of vasculitis requires the clinician to integrate clinical, radiologic, laboratory, and often histopathologic data (clinical-radiologic-pathologic correlation) and make a determination that the evidence collectively does or does not support a diagnosis of vasculitis. The practicing clinician must know when to suspect vasculitis and be familiar with the common presentations and manifestations of the individual vasculitides.

Simply raising vasculitis as a diagnostic consideration often represents a major step toward making the diagnosis. Clinical scenarios that should prompt consideration of small-vessel vasculitis include (1) alveolar hemorrhage, (2) the presence of pulmonary nodules and/or cavities, especially once malignancy and infection have been excluded, (3) glomerulonephritis (**Fig. 1**), (4) tracheal or subglottic stenosis (**Fig. 2**), (5) destructive/ulcerating upper airway disease, or longstanding refractory otitis or sinusitis, (6) mononeuritis multiplex or unexplained peripheral neuropathy, (7) retroorbital mass, (8) palpable purpura (**Fig. 3**) or other evidence of cutaneous vasculitis, and (9) maturity onset asthma with or without eosinophilia.[11,12] An interesting study by Mandl and colleagues[13] in 2002 found that among the most common presenting symptoms that prompted evaluation of autoantibody testing for vasculitis in a teaching hospital setting were dyspnea, fever of unknown origin, renal failure, and cough, but if autoantibody testing for small-vessel vasculitis was restricted to those patients who had one or more of these findings, the positive predictive value of the test improved with no loss in sensitivity and a reduction in the rate of false-positive tests.

Of particular interest to the chest physician is the evaluation and management of diffuse alveolar hemorrhage (DAH). The classic clinical triad that suggests alveolar hemorrhage of hemoptysis, anemia, and diffuse alveolar infiltrates is relatively insensitive, and indeed, up to one-third of patients lack the cardinal symptom of hemoptysis at time of presentation.[14] Therefore, any patient who presents with unexplained bilateral alveolar infiltrates may potentially have alveolar hemorrhage. Other indicators of lung hemorrhage are anemia with a recent reduction in hemoglobin of 1 to 2 g/dL, and an increase in the diffusing capacity of carbon monoxide.

A diagnosis of DAH is made at the time of bronchoscopy when with the bronchoscope in wedge position, bronchoalveolar lavage reveals increasingly hemorrhagic returns with serial lavage, or at a minimum, a hemorrhagic return that does not clear with serial lavage (**Fig. 4**). Although the presence of hemorrhage may correlate pathologically with (1) capillaritis, (2) bland hemorrhage (eg, coagulopathy, mitral stenosis), or (3) diffuse alveolar damage with hemorrhage (adult respiratory distress syndrome or acute exacerbation of fibrotic lung disease), the presence of DAH is often highly suggestive of a vasculitis or related disorder.

Table 2
Chapel Hill consensus definitions and ACR classification criteria

	ACR Criteria	Chapel Hill Definition
WG	Nasal or oral inflammation Abnormal chest radiograph Active urinary sediment Granulomatous inflammation on biopsy ≥2 of 4 criteria to meet classification as WG	Granulomatous inflammation involving the respiratory tract, and necrotizing vasculitis affecting small- to medium-sized vessels (eg, capillaries, venules, arterioles, and arteries)
CSV	Asthma Eosinophilia Mono- or polyneuropathy Pulmonary infiltrates Paranasal sinus abnormality Extravascular eosinophils ≥4 criteria to meet classification as CSV	Eosinophil-rich and granulomatous inflammation involving the respiratory tract, necrotizing vasculitis affecting small to medium sized vessels, and associated with asthma and eosinophilia
MPA	No separate classification from classic polyarteritis nodosa	Necrotizing vasculitis with few or no immune deposits, affecting small vessels (eg, capillaries, venules, or arterioles)

Data from Jennette JC, Falk RJ, Andrassy K, et al. Nomenclature of systemic vasculitides. Proposal of an international consensus conference. Arthritis Rheum 1994;37:187; Leavitt RY, Fauci AS, Bloch DA, et al. The American College of Rheumatology 1990 criteria for the classification of Wegener's granulomatosis. Arthritis Rheum 1990;33:1101; Lightfoot RW, Michel BA, Bloch DA, et al. The American College of Rheumatology 1990 criteria for the classification of polyarteritis nodosa. Arthritis Rheum 1990;33:1088; Masi AT, Hunder GG, Lie JT, et al. The American College of Rheumatology 1990 criteria for the classification of Churg-Strauss syndrome (allergic granulomatosis and angiitis). Arthritis Rheum 1990;33:1094.

The differential diagnosis for a histopathologic lesion of pulmonary capillaritis includes all of the small-vessel vasculitides (WG and MPA most commonly), Goodpasture syndrome, the primary connective tissue diseases (most commonly systemic lupus erythematosus [SLE]) drug-induced capillaritis (eg, propylthiouracil), DAH associated with bone marrow transplantation, primary antiphospholipid antibody syndrome, cryoglobulinemia, poststreptococcal disease, and idiopathic pauci-immune pulmonary capillaritis. The concomitant finding of glomerulonephritis is diagnostic of a pulmonary-renal syndrome and narrows the differential diagnosis to small-vessel vasculitis, SLE, Goodpasture syndrome, cryoglobulinemia, and poststreptococcal disease.

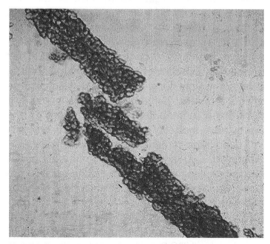

Fig. 1. Photomicrograph of a red cell cast in a patient with glomerulonephritis secondary to Wegener granulomatosis.

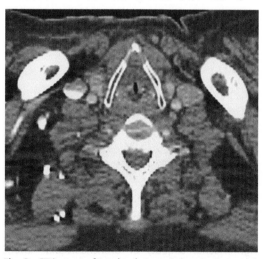

Fig. 2. CT image of tracheal stenosis in a patient with Wegener granulomatosis.

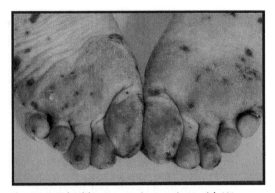

Fig. 3. A palpable purpura in a patient with Wegener granulomatosis.

Medium-vessel vasculitides such as polyarteritis nodosa and Kawasaki disease (KD) in general spare the lungs, but rare cases of DAH have been associated with polyarteritis nodosa (PAN). The Chapel Hill Criteria maintain that the co-occurrence of a small-vessel vasculitis (eg, capillaritis) with features of PAN should lead to a diagnosis of MPA.

Large-vessel vasculitides such as Takayasu arteritis (TA) may present with pulmonary artery aneurysms or stenoses that, in general, are identified via radiographic imaging obtained for the evaluation of hemoptysis, cough, chest discomfort, pulmonary hypertension, or as incidental findings. Pulmonary artery involvement occurs in approximately 50% of cases of TA[15,16] and 1% to 8% of patient's with Behcet disease.[17] Aortic or cardiac involvement may produce chest pain or shortness of breath relating to heart failure or valvular heart disease. Similarly, these patients may present in a critical care setting with aortic dissection,

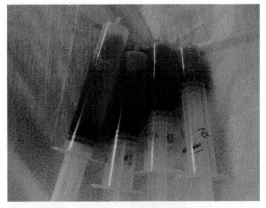

Fig. 4. Serial aliquots of bronchoalveolar lavage demonstrating a hemorrhage return that does not clear with serial lavage diagnostic for DAH.

rupture, acute valvular incompetence, myocardial infarction, pulmonary artery rupture, or stroke.

THE INDIVIDUAL VASCULITIDES

The clinical presentation of these syndromes varies depending on the size of the affected vessels, the target organs involved, and the amount of inflammation and damage associated with the disease process. Limited or incomplete presentations occur and some presentations have overlapping features of more than 1 syndrome.

WG

WG is the most common of the small-vessel AAVs, and classically is characterized by the presence of (1) upper respiratory tract disease, (2) lower respiratory tract disease, and (3) renal disease (glomerulonephritis). Upper and lower respiratory tract involvement are the most common manifestations of WG, especially at the time of onset of the disease, occurring in 75% to 95% of all patients.[18–22] Upper airway disease may manifest as epistaxis, rhinitis, sinusitis, deforming or ulcerating upper airway lesions, otitis, otalgia, tinnitus, hearing loss, laryngeal disease, subglottic stenosis, and/or tracheal stenosis. Lower respiratory disease may manifest as cough, chest pain, shortness of breath, hemoptysis, endobronchial lesions, pulmonary infiltrates, nodules, or cavities. Subglottic, tracheal, and endobronchial disease, usually absent at the time of diagnosis, often develops after a delay of months or years. Renal involvement is present in 40% of patients at the time of initial presentation but develops in 70% to 80% of patients over the course of the disease. Other common target organs include the skin (45%–60%), eyes (25%–50%), peripheral nervous system (10%–30%), musculoskeletal system (30%–70%), and heart (5%–15%).[18–22] Constitutional symptoms are common, and at least half of patients complain of fatigue malaise, anorexia, fever, or weight loss. Although cardiac disease affects a modest percentage of patients, cardiac involvement contributes disproportionally to the attributable mortality of WG, and patients with WG need to be screened carefully with electrocardiogram (ECG) and echocardiogram for occult cardiac disease including conduction delays, endomyocarditis/cardiomyopathy, valvular disease, and pericardial disease.

Chest radiographs are abnormal in most patients with WG, and high resolution computed tomography (HRCT) scanning of the chest shows 1 or more abnormalities in nearly all patients. No one pattern is suggestive of WG, and patients may present with interstitial, alveolar or mixed infiltrates, nodules, or cavities (**Fig. 5**).[23,24] The nodules or cavities may be solitary or multiple, and the infiltrates may be bilateral or unilateral, heterogeneous or homogeneous, fleeting or persistent. The presence of pulmonary nodules and cavities in patients in whom infection and malignancy have been convincingly ruled out may well represent WG (**Fig. 6**).

Pathologically, WG is characterized by the triad of a necrotizing, small- and medium-vessel vasculitis, granulomatous inflammation (often in a geographic pattern).[25] A study of surgical lung biopsy specimens by Travis and colleagues[26] found that vascular changes (ie, vasculitis) were found in 94% of biopsies, parenchymal necrosis in 84%, giant cells in 79%, microabscesses in 69%, and poorly formed granulomas in 59% (**Fig. 7**).

MPA

MPA is characterized by a prolonged prodrome of profound constitutional symptoms (fatigue, malaise, anorexia, fever, night sweats, arthralgias, myalgias, and weight loss) and glomerulonephritis.[27–31]

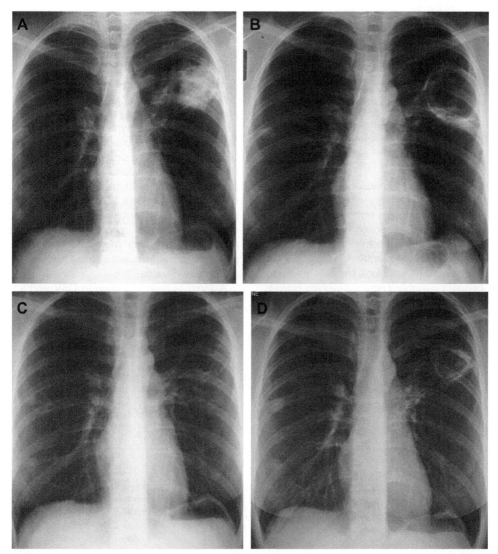

Fig. 5. Serial chest radiographs in a 21-year old patient with Wegener granulomatosis. (*A*) At the time of diagnosis, the patient had a cavitating opacity in the left upper zone. (*B*) Following 2 months of therapy, there remains a large, thin-walled residual cavity in the left upper lobe. (*C*) After achieving disease remission, there is complete resolution of the cavity. (*D*) One year later, the patient suffers a disease relapse with recurrent left upper lobe cavity and enlarging right-sided nodules.

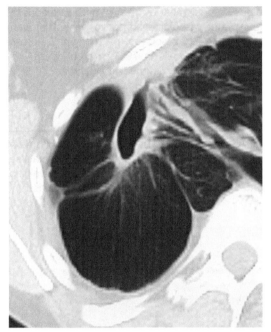

Fig. 6. HRCT image of a large pulmonary cavity secondary to Wegener granulomatosis.

A rapidly progressive glomerulonephritis is nearly universal in MPA. Pulmonary involvement occurs in only a minority of patients but manifests as alveolar hemorrhage. Thus, although only 10% to 30% of patients with MPA have pulmonary involvement, that involvement is frequently life-threatening.[32] Other target end organs include the skin, musculoskeletal system, peripheral nervous system, bowels, heart, eyes, and upper airways. Rare cases of MPA can occur without renal involvement and cause diagnostic difficulty especially if ANCA testing is negative. Overlapping presentations with polyarteritis nodosa also occur.

Chest imaging may be normal or may show heterogeneous, patchy, bilateral ground-glass abnormalities suggestive of alveolar hemorrhage in approximately one-quarter of patients.

Histopathology shows a small-vessel necrotizing vasculitis with a mixed inflammatory cell infiltrate.[25] The absence of granulomas, giant cells, or prominent eosinophilia distinguishes MPA from the other AAVs.

CSV

Churg-Strauss syndrome or CSV is characterized by the clinical triad of (1) asthma, (2) eosinophilia, and (3) vasculitis. Because of the prominence of the eosinophilia and asthma in the disease presentation, CSV often enters the differential diagnosis with other entities characterized by eosinophilia or refractory asthma such as allergic bronchopulmonary mycosis, chronic, idiopathic, eosinophlic pneumonia, parasitic infections, steroid-dependent asthma, and hypereosinophilic syndrome. Lanham and colleagues[33] classically described 3 phases of CSV: (1) a prodromal phase of asthma, rhinitis, and sinusitis followed by (2) an eosinophilic phase that in turn is ultimately followed by (3) a vasculitic phase. A recent concept has emerged of 2 overlapping CSV subsets, one ANCA positive with more frequent renal involvement, and one ANCA negative with more pronounced eosinophilia and more frequent cardiac and more severe pulmonary disease.[34]

Asthma is near universal in CSV and although the severity and duration are highly variable, on average, asthma precedes the onset of the vasculitis by 7 to 8 years and is frequently

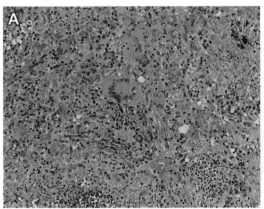
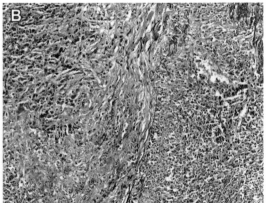

Fig. 7. Histopathologic specimen from a patient with Wegener granulomatosis. (*A*) Granulomatous inflammation with giant cell and microabscess formation; (*B*) vasculitis with disruption of the elastic lamina. (*Courtesy of* Dr Carlyne Cool, University of Colorado, CO.)

steroid-dependent.[35–37] Rhinitis, nasal polyposis, and sinusitis are also extremely common, but in contrast to WG, they are rarely ulcerating or destructive in CSV. Peripheral nervous system involvement (mononeuritis multiplex) and cutaneous involvement are common (50%–70% of cases).[29,38] Cardiac involvement occurs in 10% to 50% of patients and is responsible for 33% to 83% of CSV-related deaths.[39–43] Specifically, coronary arteritis and endomyocarditis/cardiomyopathy are common, life-threatening, and often unsuspected in patients with CSV. CSV may manifest in the heart as conduction delays, heart failure, myocardial infarction, valvular disease, pericardial disease, arrhythmias, nonspecific ECG abnormalities, or sudden death.

Chest radiographs are abnormal in 70% of patients with CSV, and HRCT of the chest shows significant findings in 90% of patients. The imaging abnormalities most commonly show patchy, bilateral, heterogeneous, ground-glass opacities that are frequently migratory but also may show air-trapping/hyperinflation, bronchial wall thickening and mosaicism of severe asthma, or interlobular septal thickening, nodules, effusions, or focal consolidation.[44–47]

Bronchoalveolar lavage can be of some use in the diagnosis of CSV if it shows eosinophilia (>25% eosinophils). The presence of eosinophil-rich infiltrates in the alveolar space can confirm the presence of eosinophilic pneumonia, which in turn is consistent with, but not diagnostic of, CSV. On the other hand, it is rare that transbronchial biopsies reveal true diagnostic histopathologic findings by which to definitively prove a diagnosis of CSV.[48,49] Histopathologic findings of CSV include a necrotizing small- to medium-vessel vasculitis, eosinophilic pneumonia (eosinophil-rich alveolar infiltrates), and extravascular granuloma formation.[9]

From a treatment perspective, the asthmatic/eosinophilic manifestations of CSV do not necessarily follow the same clinical trajectory as the vasculitic manifestations of the disease. Therefore, careful attention must be paid to the treatment of severe, often steroid-dependent asthma, and severe chronic, eosinophilic rhinosinusitis, and targeted therapies such as topical (inhaled and nasal) corticosteroids, long-acting bronchodilators, nasal saline irrigation, and allergen avoidance should be deployed.[50] This is especially true as corticosteroids are tapered, because cytotoxic steroid-sparing therapy is far more efficacious for the treatment of the vasculitic aspects of the disease than the eosinophillic aspects, whereas the corticosteroids are highly effective for both aspects. Some 30% to 40% of patients have persisting corticosteroid-dependent asthma despite control of vasculitic features. The converse of this point is underscored by concerns in the late 1990s that leukotriene antagonists might be promoting a biologic conversion of severe asthma to CSV.[51,52] It now seems that the introduction of leukotriene antagonists permitted a successful tapering of corticosteroids in patients with CSV whose rate-limiting disease manifestation was asthma, and that this corticosteroid taper led to the unmasking of vasculitic disease manifestations.[53–57] This same phenomenon of unmasking CSV has also been observed when the introduction of omalizumab (anti-IgE monoclonal antibody) therapy permitted withdrawal of oral corticosteroids.[58]

PAN

PAN is a necrotizing medium-vessel vasculitis that preferentially affects the renal and visceral beds. Coronary artery aneurysms may occur in up to half of patients,[59,60] and chest manifestations of PAN are most commonly a result of cardiac involvement. However, DAH, pleural effusion, and pulmonary infiltrates have all been reported in case reports.[61]

KD

KD is a medium-vessel vasculitis that almost exclusive affects children, and although KD in general spares the lungs, patients with KD may present with pulmonary symptoms (eg, shortness of breath) from the cardiac complications of KD such as coronary artery aneurysms, myocarditis, pericarditis, and valvular heart disease.

TA

As discussed earlier, TA is complicated by pulmonary vascular involvement in approximately half of cases and may manifest as pulmonary artery aneurysms, stenoses, occlusions, rupture, or pulmonary hypertension.[15,16,62–64] Aortic involvement, coronary arteritis and heart failure are also fairly common chest manifestations of TA.

Giant Cell Arteritis

Giant cell arteritis is a granulomatous vasculitis that preferential affects the aorta, the carotid arteries, and the major branches thereof. Most chest complications of giant cell arteritis relate to aortitis and include aortic dissection, rupture, aortic regurgitation, and heart failure. Pulmonary complications are rare, but include cough, hoarseness, pleural effusions, pulmonary artery stenosis, alveolar hemorrhage, and pulmonary nodules.[61]

VASCULITIS OCCURRING IN THE CONTEXT OF OTHER LUNG DISEASES

Chronic infections, such as those seen with infective endocarditis, bronchiectasis, or cystic fibrosis can induce a secondary vasculitis that may rarely be MPO-ANCA positive and/or include renal disease. Because immunosuppressive treatment exacerbates the underlying infection, it is important that infectious drives for vasculitis are identified. Tuberculosis is an important competing consideration within the differential diagnosis of vasculitis, especially when considering a diagnosis of WG, however immune stimulation caused by mycobacterial infection can also be a cause of a secondary vasculitis.

CLINICAL EVALUATION

Investigation of a patient with suspected vasculitis requires exclusion of mimics of vasculitic presentations, detection of causes of secondary vasculitic syndromes, determination of the extent and severity of disease, and identification of comorbidities.

History and Examination

The evaluation of the patient with suspected or known vasculitis begins with a thorough history and physical examination. Although often managed by subspecialists, the clinicians who care for patients with vasculitis are best served by being consummate internists. A careful review of systems and a physical examination is required to identify all potential manifestations of a given vasculitis and to direct further laboratory testing and imaging studies. Infection, malignancy, drug reactions, and thromboembolic disease may all present with a secondary vasculitis (especially a cutaneous leukocytoclastic vasculitis), and need to be either identified or convincingly ruled out before treating the patient with immunosuppressive agents. Other potential competing diagnostic possibilities commonly include connective tissue diseases, sarcoidosis, interstitial lung diseases, and poststreptococcal disease.

Laboratory Testing

Laboratory testing should be targeted toward assisting with the diagnosis of vasculitis, fully characterizing the disease manifestations of a patient who potentially or definitively has vasculitis, and/or monitoring the disease activity (and associated end-organ damage) in a patient with known vasculitis. Complete blood count, liver function testing, renal function testing, electrocardiogram, and inflammatory markers such as sedimentation rate and C-reactive protein are helpful. Connective tissue disease serologies (antinuclear antibodies, rheumatoid factor, anticyclic citrullinated peptide, antitopoisomerase (Scl-70), anti-SS-A/Ro and anti-SS-B/La), hepatitis serologies, antiphospholipid antibody testing, antiglomerular basement membrane antibodies, and cryoglobulins are all useful in addressing competing diagnostic possibilities.

ANCAs have a prominent role in the pathogenesis of the small-vessel, pauci-immune or ANCA-associated vasculitides of WG, MPA, and CSV. Neutrophil-specific autoantibodies were first identified in the late 1950s, but it was not until the 1980s that their role in small-vessel vasculitis became apparent.[65] Antineutrophil antibodies occur in 3 staining patterns: cytoplasmic or c-ANCA, perinuclear or p-ANCA, and most recently atypical or a-ANCA (**Fig. 8**).

The c-ANCA staining pattern tends to correspond with autoantibodies directed against proteinase-3 and is commonly seen in patients with WG. Specific enzyme-linked immunosorbent assays (ELISAs) that directly measure antiproteinase-3 (PR3) antibodies are now also widely available. c-ANCA or antiproteinase-3 ELISAs have an

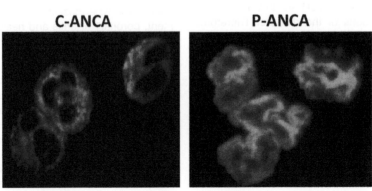

Fig. 8. Photomicrograph demonstrating the indirect immunofluorescence staining patterns associated with ANCAs.

85% to 90% sensitivity and 95% specificity for generalized active WG.[66–68] However, patients who have organ-limited disease or whose disease is in remission have much lower rates of ANCA positivity (60% and 40%, respectively).[69] False-positive c-ANCAs are relatively uncommon but may be seen in *Pseudomonas* sp infections and other autoimmune diseases, albeit rarely.[70]

p-ANCA corresponds predominantly with auto-antibodies against MPO but may also reflect auto-antibodies against elastase, lactoferrin, cathepsin, azurocidin, lysozyme, and bacterial permeability–increasing protein (BPI). p-ANCAs are frequently positive in patients with generalized active MPA and CSV, but are less sensitive and less specific than c-ANCA/PR3 are for WG. Other diseases that may be p-ANCA positive include rheumatoid arthritis, ulcerative colitis, autoimmune hepatitis, endocarditis, and other autoimmune disorders.[70] p-ANCA/anti-MPO ELISA testing has approximately 50% to 75% sensitivity for active MPA and only 35% to 50% sensitivity for CSV.[71–74]

The indirect immunofluorescence test (IIF, yielding a c-ANCA or p-ANCA if positive) is often used as a screening test because it tends to have a higher sensitivity but relatively low specificity. On the other hand, PR3-ANCA and MPO-ANCA ELISA testing have been shown to have greater diagnostic importance, as they are less sensitive, but more specific than IIF. Thus, a positive c-ANCA or p-ANCA requires confirmation by ELISA; however, it is preferable for all 3 assays to be performed when ANCA testing is first requested. Crucially, a negative ANCA is of no diagnostic value because ANCA is not always present in ANCA-associated vasculitis and ANCA is negative in other vasculitic subgroups. Ultimately, the diagnosis of vasculitis rests on the clinician integrating the clinical, laboratory, radiologic, and pathologic information, not the results of a single serology.

Several investigators have evaluated ANCA titers as a biomarker for predicting disease relapse. However, the test is insufficiently sensitive or specific to predict disease relapse, and as with the initial diagnosis, the diagnosis of a disease flare remains a clinical diagnosis.[75–78] Monitoring ANCA after diagnosis still has value as those remaining ANCA positive after induction therapy, or becoming positive again, have a higher relapse risk than those remaining ANCA negative and this information is of value when treatment withdrawal is being considered.[79]

Imaging

As with the clinical and laboratory evaluation, imaging in the patient with suspected vasculitis is directed toward making a diagnosis of vasculitis and/or delineating all the manifestations and end-organ involvement of a patient with known vasculitis. Thus, the clinician should have a low threshold for imaging organs that (1) are implicated by signs, symptoms, or laboratory abnormalities, (2) epidemiologically have a high prevalence of involvement in a specific vasculitis, or (3) have a high morbidity or mortality associated with their involvement. Commonly obtained studies include HRCT of the chest, CT of the sinuses, and echocardiogram. Other studies that may be indicated depending on clinical circumstances may include magnetic resonance imaging of the brain or heart, CT of the abdomen, or angiography.

Invasive Studies and Biopsy

Although it is sometime possible to make a diagnosis of vasculitis based on a characteristic clinical course, imaging and/or laboratory (autoantibody) findings, a histopathologic demonstration of vasculitis is frequently required to confirm the diagnosis. The choice of biopsy site depends on (1) the pattern of end-organ involvement, (2) the accessibility of the biopsy site, (3) the morbidity associated with biopsy at a specific site, and (4) the likelihood of obtaining diagnostic tissue.

The role of bronchoscopy in the diagnosis of vasculitis focuses on (1) the diagnosis of DAH (discussed earlier), (2) sampling the lower airways for complicating respiratory infections, and (3) assessing the large airways for endobronchial lesions such as those seen in WG. Lower respiratory tract sampling is frequently indicated in patients with new pulmonary signs or symptoms who are on immunosuppressive therapies, and who have underlying immune dysfunction and abnormal lung architecture. Hence, bronchoscopy with bronchoalveolar lavage is frequently part of the infectious workup of the patient with vasculitis. As outlined later, infection is a frequent cause of morbidity and mortality in vasculitis, and a drive to ongoing vasculitis, thus the need to aggressively exclude infection in a sick patient with vasculitis cannot be overemphasized. Airway lesions are relatively common in WG. Airway inspection, endobronchial biopsy, and/or virtual bronchoscopy may assist with diagnosis and management.[80] Transbronchial biopsies, however, are rarely useful in the diagnosis of pulmonary vasculitis, as diagnostic tissue is obtained in less than 20% of cases.[81]

Nerve conduction studies (NCV) are useful for the evaluation of peripheral nervous system involvement and can confirm the presence of the neuropathy; however, the findings on NCV are rarely diagnostic of the vasculitis itself.

Skin and sinus are easily accessible sites for sampling; however, the diagnostic yield is considerably less than it is for renal or surgical lung biopsies. A study by Devaney and colleagues[82] of 126 upper airway biopsy specimens form 70 patients found the characteristic combination of vasculitis, necrosis, and granulomatous inflammation together were seen in only 16% of specimens. Similarly, skin biopsies frequently showed a nonspecific leukocytoclastic vasculitis, but not the more specific features that would permit a definitive diagnosis. On the other hand, the additional information garnered from these sites may still confirm a diagnosis in a patient with a high pretest probability for vasculitis.

Percutaneous renal biopsy is commonly performed in patients with acute glomerulonephritis. Histopathologically, the finding of a segmental, necrotizing glomerulonephritis is consistent with a diagnosis of vasculitis, and immunofluorescence studies can then further refine the diagnosis. An absence of immune deposits on immunofluorescence is by definition a pauci-immune glomerulonephritis, and this is consistent with an ANCA-associated small-vessel vasculitis.[83–86] Linear IgG deposits, however, suggest Goodpasture syndrome; irregular, clumped IgG deposits are found in SLE, and IgA deposits are found in Henoch-Schönlein purpura.

Surgical lung biopsy is a high-yield diagnostic procedure and extremely valuable in making a diagnosis of pulmonary vasculitis. Although surgical lung biopsies require general endotracheal anesthesia and carry a higher risk of complications than any of the aforementioned procedures, it is still generally safe and well tolerated. Moreover, many of these biopsies are now done via video-assisted thorascopic surgery, which reduces the pain, recovery time, and risk of complications relative to an open lung biopsy. When performing a diagnostic biopsy, there must be close coordination between the surgeon, pathologist, and pulmonologist, as the sample must be processed not only using formalin fixation and conventional histopathology but also taken immediately for frozen sections for immunofluorescence and placed in saline for cultures.

TREATMENT

Treatment of vasculitis regularly involves the use of corticosteroids and cytotoxic agents, all of which have the potential for serious toxicity and adverse events. Therapy needs to be carefully titrated to disease activity because over treating carries the real risk of precipitating an adverse event, whereas under treating may permit a potentially life-threatening process to evolve and progress. Objective disease classification instruments have been developed to assist the clinician in categorizing disease severity so that therapies may be appropriately titrated to disease activity and the associated risk of end-organ injury and/or mortality. The most clinically useful of these remains the European Vasculitis Study Group (EUVAS) classification, which divides disease activity into 1 of 5 categories: (1) localized disease, (2) early generalized disease, (3) generalized, active disease, (4) severe/life-threatening disease, and (5) refractory disease (**Table 3**). More aggressive immunosuppressive regimens are used to induce a remission in patients with active disease, and in patients whose disease activity is of greater severity; less aggressive regimens with more favorable side-effect profiles are used for maintenance of remission.

Localized Disease

Localized disease refers to isolated upper airway disease and a complete absence of other end-organ involvement or constitutional symptoms. In general, patients in this category can be managed with topical therapy, corticosteroids, and/or a single moderate potency cytotoxic agent such as methotrexate or azathioprine. The role of trimethoprim/sulfamethoxazole as adjunctive therapy or even monotherapy for localized upper airways disease remains controversial.[87,88] In patient's who have progressive or refractory localized disease, escalation of therapy is generally recommended as outlined later.

Early Generalized Disease

Early generalized disease is defined by the presence of constitutional symptoms and active vasculitis but without any specific threat to organ function. Although cyclophosphamide-based regimens have been and continue to be used for early generalized disease, agents with less toxicity have been studied for induction of remission in this subgroup of patients. For example, the Non-Renal Alternative with Methotrexate (NORAM) trial compared methotrexate with cyclophosphamide for the induction of remission in early disease.[89] Although the time to remission (5 months vs 3 months) and relapse rate (74% vs 42%) favored cyclophosphamide, the methotrexate was better tolerated and had a more favorable side-effect profile than the cyclophosphamide. Although methotrexate is now considered an acceptable alternative to cyclophosphamide for early disease,

Table 3
EUVAS disease classification criteria and recommended first-line therapy options

Disease Severity	Constitutional Symptoms	Renal Function	Threatened Organ Function	Treatment Options for Induction
Limited	No	Serum creatinine <120 μmol/L (1.4 mg/dL)	No	Corticosteroids or methotrexate or azathioprine +/− topical therapies
Early generalized	Yes	Serum creatinine <120 μmol/L (1.4 mg/dL)	No	Cyclophosphamide + corticosteroids or methotrexate + corticosteroids (mycophenolate + corticosteroids is currently under investigation)
Active generalized	Yes	Serum creatinine <500 μmol/L (5.7 mg/dL)	Yes	Cyclophosphamide + corticosteroids
Severe	Yes	Serum creatinine >500 μmol/L (5.7 mg/dL)	Yes	Cyclophosphamide + corticosteroids + plasma exchange
Refractory	Yes	Any	Yes	Consider investigational or compassionate use agents (eg, rituximab)
Remission	No	Serum creatinine <120 μmol/L (1.4 mg/dL)	No	Azathioprine +/− low-dose corticosteroids Mycophenolate +/− low-dose corticosteroids Leflunomide +/− low-dose corticosteroids

there is considerable interest in mycophenolate mofetil, and to a lesser extent, azathioprine, as moderate potency alternatives to either cyclophosphamide or methotrexate in this group of patients. In particular, the EUVAS sponsored Randomized Clinical Trial of Mycophenolate Mofetil Versus Cyclophosphamide for Remission Induction in ANCA Associated Vasculitis (MYCYC) trial comparing mycophenolate mofetil with cyclophosphamide for the induction of remission in AAV is currently underway and should better inform on this question when complete.

Generalized Active Disease

Generalized active disease is defined by the presence of constitutional symptoms and threatened organ function caused by vasculitic activity. Cyclophosphamide plus oral corticosteroids have represented first-line therapy for generalized active disease since the 1980s and remains so today. Although patients were traditionally treated with daily oral cyclophosphamide, recent data suggest that intermittent intravenous cyclophosphamide therapy may offer equally efficacious therapy with a more favorable side-effect profile.[90] In the Daily Oral Versus Pulse Cyclophosphamide

for Renal Vasculitis (CYCLOPS) trial, 149 patients with newly diagnosed generalized active AAV were randomized to pulse intravenous cyclophosphamide (15 mg/kg every 2–3 weeks) or daily oral cyclophosphamide (2 mg/kg/d) plus prednisolone.[91] No difference in time to remission or the proportion of patients who achieved remission (88.1% vs 87.7% at 9 months) was identified, however, the pulse group had a lower rate of leukopenia and received a lower total cumulative dosage of cyclophosphamide compared with the oral therapy group.

Severe Disease

Severe disease is defined by the threat of immediate organ failure and/or death. Most commonly, this manifests as rapidly progressive glomerulonephritis and renal failure (creatinine >5.7 mg/dL) or alveolar hemorrhage associated with respiratory failure; however, cardiomyopathy with heart failure, life-threatening arrhythmias, central nervous system disease, and gastrointestinal disease with bowel ischemia or life-threatening hemorrhage may also require maximal therapy on an urgent basis. At present, the combination of corticosteroids, plasma exchange, and cyclophosphamide is recommended for the treatment of severe disease. The addition of plasma exchange is supported by the Randomized Trial of Plasma Exchange or High-Dosage Methylprednisolone as Adjunctive Therapy for Severe Renal Vasculitis (MEPEX) study.[92] In this trial of 137 patients with a new diagnosis of AAV and a serum creatinine level greater than 500 μmol/L (5.8 mg/dL), all patients received standard therapy with oral cyclophosphamide and oral prednisolone and were then randomized to either 7 plasma exchanges or 3000 mg of intravenous methylprednisolone. At 3 months, 69% of patients treated with plasma exchange plus were alive and independent of dialysis compared with only 49% in the high-dose intravenous methylprednisolone group. The extrapolation of these data to other life-threatening manifestations of vasculitis is supported by a 20-patient case series that showed the efficacy of this treatment strategy in alveolar hemorrhage.[93] The timing of initiation of cyclophosphamide administration in the critical care setting, especially in patients with concomitant infection, respiratory failure requiring mechanical ventilation, bowel ischemia/perforation, or attended by other serious complications does still remain controversial and subject to the discretion of the physicians caring for the patient.

Refractory Disease

By definition, refractory disease is disease that does not respond to conventional accepted therapy. Investigational therapies are considered for the treatment of refractory disease.

Recent data evaluating rituximab, a monoclonal antibody targeted against the CD20 antigen that is expressed B cell precursors, approved for use in B cell lymphoma and rheumatoid arthritis, are encouraging. Several small case series have found rituximab to be effective at inducing disease remission in patients who were either refractory to or intolerant of cyclophosphamide.[94–97] A larger, multicenter, retrospective, cohort study of 65 patients treated with varying regimens of rituximab reported a 98% response rate (75% complete remission, 23% partial remission) for relapsing or refractory AAV.[98] Although still experimental and the subject of 2 prospective randomized control trials, the Rituximab for ANCA-associated Vasculitis (RAVE) trial in the United States and the RITUXVAS trial in Europe, rituximab seems to be the leading candidate among the investigational therapies.

Other agents considered for the treatment of refractory disease have included antithymocyte globulin, alemtuzumab, deoxyspergualin, intravenous immunoglobulin, and the tumor necrosis factor (TNF) antagonist infliximab. Two small clinical trials with infliximab, a chimeric IgGk monoclonal antibody against soluble and membrane-bound TNF approved for use in rheumatoid arthritis, for the induction of remission in refractory disease have reported a positive signal.[99,100] However, this agent has yet to undergo more rigorous evaluation in prospective randomized controlled trial(s).

Antithymocyte globulin was the subject of the EUVAS Sponsored Anti-Thymocyte Globulin (ATG) Trial for Therapy of Refractory ANCA-Associated Vasculitis. In this study 15 patients received open-label ATG for refractory vasculitis, and although partial disease remission was induced in 9/15 and complete disease remission was induced in 4/15, 2 patients died after drug administration, 1 of pulmonary hemorrhage and another of infection. Serum sickness and nonfatal infections were also among the notable complications.

Intravenous immunoglobulin (IVIg) has also been tried on a compassionate use basis and studied in small clinical trials. Although IVIg may reduce disease activity acutely in patients who have persistent disease after standard therapy, this effect is generally short-lived and this intervention is most appropriate in acute situations where conventional therapy is contraindicated especially if severe infection is present.[101]

For patients with life-threatening, refractory alveolar hemorrhage, the administration of recombinant, activated factor VII has been reported in case reports to control otherwise uncontrollable alveolar hemorrhage.[102,103] Although this intervention has not been rigorously studied, the clinical experience is worth noting given the high mortality associated with hemorrhage refractory to IV steroids, plasmapheresis, and supportive care. Similarly, there are case reports of extracorporeal membrane oxygenation (ECMO) for refractory hypoxemia secondary to uncontrollable alveolar hemorrhage to buy time until other interventions have a chance to control the disease; however, ECMO in adult patients remains experimental and controversial.[104]

Tracheobronchial disease can be a refractory manifestation of pulmonary disease in WG. Progressive stenotic lesions can cause segmental, lobar, or lung collapse and/or acute stridor. Management of these complications of the disease requires a combination of direct techniques to enlarge the airway, including balloon dilatation, laser or cryotherapy, and local administration of corticosteroids or mitomicin C to reduce the risk of recurrence. Systemic therapy is then required to control Wegener activity as well as microbial surveillance and treatment of infection. Endobronchial stenting should be avoided if possible as it results in exuberant epithelial overgrowth and re-stenosis.

Maintenance of Remission

In principle, less aggressive cytotoxic/immunosuppressive regimens are used for maintenance of disease remission compared with the regimen(s) used for the induction of remission. The timing of this transition from induction therapy to maintenance therapy had been the subject of considerable debate until the results of the Cyclophosphamide versus Azathioprine for Remission in Generalized Vasculitis (CYCAZAREM) trial were published in 2003.[105] In this landmark trial, patients with generalized active vasculitis were treated with cyclophosphamide to induce disease remission. Patients were then either continued on cyclophosphamide to complete 12 months of empiric therapy before transitioning to the more moderate potency azathioprine, or were transitioned to azathioprine once a clinical remission was achieved. Clinical remission was achieved in 93% of patients and no differences in the relapse rate or disease activity scores were identified at 18 months between the 2 groups. Therefore, patients are now routinely transitioned to maintenance therapy once a clinical remission occurs.

With regard to specific agents, azathioprine remains the most commonly used first-line agent. However, mycophenolate mofetil, methotrexate, and leflunomide are also used for the maintenance of remission. The International Mycophenolate Mofetil to Reduce Outbreaks of Vasculitides (IMPROVE) trial directly compares mycophenolate mofetil with azathioprine head-to-head for the maintenance of remission in renal vasculitis and data collection for this trial is complete. However, the results of this study have not yet been published, but the reader is advised to review the data when they become available. A small trial comparing leflunomide with methotrexate showed superiority in the leflunomide arm,[106] but leflunomide has not been directly compared with azathioprine or mycophenolate mofetil. The addition of the soluble TNF receptor etanercept to maintenance immunosuppression and corticosteroids did not increase the proportion of patients with WG achieving a sustained remission in the Wegener's Granulomatosis Etanercept (WGET) study.[107]

Although corticosteroids are used as adjunctive therapy for the induction of remission, the role of corticosteroids as concomitant therapy for maintenance of remission is unclear. A meta-analysis of 7 randomized control trials and 3 observational studies found that continuation of low-dose corticosteroids (5–7.5 mg/d) may be associated with lower rates of relapse.[108] However, given the heterogeneity of the clinical populations and potential confounders, these data should be used to inform clinical trial design rather than informing clinical practice.

The question of when therapy can safely be discontinued also remains a significant controversy in the management of vasculitis. Again, the key question is whether the risks associated with pharmacologic therapy are greater or less than the risk of disease relapse in a patient who has been in remission for a prolonged period of time. Factors increasing the risk of relapse include treatment withdrawal, persistent ANCA positivity, a diagnosis of WG, respiratory tract disease, nasal carriage of *Staphylococcus aureus* and the absence of renal disease. The Randomized Trial of Prolonged Remission-Maintenance Therapy in Systemic Vasculitis (REMAIN) will compare 24 months of therapy with 48 months of therapy as regards disease relapse rates. Until the results of this trial are known, the optimal duration of maintenance therapy will remain the subject of debate.

LONGITUDINAL MONITORING AND DIAGNOSIS OF FLARES AND COMPLICATIONS

Commonly, vasculitis is characterized by a waxing and waning disease course, and two-thirds of patients with WG and one-third of patients with MPA will have one or more relapses of their underlying disease by 5 years. Careful longitudinal monitoring of disease activity to identify potential relapses as early as possible is recommended. In general, this includes a thorough history, physical examination, and review of systems directed toward known manifestations of vasculitis. Complete blood count, renal function, liver function, electrocardiogram, echocardiogram, imaging studies, and ANCA testing at regular intervals provide additional data regarding end-organ disease activity and/or damage. An important caveat to this assessment is the need to distinguish between disease activity and vasculitic damage, as disease activity requires escalation in therapy, whereas this same escalation is counterproductive if targeted to chronic irreversible damage. The Birmingham Vasculitis Activity Score is a validated objective instrument by which disease activity may be graded, but its use is generally limited to clinical investigation, although some vasculitis centers regularly use this instrument as part of clinical care.[109] The EUVAS grading is useful for guiding therapy but does not adjudicate which signs or symptoms constitute a relapse.

In addition to disease flares, new signs or symptoms in a patient with a history of vasculitis may also represent infection, drug toxicity, thromboembolic disease, or a disease process that is independent from the underlying vasculitis.

Infection has been shown to be a common cause of morbidity and mortality in patients with known vasculitis. Indeed, 13% to 26% of deaths in patients with vasculitis are caused by infectious complications.[27,110] Only the vasculitis itself is responsible for more attributable mortality than infection in patients with AAV. Patients with vasculitis, and especially patients maintained on high-dose corticosteroids and/or cytotoxic agents are at risk for atypical organisms (fungi, mycobacteria, *Pneumocystis jiroveci*, and *Nocardia* sp, as well as routine bacterial and viral agents) and atypical presentations of their infections. The practicing clinical must always remain hypervigilant in observing for and working up possible infectious complications. Damage to the respiratory tract caused by vasculitis results in impaired ciliary function and increased susceptibility to infection. A vicious circle of repeated infections driving vasculitic activity and further damage is then set up. Unfortunately immunosuppressive therapy only addresses the immune dysregulation and potentially exacerbates underlying infections. In consequence, disease control of relapsing respiratory tract vasculitis requires careful attention to bacterial, fungal, and viral colonization and infection, and may require prolonged antibiotic therapy.

Thromboembolic disease in the setting of AAV was under appreciated until the Wegener's Clinical Occurrence of Thrombosis (WeCLOT) investigators identified that the incidence of thromboembolic disease in patients with WG was 7.0 per 100 person-years, which is the same rate of venous thromboembolic (VTE) disease as for patients with a known prior history of VTE.[111] Although rates of VTE in other vasculitides remain unknown, clinicians should consider patients with AAV to be at higher risk for VTE.

Drug toxicity also remains a major cause of morbidity in patients with vasculitis and clinicians caring for these patients must routinely screen for adverse side effects potentially associated with a patient's course of therapy. Such screening should be a regular component of the vasculitis evaluation and includes laboratory and clinical evaluations. Implicit in this is a familiarity with the potential complications of the various pharmacologic agents used for the management of vasculitis.

SUMMARY

The vasculitides represent a spectrum of disorders characterized by inflammation and destruction of the blood vessel wall, and these entities commonly affect the respiratory system. Although challenging to diagnose and manage, recent advances in the treatment of these disorders has greatly improved the prognosis for patients with vasculitis, and with the advent of increasingly less toxic therapies, the future for these patients is brighter still.

REFERENCES

1. Gatenby PA, Lucas RM, Engelsen O, et al. Antineutrophil cytoplasmic antibody-associated vasculitides: could geographic patterns be explained by ambient ultraviolet radiation? Arthritis Rheum 2009;61:1417.
2. Watts RA, Scott DG, Jayne DR, et al. Renal vasculitis in Japan and the UK–are there differences in epidemiology and clinical phenotype? Nephrol Dial Transplant 2008;23:3928.
3. Cotch MF, Hoffman GS, Yerg DE, et al. The epidemiology of Wegener's granulomatosis: estimates of the five-year period prevalence, annual mortality, and geographic disease distribution from population based data sources. Arthritis Rheum 1996; 39:87.
4. Reinhold-Keller E, Herlyn K, Wagner-Bastmeyer R, et al. Stable incidence of primary systemic vasculitides over five years: results from the German Vasculitis Register. Arthritis Rheum 2005;53:93.
5. Watts RA, Lane SE, Bentham G, et al. Epidemiology of systemic vasculitis: a ten-year study in the United Kingdom. Arthritis Rheum 2000;43:414.
6. Leavitt RY, Fauci AS, Bloch DA, et al. The American College of Rheumatology 1990 criteria for the classification of Wegener's granulomatosis. Arthritis Rheum 1990;33:1101.
7. Lightfoot RW, Michel BA, Bloch DA, et al. The American College of Rheumatology 1990 criteria for the classification of polyarteritis nodosa. Arthritis Rheum 1990;33:1088.
8. Masi AT, Hunder GG, Lie JT, et al. The American College of Rheumatology 1990 criteria for the classification of Churg-Strauss syndrome (allergic granulomatosis and angiitis). Arthritis Rheum 1990;33:1094.
9. Jennette JC, Falk RJ, Andrassy K, et al. Nomenclature of systemic vasculitides. Proposal of an international consensus conference. Arthritis Rheum 1994;37:187.
10. Rao JK, Allen NB, Pincus T. Limitations of the 1990 American College of Rheumatology classification criteria in the diagnosis of vasculitis. Ann Intern Med 1998;129:345.
11. Hagen EC, Daha MR, Hermans J, et al. Diagnostic value of standardized assays for anti-neutrophil cytoplasmic antibodies in idiopathic systemic vasculitis. EC/BCR Project for ANCA Assay Standardization. Kidney Int 1998;53:743.

12. Savige J, Gillis D, Benson E, et al. International consensus statement on testing and reporting of antineutrophil cytoplasmic antibodies (ANCA). Am J Clin Pathol 1999;111:507.

13. Mandl LA, Solomon DH, Smith EL, et al. Using antineutrophil cytoplasmic antibody testing to diagnose vasculitis. Arch Intern Med 2002;162:1509.

14. Zamora MR, Warner ML, Tuder R, et al. Diffuse alveolar hemorrhage and systemic lupus erthematosus (SLE): clinical presentation, histology, survival and outcome. Medicine 1997;76:192.

15. Vanoli M, Castellani M, Bacchiani G, et al. Non-invasive assessment of pulmonary artery involvement in Takayasu's arteritis. Clin Exp Rheumatol 1999;17:215.

16. Yamada I, Shibuya H, Matsubara O, et al. Pulmonary artery disease in Takayasu's arteritis: angiographic findings. Am J Roentgenol 1992; 159:263.

17. Erkan F, Gul A, Tasali E. Pulmonary manifestations of Behcet's disease. Thorax 2001;56:572.

18. Anderson G, Coles ET, Crane M, et al. Wegener's granulomatosis: a series of 265 British cases seen between 1975 and 1985. A report by a subcommittee of the British Thoracic Society Research Committee. Q J Med 1992;83:427.

19. Fauci AS, Haynes BF, Katz P, et al. Wegener's granulomatosis: prospective clinical and therapeutic experience with 85 patients for 21 years. Ann Intern Med 1983;98:76.

20. Hoffman GS, Kerr GS, Leavitt RY, et al. Wegener's granulomatosis: an analysis of 158 patients. Ann Intern Med 1992;116:488.

21. Reinhold-Keller E, Beuge N, Latza U, et al. An interdisciplinary approach to the care of patients with Wegener's granulomatosis. Arthritis Rheum 2000; 43:1021.

22. Romas E, Murphy BF, d'Apice AJ, et al. Wegener's granulomatosis: clinical features and prognosis in 37 patients. Aust N Z J Med 1993;23:168.

23. Cordier J-F, Valeyre D, Guillevin L, et al. Pulmonary Wegener's granulomatosis. A clinical and imaging study of 77 cases. Chest 1990;97:906.

24. Reuter M, Schnabel A, Wesner F, et al. Pulmonary Wegener's granulomatosis: correlation between high-resolution CT findings and clinical scoring of disease activity. Chest 1998;114:500.

25. Lie JT. Illustrated histopathologic classification criteria for selected vasculitic syndromes. Arthritis Rheum 1990;33:1074.

26. Travis WD, Hoffman GS, Leavitt RY, et al. Surgical pathology of the lung in Wegener's granulomatosis. Am J Surg Pathol 1991;15:315.

27. Gayraud M, Guillevin L, le Toumelin P, et al. Long-term followup of polyarteritis nodosa, microscopic polyangiitis, and Churg-Strauss syndrome: analysis of four prospective trials including 278 patients. Arthritis Rheum 2001;44:666.

28. Guillevin L, Durand-Gasselin B, Cevallos R, et al. Microscopic polyangiitis: clinical and laboratory findings in eighty-five patients. Arthritis Rheum 1999;42:421.

29. Guillevin L, Lhote F, Gherardi R. Polyarteritis nodosa, microscopic polyangiitis, and Churg-Strauss syndrome: clinical aspects, neurologic manifestations, and treatment. Neurol Clin 1997;15:865.

30. Lhote F, Guillevin L. Polyarteritis nodosa, microscopic polyangiitis and Churg-Strauss syndrome. Semin Respir Crit Care Med 1998;19:27.

31. Lhote F, Guillevin L. Polyarteritis nodosa, microscopic polyangiitis, and Churg-Strauss syndrome. Clinical aspects and treatment. Rheum Dis Clin North Am 1995;21:911.

32. Lauque D, Cadranel J, Lazor R, et al. Microscopic polyangiitis with alveolar hemorrhage. A study of 29 cases and review of the literature. Groupe d'Etudes et de Recherche sur les Maladies "Orphelines" Pulmonaires (GERM"O"P). Medicine (Baltimore) 2000;79:222.

33. Lanham J, Elkon K, Pusey C, et al. Systemic vasculitis with asthma and eosinophilia: a clinical approach to the Churg-Strauss syndrome. Medicine 1984;63:65.

34. Sinico RA, Di Toma L, Maggiore U, et al. Prevalence and clinical significance of antineutrophil cytoplasmic antibodies in Churg-Strauss syndrome. Arthritis Rheum 2005;52:2926.

35. Guillevin L, Cohen P, Gayraud M, et al. Churg-Strauss syndrome. Clinical study and long-term follow-up of 96 patients. Medicine 1999;78:26.

36. Guillevin L, Lhote F, Gayraud M, et al. Prognostic factors in polyarteritis nodosa and Churg-Strauss syndrome. A prospective study in 342 patients. Medicine 1996;75:17.

37. Solans R, Bosch JA, Perez-Bocanegra C, et al. Churg-Strauss syndrome: outcome and long-term follow-up of 32 patients. Rheumatology 2001;40:763.

38. Sehgal M, Swanson JW, DeRemee RA, et al. Neurologic manifestations of Churg-Strauss syndrome. Mayo Clin Proc 1995;70:337.

39. Fong C, Schmidt G, Cain N, et al. Churg-Strauss syndrome, cardiac involvement and life threatening ventricular arrhythmias. Aust N Z J Med 1992;22:167.

40. Morgan JM, Raposo L, Gibson DG. Cardiac involvement in Churg-Strauss syndrome shown by echocardiography. Br Heart J 1989;62:462.

41. Pagnoux C, Guillevin L. Cardiac involvement in small and medium-sized vessel vasculitides. Lupus 2005;14:718.

42. Smedema JP, van Paassen P, van Kroonenburgh MJ, et al. Cardiac involvement of Churg Strauss syndrome demonstrated by magnetic resonance imaging. Clin Exp Rheumatol 2004;22:S75.

43. Val-Bernal JF, Mayorga M, Garcia-Alberdi E, et al. Churg-Strauss syndrome and sudden cardiac death. Cardiovasc Pathol 2003;12:94.

44. Buschman DL, Waldron JA, King TE. Churg Strauss pulmonary vasculitis: high resolution computed tomography scanning and pathologic findings. Am Rev Respir Dis 1990;142:458.

45. Choi YH, Im J-G, Han BK, et al. Thoracic manifestations of Churg-Strauss syndrome. Chest 2000; 117:117.

46. Staples CA. Pulmonary angiitis and granulomatosis. Radiol Clin North Am 1991;29:973.

47. Worthy SA, Muller NL, Hansell DM, et al. Churg-Strauss syndrome: the spectrum of pulmonary CT findings in 17 patients. AJR Am J Roentgenol 1998;170:297.

48. Schnabel A, Csernok E, Braun J, et al. Inflammatory cells and cellular activation in the lower respiratory tract in Churg-Strauss syndrome. Thorax 1999;54:771.

49. Wallaert B, Gosset P, Prin L, et al. Bronchoalveolar lavage in allergic granulomatosis and angiitis. Eur Respir J 1993;6:413.

50. Le Gall C, Pham S, Vignes S, et al. Inhaled corticosteroids and Churg-Strauss syndrome: a report of five cases. Eur Respir J 2000;15:978.

51. Weschler ME, Finn D, Gunawardena D, et al. Churg-Strauss syndrome in patients receiving montelukast as treatment for asthma. Chest 2000;117:708.

52. Weschler ME, Garpestad E, Flier SR, et al. Pulmonary infiltrates, eosinophilia, and cardiomyopathy following corticosteroid withdrawal in patients with asthma receiving zafirlukast. JAMA 1998;279:455.

53. Coulter D. Pro-active safety surveillance. Pharmacoepidemiol Drug Saf 2000;9:273.

54. Jamaleddine G, Diab K, Tabbarah Z, et al. Leukotriene antagonists and the Churg-Strauss syndrome. Semin Arthritis Rheum 2002;31:218.

55. Keogh KA, Specks U. Churg-Strauss syndrome: clinical presentation, antineutrophil cytoplasmic antibodies, and leukotriene receptor antagonists. Am J Med 2003;115:284.

56. Lilly CM, Churg A, Lazarovich M, et al. Asthma therapies and Churg-Strauss syndrome. J Allergy Clin Immunol 2002;109:S1.

57. Weller PF, Plaut M, Taggart V, et al. The relationship of asthma therapy and Churg-Strauss syndrome: NIH workshop summary report. J Allergy Clin Immunol 2001;108:175.

58. Wechsler ME, Wong DA, Miller MK, et al. Churg-Strauss syndrome in patients treated with omalizumab. Chest 2009;136:507.

59. Holsinger DR, Osmundson PJ, Edwards JE. The heart in periarteritis nodosa. Circulation 1962;25:610.

60. Schrader ML, Hochman JS, Bulkley BH. The heart in polyarteritis nodosa: a clinicopathologic study. Am Heart J 1985;109:1353.

61. Frankel SK, Schwarz MI. Cardiopulmonary manifestations of vasculitis. In: Ball GV, Bridges SL, editors. Vasculitis. 2nd edition. Oxford (UK): Oxford University Press; 2008. p. 149–60.

62. Lie JT. Isolated pulmonary Takayasu arteritis: clinicopathologic characteristics. Mod Pathol 1996;9:469.

63. Lie JT. Pathology of isolated nonclassical and catastrophic manifestations of Takayasu arteritis. Int J Cardiol 1998;66:S11.

64. Yamada I, Numano F, Suzuki S. Takayasu's arteritis: evaluation with MR imaging. Radiology 1993;188:89.

65. Van der Woude FJ, Rasmussen N, Lobatto S, et al. Autoantibodies against neutrophils and monocytes: tool for diagnosis and marker of disease activity in Wegener's granulomatosis. Lancet 1985;1:425.

66. Cohen-Tervaert JW, van der Woude FJ, Fauci AS, et al. Association between active Wegener's granulomatosis and anticytoplasmic antibodies. Arch Intern Med 1989;149:2461.

67. Gross WL. Antineutrophil cytoplasmic autoantibody testing in vasculitides. Rheum Dis Clin North Am 1995;21:987.

68. Nolle B, Specks U, Ludemann J, et al. Anticytoplasmic autoantibodies: their immunodiagnostic value in Wegener granulomatosis. Ann Intern Med 1989;111:28.

69. Cohen P, Guillevin L, Baril L, et al. Persistence of antineutrophil cytoplasmic antibodies (ANCA) in asymptomatic patients with systemic polyarteritis nodosa or Churg-Strauss syndrome: follow-up of 53 patients. Clin Exp Rheumatol 1995;13:193.

70. Schonermarck U, Lamprecht P, Csernok E, et al. Prevalence and spectrum of rheumatic diseases associated with proteinase-3-antineutrophil cytoplasmic antibodies (ANCA) and myeloperoxidase-ANCA. Rheumatology (Oxford) 2001;40:178.

71. Ara J, Mirapeix E, Rodriguez R, et al. Relationship between ANCA and disease activity in small vessel vasculitis patients with anti-MPO ANCA. Nephrol Dial Transplant 1999;14:1667.

72. Choi HK, Liu S, Merkel PA, et al. Diagnostic performance of antineutrophil cytoplasmic antibody tests for idiopathic vasculitides: metaanalysis with a focus on myeloperoxidase antibodies. J Rheumatol 2001;28:1584.

73. Cohen Tervaert JW, Goldschmeding R, Elema JD, et al. Association of autoantibodies to myeloperoxidase with different forms of vasculitis. Arthritis Rheum 1990;33:1264.

74. Cohen-Tervaert JW, Goldschmeding R, Elema JD, et al. Antimyeloperoxidase antibodies in the Churg-Strauss syndrome. Thorax 1991;46:70.

75. Boomsma MM, Stegeman CA, van der Leij MJ, et al. Prediction of relapses in Wegener's granulomatosis by measurement of antineutrophil cytoplasmic antibody levels: a prospective study. Arthritis Rheum 2000;43:2025.

76. Jayne DR, Gaskin G, Pusey CD, et al. ANCA and predicting relapse in systemic vasculitis. Q J Med 1995;88:127.

77. Kerr GS, Fleisher TA, Hallahan CW, et al. Limited prognostic value of changes in antineutrophil cytoplasmic antibody titers in patients with Wegener's granulomatosis. Adv Exp Med Biol 1993;336:411.

78. Segelmark M, Phillips BD, Hogan SL, et al. Monitoring proteinase 3 antineutrophil cytoplasmic antibodies for detection of relapses in small vessel vasculitis. Clin Diagn Lab Immunol 2003;10:769.

79. Sanders JS, Huitma MG, Kallenberg CG, et al. Prediction of relapses in PR3-ANCA-associated vasculitis by assessing responses of ANCA titres to treatment. Rheumatology (Oxford) 2006;45:724.

80. Summers RM, Aggarwal NR, Sneller MC, et al. CT virtual bronchoscopy of the central airways in patients with Wegener's granulomatosis. Chest 2002;121:242.

81. Schnabel A, Holl-Ulrich K, Dalhoff K, et al. Efficacy of transbronchial biopsy in pulmonary vasculitides. Eur Respir J 1997;10:2738.

82. Devaney KO, Travis WD, Hoffman G, et al. Interpretation of head and neck biopsies in Wegener's granulomatosis. A pathologic study of 126 biopsies in 70 patients. Am J Surg Pathol 1990;14:555.

83. Hauer HA, Bajema IM, van Houwelingen HC, et al. Renal histology in ANCA-associated vasculitis: differences between diagnostic and serologic subgroups. Kidney Int 2002;61:80.

84. Jennette JC, Falk RJ. Diagnosis and management of glomerulonephritis and vasculitis presenting as acute renal failure. Med Clin North Am 1990;74:893.

85. Weiss MA, Crissman JD. Renal biopsy findings in Wegener's granulomatosis: segmental necrotizing glomerulonephritis with glomerular thrombosis. Hum Pathol 1984;15:943.

86. Weiss MA, Crissman JD. Segmental necrotizing glomerulonephritis: diagnostic, prognostic, and therapeutic significance. Am J Kidney Dis 1985;6:199.

87. De Remee RA. Wegener's granulomatosis. Ann Intern Med 1992;117:619.

88. De Remee RA, McDonald TJ, Weiland LH. Wegener's granulomatosis: observations on treatment with antimicrobial agents. Mayo Clin Proc 1985;60:27.

89. de Groot K, Rasmussen N, Bacon PA, et al. Randomized trial of cyclophosphamide versus methotrexate for induction of remission in early systemic antineutrophil cytoplasmic antibody-associated vasculitis. Arthritis Rheum 2005;52:2461.

90. de Groot K, Adu D, Savage CO. The value of pulse cyclophosphamide in ANCA-associated vasculitis: meta-analysis and critical review. Nephrol Dial Transplant 2001;16:2018.

91. de Groot K, Harper L, Jayne DR, et al. Pulse versus daily oral cyclophosphamide for induction of remission in antineutrophil cytoplasmic antibody-associated vasculitis: a randomized trial. Ann Intern Med 2009;150:670.

92. Jayne DRW, Gaskin G, Rasmussen N, et al. Randomised trial of plasma exchange or high dose methyl prednisolone as adjunctive therapy for severe renal vasculitis. J Am Soc Nephrol 2007;18:2180.

93. Klemmer PJ, Chalermskulrat W, Reif MS, et al. Plasmapheresis therapy for diffuse alveolar hemorrhage in patients with small vessel vasculitis. Am J Kidney Dis 2003;42:1149.

94. Brihaye B, Aouba A, Pagnoux C, et al. Adjunction of rituximab to steroids and immunosuppressants for refractory/relapsing Wegener's granulomatosis: a study on 8 patients. Clin Exp Rheumatol 2007;25:S23.

95. Ferraro AJ, Day CJ, Drayson MT, et al. Effective therapeutic use of rituximab in refractory Wegener's granulomatosis. Nephrol Dial Transplant 2005;20:622.

96. Keogh KA, Wylam ME, Stone JH, et al. Induction of remission by B lymphocyte depletion in eleven patients with refractory antineutrophil cytoplasmic antibody-associated vasculitis. Arthritis Rheum 2005;52:262.

97. Keogh KA, Ytterberg SR, Fervenza FC, et al. Rituximab for refractory Wegener's granulomatosis: report of a prospective, open-label pilot trial. Am J Respir Crit Care Med 2006;173:180.

98. Jones RB, Ferraro AJ, Chaudhry AN, et al. A multicenter survey of rituximab therapy for refractory antineutrophil cytoplasmic antibody-associated vasculitis. Arthritis Rheum 2009;60:2156.

99. Bartolucci P, Ramanoelina J, Cohen P, et al. Efficacy of the anti-TNF-alpha antibody infliximab against refractory systemic vasculitides: an open pilot study on 10 patients. Rheumatology (Oxford) 2002;41:1126.

100. Booth A, Harper L, Hammad T, et al. Prospective study of TNFa blockade with infliximab in antineutrophil cytoplasmic antibody-associated systemic vasculitis. J Am Soc Nephrol 2004;15:717.

101. Jayne DR, Chapel H, Adu D, et al. Intravenous immunoglobulin for ANCA-associated systemic vasculitis with persistent disease activity. QJM 2000;93:433.

102. Betensley AD, Yankaskas JR. Factor viia for alveolar hemorrhage in microscopic polyangiitis. Am J Respir Crit Care Med 2002;166:1291.

103. Henke DC, Falk RJ, Gabriel DA. Successful treatment of diffuse alveolar hemorrhage with activated factor VII. Ann Intern Med 2004;140:493.

104. Ahmed SH, Aziz T, Cochran J, et al. Use of extracorporeal membrane oxygenation in a patient

with diffuse alveolar hemorrhage. Chest 2004;126:305.

105. Jayne D, Rasmussen N, Andrassy K, et al. A randomized trial of maintenance therapy for vasculitis associated with antineutrophil cytoplasmic autoantibodies. N Engl J Med 2003; 349:36.

106. Metzler C, Miehle N, Manger K, et al. Elevated relapse rate under oral methotrexate versus leflunomide for maintenance of remission in Wegener's granulomatosis. Rheumatology (Oxford) 2007;46:1087.

107. WGET Investigators. Etanercept plus standard therapy for Wegener's granulomatosis. N Engl J Med 2005;352:351.

108. Walsh M, Merkel PA, Jayne D. The effect of low-dose corticosteroids on risk of relapse in ANCA-associated vasculitis: a systematic review and meta-analysis of clinical trials [abstract 2012].

2007 American College of Rheumatology/National Scientific Meeting Highlights. Boston, November 6–11, 2007.

109. Mukhtyar C, Lee R, Brown D, et al. Modification and validation of the Birmingham vasculitis activity score (version 3). Ann Rheum Dis 1827;68:2009.

110. Bourgarit A, Le Toumelin P, Pagnoux C, et al. Deaths occurring during the first year after treatment onset for polyarteritis nodosa, microscopic polyangiitis, and Churg-Strauss syndrome: a retrospective analysis of causes and factors predictive of mortality based on 595 patients. Medicine (Baltimore) 2005;84:323.

111. Merkel PA, Lo GH, Holbrook JT, et al. Brief communication: high incidence of venous thrombotic events among patients with Wegener granulomatosis: the Wegener's Clinical Occurrence of Thrombosis (WeCLOT) Study. Ann Intern Med 2005; 142:620.

Pulmonary Manifestations of the Antiphospholipid Antibody Syndrome

H. James Ford, MD[a,*], Robert A.S. Roubey, MD[b]

KEYWORDS

- Antiphospholipid • Lupus • Pulmonary embolism
- Pulmonary hypertension

The antiphospholipid syndrome (APS) is an auto-immune condition in which autoantibodies directed against certain phospholipid-binding plasma proteins are associated with an increased risk of thrombosis (both venous and arterial), pregnancy loss and morbidity.[1] Additional clinical manifestations associated with antiphospholipid antibodies (aPLs) include livedo reticularis, cardiac valvular disease, nephropathy, thrombocytopenia, and Coombs' positive hemolytic anemia.[2] APS may occur in the absence of other autoimmune diseases, in which case it is termed *primary APS*. APS in patients with systemic lupus erythematosus (SLE) or other autoimmune diseases is termed *secondary APS*. Catastrophic APS is a severe form of the syndrome in which widespread thromboses of small- and medium-sized blood vessels lead to multiorgan system dysfunction.[3] The commonly used clinical laboratory tests for aPL are anticardiolipin antibody tests (immunoassays which detect, primarily, antibodies to β_2-glycoprotein I [β2GPI]), anti-β2GPI immunoassays, and lupus anticoagulant assays (clotting tests that can detect both antibodies to prothrombin and some anti-β2GPI antibodies).[4]

APS is one of the most common causes of acquired thrombophilia. Although studies differ, it is estimated that 15% or more of all cases of deep vein thrombosis with or without pulmonary embolism are associated with moderate to high levels of aPL.[5] APS accounts for approximately 10% to 20% of otherwise unexplained recurrent pregnancy loss.[6] A broad spectrum of pulmonary disease may occur in APS (**Fig. 1**). The most common pulmonary manifestations are pulmonary thromboembolism and pulmonary hypertension. In this article we review these manifestations, as well as less common findings including acute respiratory distress syndrome (ARDS), alveolar hemorrhage, and pulmonary capillaritis.

ACUTE PULMONARY EMBOLISM

The pulmonary manifestations of APS can be quite variable, but the overwhelming majority of complications in the lung involve venous thromboembolism and its associated sequelae. Approximately 40% of patients with APS suffer pulmonary embolism (PE) during the course of the disease, with up to 55% having documented deep venous thrombosis (DVT) of the extremities.[7] PE was the first significant pulmonary complication of APS reported in the medical literature. In fact, pulmonary embolism is often the initial clinical manifestation of APS. Among all patients who develop DVT, it is estimated that 5% to 20% of them have detectable antiphospholipid antibodies (aPLs). Interestingly, Cervera and colleagues[8] prospectively examined the incidence of complications of APS in a multicenter cohort of 1000 patients with APS

[a] Division of Pulmonary and Critical Care Medicine, University of North Carolina at Chapel Hill, 130 Mason Farm Road, CB 7020, Chapel Hill, NC 27599, USA
[b] Division of Rheumatology, Allergy, and Immunology, and Thurston Arthritis Research Center, University of North Carolina at Chapel Hill, Chapel Hill, NC, USA
* Corresponding author.
E-mail address: hubert_ford@med.unc.edu

Clin Chest Med 31 (2010) 537–545
doi:10.1016/j.ccm.2010.05.005

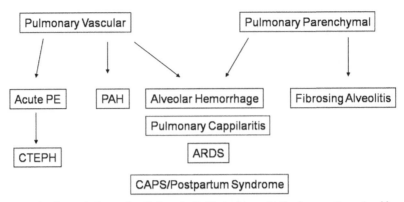

Fig. 1. Various recognized associations of antiphospholipid syndrome in the lung, categorized by vascular and/or parenchymal involvement. ARDS, acute respiratory distress syndrome; PE, pulmonary embolism; PAH, pulmonary arterial hypertension; CAPS, catastrophic antiphospholipid syndrome; CTEPH, chronic thromboembolic pulmonary hypertension.

and found that 2.1% of patients developed pulmonary embolism over the 5-year period of the study.

The clinical presentation, course, and treatment of patients with acute PE in the setting of APS do not differ appreciably from those who suffer PE in the general population. Ventilation-perfusion (V/Q) scanning, spiral computed tomographic (CT) angiography of the thorax, or pulmonary angiography are the diagnostic modalities of choice, with pulmonary angiography reserved for situations where clinical suspicion is high, but V/Q scan or CT angiography results are equivocal. Lower extremity doppler and D-dimer studies are equally useful in patients with APS as ancillary tools in the diagnosis of acute PE. Acute therapy with unfractionated or low-molecular weight heparin is recommended, with the use of argatroban, lepirudin, or fondaparinux reserved for patients with adverse reactions or other contraindications to heparins. In addition, placement of inferior vena caval filters may be clinically indicated in patients with APS patients who have persistent lower extremity DVT. Thrombolytic therapy in this subset of patients, as in all patients with acute PE, is generally reserved for those with significant hemodynamic instability owing to severe, acute right ventricular failure. As is true of any case of acute PE, segmental pulmonary infarction can occur in a small number of patients.

The long-term anticoagulation approach in patients with APS and documented thrombotic events, specifically the goals of intensity of anticoagulation with vitamin K antagonists (warfarin), had been an area of some controversy. Many clinicians followed earlier guidelines for anticoagulation in APS that targeted international normalized ratio (INR) values of greater than 3.0 for prevention of recurrent thrombotic events. However, recent prospective randomized trials in patients with APS have shown no benefit in maintaining the INR above traditionally targeted levels of 2.0 to 3.0, as used in other disease states that pose elevated thrombosis risk.[9,10]

CHRONIC PULMONARY THROMBOEMBOLIC DISEASE AND ASSOCIATED PULMONARY HYPERTENSION

It is important to note that approximately 3% of patients who suffer acute pulmonary emboli will develop permanent pulmonary vascular changes and chronic thromboembolic pulmonary hypertension (CTEPH).[11] The precise mechanisms for the development of CTEPH are unclear, but are postulated to be attributable to incomplete resolution of acute clot and endothelial damage precipitated by acute PE that sets off a cascade of vascular remodeling events that likely include the development of in situ microthrombosis.[12] It is not known whether the presence aPL alone predisposes one to the development of CTEPH, although aPLs have been observed in 20% of patients with CTEPH.[13] Patients with CTEPH do not, however, have a higher prevalence of extrapulmonary thrombophilic disorders; rather, the development of CTEPH appears to be a result of a deranged vascular response to the acute pulmonary embolism.

The manifestations of CTEPH are the same as those of pulmonary hypertension attributable to any etiology. Progressive exertional dyspnea is common, and as right heart failure progresses, lower extremity edema, ascites, dizziness with exertion, and syncope may develop. Chest pain and palpitations may be present as well, but are less common. The absence of a documented history of acute PE does not rule out the presence of CTEPH, as most patients do not have a clear history of this diagnosis.[14] Elevation of the triscuspid regurgitant jet, or signs of right ventricular and/or right atrial volume or pressure overload on echocardiography are often the first clue to the presence of pulmonary hypertension. Pulmonary hypertension must be confirmed via right heart catheterization.

All patients with pulmonary hypertension should undergo V/Q scanning to screen for chronic thromboemboli, and if significant ventilation perfusion mismatching is detected, formal pulmonary angiography should be performed (**Fig. 2**). Pulmonary angiography is important in that it allows for the determination of the extent of the disease (major vessel, segmental, or subsegmental pulmonary artery branches) and thus provides information as to the feasibility of surgical resection of the diseased vasculature via pulmonary thromboendarterectomy (PTE). Furthermore, pulmonary angiography will be normal even if V/Q scanning is abnormal in patients who have pulmonary veno-occlusive disease, an entity not amenable to surgical intervention or anticoagulation.

Pulmonary thromboendarterectomy (PTE) is the treatment of choice for CTEPH, with overall low mortality in experienced centers. The procedure was pioneered by Jamieson and colleagues and their program has performed more than 2000 PTE procedures.[15,16] Other centers worldwide have developed proficiency in this area as well, as clinicians have become more adept at recognizing this treatable form of PH. Significant improvements in pulmonary hemodynamics are usually observed, as pulmonary vascular resistance (PVR) is reduced by the removal of chronic clot, which is fibrotic material that is deeply incorporated into the vessel wall.[16] The procedure is exceedingly complex and intricate, and requires the creation of a bloodless surgical field via cardiopulmonary bypass with intermittent circulatory arrest, such that appropriate visualization and adequate dissection of thromboembolic material can be achieved. The more distal the vascular changes of CTEPH, the more challenging it is to resect the lesions thoroughly enough to effect meaningful improvements in PVR. With respect to the presence of circulating aPL, the outcomes of PTE in patients with high aPL titers were examined prospectively by D'Armini and colleagues.[17] No significant difference in postoperative mortality or major complications were observed between a group with low aPL titers (n = 156, aPL IgG titer ≤10 U/mL) and a smaller group with high aPL titers (n = 28, aPL IgG titer >10 U/mL). High aPL titer was associated with a increased incidence of postoperative transient neurologic impairment.

PULMONARY ARTERIAL AND PULMONARY VENOUS HYPERTENSION

The development of pulmonary arteriopathy and associated increase in pulmonary vascular resistance and pressure has long been recognized in association with connective tissue disease, frequently in the setting of scleroderma or SLE. Left-sided mitral or aortic valvulopathy can also exist in patients with aPL and thus lead to left ventricular (LV) dysfunction and pulmonary venous hypertension. The most recent Fourth World Symposium on Pulmonary Hypertension, provides the latest classification scheme for pulmonary hypertension (**Box 1**).[18] This classification system provides a useful construct for approaching the different types of pulmonary hypertension that can exist in patients with detectable aPL. It groups together patients who have pulmonary

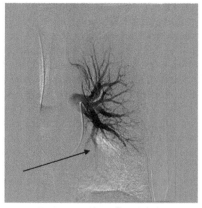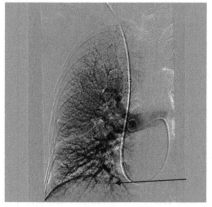

Fig. 2. Pulmonary angiogram images showing chronic pulmonary thromboembolism in a patient with antiphospholipid syndrome. The image on the left shows occlusion of the descending branch of the left pulmonary artery. The image on the right shows tapered occlusion of basilar segmental arteries in the right lung.

Box 1
World Health Organization 4th World Symposium Clinical Classification of Pulmonary Hypertension (Dana Point, 2008)[a]

1. **Pulmonary arterial hypertension (PAH)**

    1.1 Idiopathic PAH

    1.2 Heritable

    1.3 Drug- and toxin-induced

    1.4 Associated with

    1.4.1 Connective tissue diseases

    1.4.2 HIV infection

    1.4.3 Portal hypertension

    1.4.4 Congenital heart diseases

    1.4.5 Schistosomiasis

    1.4.6 Chronic hemolytic anemia

    1.5 Persistent pulmonary hypertension of the newborn

    1' Pulmonary veno-occlusive disease (PVOD) and/or pulmonary capillary hemangiomatosis (PCH)

2. **Pulmonary hypertension owing to left heart disease**

    2.1 Systolic dysfunction

    2.2 Diastolic dysfunction

    2.3 Valvular disease

3. Pulmonary hypertension owing to lung diseases and/or hypoxia

    3.1 Chronic obstructive pulmonary disease

    3.2 Interstitial lung disease

    3.3 Other pulmonary diseases with mixed restrictive and obstructive pattern

    3.4 Sleep-disordered breathing

    3.5 Alveolar hypoventilation disorders

    3.6 Chronic exposure to high altitude

    3.7 Developmental abnormalities

4. **Chronic thromboembolic pulmonary hypertension (CTEPH)**

5. Pulmonary hypertension with unclear multifactorial mechanisms

    5.1 Hematologic disorders: myeloproliferative disorders, splenectomy

    5.2 Systemic disorders: sarcoidosis, pulmonary Langerhans cell histiocytosis: lymphangioleiomyomatosis, neurofibromatosis, vasculitis

    5.3 Metabolic disorders: glycogen storage disease, Gaucher disease, thyroid disorders

    5.4 Others: tumoral obstruction, fibrosing mediastinitis, chronic renal failure on dialysis

[a] Subtypes in which antiphospholipid antibody may play a role in disease development are highlighted in bold.

Data from Simonneau G, Robbins IM, Beghetti M, et al. Updated clinical classification of pulmonary hypertension. J Am Coll Cardiol 2009;54(Suppl 1): S43–54.

---

hypertension subtypes with similar clinical and histopathologic characteristics. We have previously discussed the potential role of aPL in the evolution of CTEPH (see Group 4, **Box 1**) after acute PE, and will now further discuss patients in WHO groups 1 and 2.

WHO Group 1 PH, termed pulmonary *arterial* hypertension (PAH), represents those disorders in which there is evidence of intrinsic, progressive pulmonary vasculopathy. On the microscopic level, this is characterized by vascular endothelial and smooth muscle proliferation, in situ thrombosis, and the development of advanced plexiform lesions. The end result is decreased pulmonary vascular cross-sectional area and increased resistance to flow, causing right ventricular strain and failure. A relative excess of endothelin-1 (ET-1), the most potent vasoconstrictor substance known, as well as a relative deficiency of circulating nitric oxide and a prostaglandin-deficient state drive this process. Treatments approved by the United States Food and Drug Administration (FDA) available for PAH include agents that target these 3 pathways: endothelin receptor antagonists, phosphodiesterase-5 inhibitors, and prostacyclin analogs. Other emerging therapies target pathways that are becoming increasingly implicated as key in the development of PAH, such as platelet-derived growth factor, Rho-kinase, and serotonin transport proteins.[19–21]

The role of aPL in the pathogenesis of idiopathic PAH is unclear, but there is evidence that aPL may contribute. In a small series of patients, most with SLE and PH that phenotypically resembled IPAH (in that there was no parenchymal lung disease or identified thromboembolic disease), circulating aPL was detected in 68%.[22] This is higher than the prevalence of aPL in SLE overall, which is 30% to 50%.[23] There is also a clear association between the development of PAH and connective tissue diseases, particularly scleroderma and SLE (see Group 1.4.1 in **Box 1**), even in the absence of circulating aPL. Atsumi and colleagues[24] measured ET-1 in a small group of patients with APS and history of arterial thrombosis and found ET-1 levels were elevated in this cohort. It is thus postulated that aPL induces the expression of ET-1, and in this way contributes to vascular injury, remodeling, and thrombosis. This provides a plausible role for aPL in the pathogenesis of PAH in some patients.

Pulmonary venous hypertension (PVH), WHO Group 2 in the classification scheme in **Box 1**, represents the group of pulmonary hypertension in which pulmonary vascular pressures are largely passively elevated owing to elevated left heart filling pressures. This can be seen in the context of systolic or diastolic LV dysfunction or in the setting of significant valvulopathy. Libman and Sacks[25] first described patients with SLE who developed nonbacterial endocarditis of the mitral or aortic valves. Significant regurgitation as a result of the diseased valve can develop and lead to PVH. It is approximated that 20% to 30% of patients with SLE develop this Libman-Sacks endocarditis, whereas it is present in about 30% of patients with primary APS.[26–29] It is unclear precisely how aPL may affect the development of Libman-Sacks valvulopathy. One hypothesis is that aPLs interact with antigens on the surface of the valve and lead to valvular inflammation and verrucous vegetations. It is important to point out that the development of pulmonary hypertension in this group of patients is not attributable to the development of intrinsic pulmonary vascular disease. However, there is some evidence that long-standing PVH can lead to secondary remodeling of the pulmonary vasculature.[30] The optimal therapeutic approach to Libman-Sacks endocarditis is unclear, with a few reports suggesting that immunomodulatory therapies may be of benefit.[31] Ultimately, valve replacement may be necessary if LV dysfunction becomes severe. Anticoagulation is usually recommended in such patients because of the risk of valvular thrombosis and subsequent systemic embolic phenomenon.

The diagnostic approach to pulmonary hypertension involves screening echocardiography when the disease is suspected. If there are signs of elevated right heart and/or pulmonary artery pressures, then right heart catheterization should be performed. This is critical in differentiating between PAH and PVH, as pulmonary vascular resistance can be determined. PAH is present if the mean pulmonary artery pressure (mPAP) is 25 mm Hg or higher, the pulmonary capillary wedge pressure (PCWP) is 15 mm Hg or lower, and the pulmonary vascular resistance (PVR) is 3.0 or more Wood units.[32] PVR is determined by dividing the transpulmonary gradient (mPAP – PCWP) by the cardiac output determined by either Fick or thermodilution methods. Provocative testing such as inhalation of nitric oxide, exercise challenges, or administration of fluid boluses or systemic vasodilators can also help to assess for vasoreactivity and to differentiate PAH from PVH.

CATASTROPHIC ANTIPHOSPHOLIPID SYNDROME

A relatively rare and fulminant presentation of APS, termed catastrophic antiphospholipid syndrome (CAPS), was first described in 1992.[3] It was characterized by rapidly progressive multiorgan dysfunction, multiple small-vessel occlusions on tissue biopsy, and circulating aPLs. This syndrome only occurs in about 1% of patients with APS, but carries a 50% mortality[33]; 70% of cases occur in women. Usually there is a precipitating illness, such as infection, in 60% of cases and empiric antibiotic therapy is recommended. The main pulmonary complication is ARDS, and it occurs in the setting of multiorgan dysfunction that is driven by vascular thrombosis. Pulmonary embolism and alveolar hemorrhage are less common pulmonary manifestations. Cytokine activation creates a proinflammatory state that clinically is much like systemic inflammatory response syndrome (SIRS). Overall, the disease process bears significant similarity to more common intensive care unit illnesses, namely septic shock with associated ARDS. Clinicians must carefully consider the possibility of CAPS in such patients, especially given that it can occur with no prior history of thrombotic event or prior documentation of circulating aPL.

Laboratory features are reflective of microangiopathy. Thrombocytopenia is a frequent finding, as is the presence of schistocytes on peripheral blood smear.[34,35] Schistocyte burden is less than that seen in thrombotic thrombocytopenic purpura. CAPS may be associated with either IgG or IgM anticardiolipin antibodies. By definition, three organ systems must be involved and small-vessel occlusion proven on tissue biopsy from one organ system. Once correctly identified, treatment of CAPS centers around anticoagulation with heparin and corticosteroid therapy. In more severe cases, plasma exchange and intravenous immunoglobulin (IVIG) are used.[34] Cyclophosphamide has been used with success in patients with SLE and APS who develop CAPS.[36] There is also an ongoing trial looking at the utility of rituximab in anticoagulant-resistant manifestations of APS[37] that may ultimately shed light on the management of refractory CAPS.

ACUTE RESPIRATORY DISTRESS SYNDROME

ARDS is a syndrome defined as the presence of bilateral alveolar pulmonary infiltrates with a partial pressure arterial oxygen (PaO2) to fraction of inspired oxygen (FiO2) ratio of less than 200.[38]

This must occur in the setting of normal left atrial/ventricular filling pressures, and thus represents noncardiogenic pulmonary edema. In most cases, ARDS is associated with primary pulmonary or systemic infection (sepsis), trauma, inhalational injury, blood product transfusion, or other systemic inflammatory state. There have been numerous reports of ARDS in association with APS. This occurs most often in the setting of CAPS, as described previously. In a large registry of 220 patients with CAPS, it was determined that ARDS was present as a pulmonary complication not attributable to primary pulmonary infection in 21% of the patients.[39] Interestingly, there was no difference in mortality in this cohort of patients when comparing those with and without ARDS.

It is unclear whether aPL itself directly causes ARDS, or whether the illness that precipitates CAPS is the cause. Because the acute phase of ARDS is characterized by increased permeability of the alveolar-capillary membrane, and thus extravasation of proteinaceous edema fluid, red blood cells, and neutrophils, it is known that immunoglobulins may also enter the alveolus.[40,41] Maneta-Peyret and colleagues[42] demonstrated the presence of aPL in the bronchoalveolar lavage (BAL) fluid of patients with ARDS compared with non-ARDS mechanically ventilated controls. It is not known whether such antibodies are locally produced or are introduced to the alveolus simply as a result of loss of interface integrity. A case report of a patient with ARDS and CAPS also demonstrated the presence of aPL in the BAL fluid.[43] These studies led to the hypothesis that aPL could drive the process of ARDS in APS. It is also possible that the surge of inflammatory cytokines seen in CAPS is the major inciting event in the development of ARDS by increasing neutrophil migration and alveolar permeability.

ALVEOLAR HEMORRHAGE SYNDROMES AND PULMONARY CAPILLARITIS

Diffuse alveolar hemorrhage (DAH) is characterized by the presence of diffuse alveolar infiltrates that are associated with dyspnea, cough, and fever and often progresses to hypoxemic respiratory failure. Hemoptysis may be present, but is absent in 33% of cases. Depending on the extent of hemorrhage, anemia is usually present as well. The diagnosis is made by serial bronchoalveolar lavages showing increasingly hemorrhagic appearance on direct visualization. Further confirmatory testing of BAL fluid for hemosiderin-laden macrophages and serial increase in red blood cell counts can also be performed. Biopsy is usually not required, but if performed, alveolar hemorrhage is observed with microvascular thrombosis. Pulmonary capillaritis may be present as well.[44] The exact incidence of DAH in patients with secondary or primary APS is unclear. There is a relative paucity of reported cases, but the disease can be easily missed, owing in large part to the similarity of radiographic findings to other disease processes, as well as the frequent lack of hemoptysis, even in cases where there are large amounts of intra-alveolar bleeding.[45]

The mainstay of treatment of DAH is high-dose corticosteroid therapy, usually on the order of 1 g methylprednisolone intravenously on a daily basis for 3 to 5 days. Recurrence of the disease process with cessation of steroids is not uncommon, and often requires the initiation of other immunomodulatory therapy such as cyclophosphamide, cyclosporine, or mycophenolate. When immunosuppressive therapy is ineffective, intravenous immunoglobulin or plasmapheresis can be used with improvement in regression of DAH.[46,47]

Pulmonary capillaritis appears to be the histopathologic hallmark of DAH in the setting of circulating aPL. It is characterized by infiltration of neutrophils into the lung interstitium, causing structural necrosis and loss of capillary integrity. This, in turn, leads to extravasation of red blood cells into the alveolus.[48] It is speculated that aPL induces an up-regulation of vascular endothelial cell adhesion molecules and thus incites neutrophil migration to the interstitium, leading to the changes described earlier and subsequent hemorrhage.[46] Complement C5 activation, leading to neutrophil activation and mobilization to the alveolar septum, may also contribute to DAH in the setting of APS, a hypothesis extrapolated from studies on the role of complement in aPL-mediated pregnancy loss.[49]

RARER ENTITIES
Fibrosing Alveolitis

Fibrosing alveolitis in the setting of aPL is an entity reported only twice in the medical literature.[50,51] In fact, it is unclear if this represents a fibrotic process uniquely associated with APS. Both patients had APS and documented alveolitis and interstitial fibrosis on pathology. In one of the cases, concomitant pulmonary embolism and pneumonia were present as well. Future prospective characterizations of lung disease in APS, as well as postmortem studies may help to shed light on the true frequency of this fibrotic process and determine how closely it is associated with aPL.

Postpartum Syndrome

Postpartum syndrome was first described in a series of 3 obstetric patients in 1987 by Kochenour and colleagues.[52] The clinical syndrome was characterized by cyclic fevers, pleuritis, and dyspnea. Chest radiographs showed diffuse, patchy pulmonary infiltrates and pleural effusions. Each of the patients had abnormal electrocardiographic findings and one developed cardiomyopathy with extensive immunoglobulin and complement C3 deposition in the myocardium. Kuperminc and colleagues[53] described a patient with similar manifestations, further complicated by renal insufficiency with preeclampsia. There was no infectious or thrombotic etiology identified to explain these patients' clinical courses. All 4 of the patients described in these 2 reports had circulating aPL. It is thus postulated that certain rare obstetric patients with aPL are predisposed to a CAPS-like syndrome characterized by multiorgan system dysfunction driven by microangiopathy, including the lung parenchyma and vasculature.

SUMMARY

The presence of aPL in a wide spectrum of pulmonary diseases is undeniable, with most of the associations occurring in the pulmonary vasculature in the form of acute and chronic thromboembolic disease and pulmonary hypertension. Although direct causative and pathophysiologic mechanisms implicating aPL have not been elucidated in many of these processes, clinicians should be aware of the need to consider primary or secondary APS in patients who present with pulmonary vascular disease or diffuse alveolar filling processes such as ARDS and DAH. This should prompt appropriate serologic testing and rheumatologic consultation when needed. Further prospective characterization of APS and treatment trials should help to better define the underpinnings of the development of pulmonary disease in this patient population, as well as to define the optimal treatment regimens.

REFERENCES

1. George D, Erkan D. Antiphospholipid syndrome. Prog Cardiovasc Dis 2009;52(2):115–25.
2. Miyakis S, Lockshin MD, Atsumi T, et al. International consensus statement on an update of the classification criteria for definite antiphospholipid syndrome (APS). J Thromb Haemost 2006;4(2):295–306.
3. Asherson RA. The catastrophic antiphospholipid syndrome. J Rheumatol 1992;19:508–12.
4. Roubey RA. Antiphospholipid syndrome: antibodies and antigens. Curr Opin Hematol 2000;7(5):316–20.
5. Ginsburg KS, Liang MH, Newcomer L, et al. Anticardiolipin antibodies and the risk for ischemic stroke and venous thrombosis. Ann Intern Med 1992;117: 997–1002.
6. Branch DW, Khamashta MA. Antiphospholipid syndrome: obstetric diagnosis, management, and controversies. Obstet Gynecol 2003;101(6): 1333–44.
7. Ordi Ros J, O'Callaghan AS, Vilardell M. Thrombotic manifestations in the antiphospholipid syndrome. In: Asherson RA, Cervera R, Piette J-C, et al, editors. The antiphospholipid syndrome II: autoimmune thrombosis. Amsterdam: Elsevier Science; 2002. p. 145–54.
8. Cervera R, Khamashta MA, Shoenfeld Y, et al. Morbidity and mortality in the antiphospholipid syndrome during a 5-year period: a multicentre prospective study of 1000 patients. Ann Rheum Dis 2009;68(9):1428–32.
9. Crowther MA, Ginsberg JS, Julian J, et al. A comparison of two intensities of warfarin for the prevention of recurrent thrombosis in patients with the antiphospholipid antibody syndrome. N Engl J Med 2003;349(12):1133–8.
10. Finazzi G, Marchioli R, Brancaccio V, et al. A randomized clinical trial of high-intensity warfarin vs. conventional antithrombotic therapy for the prevention of recurrent thrombosis in patients with the antiphospholipid syndrome (WAPS). J Thromb Haemost 2005;3(5):848–53.
11. Tapson VF, Humbert M. Incidence and prevalence of chronic thromboembolic pulmonary hypertension: from acute to chronic pulmonary embolism. Proc Am Thorac Soc 2006;3(7):564–7.
12. Hoeper MM, Mayer E, Simonneau G, et al. Chronic thromboembolic pulmonary hypertension. Circulation 2006;113(16):2011–20.
13. Wolf M, Boyer-Neumann C, Parent F, et al. Thrombotic risk factors in pulmonary hypertension. Eur Respir J 2000;15(2):395–9.
14. Lang IM. Chronic thromboembolic pulmonary hypertension–not so rare after all. N Engl J Med 2004; 350(22):2236–8.
15. Jamieson SW, Kapelanski DP, Sakakibara N, et al. Pulmonary endarterectomy: experience and lessons learned in 1,500 cases. Ann Thorac Surg 2003; 76(5):1457–62.
16. Auger WR, Kim NH, Kerr KM, et al. Chronic thromboembolic pulmonary hypertension. Clin Chest Med 2007;28(1):255–69, x.
17. D'Armini AM, Totaro P, Nicolardi S, et al. Impact of high titre of antiphospholipid antibodies on postoperative outcome following pulmonary endarterectomy. Interact Cardiovasc Thorac Surg 2010;10(3): 418–22.

18. Simonneau G, Robbins IM, Beghetti M, et al. Updated clinical classification of pulmonary hypertension. J Am Coll Cardiol 2009;54(Suppl 1):S43–54.

19. Perros F, Montani D, Dorfmuller P, et al. Platelet-derived growth factor expression and function in idiopathic pulmonary arterial hypertension. Am J Respir Crit Care Med 2008;178(1):81–8.

20. Abe K, Shimokawa H, Morikawa K, et al. Long-term treatment with a Rho-kinase inhibitor improves monocrotaline-induced fatal pulmonary hypertension in rats. Circ Res 2004;94(3):385–93.

21. Maclean MR. Pulmonary hypertension and the serotonin hypothesis: where are we now? Int J Clin Pract Suppl 2007;156:27–31.

22. Asherson RA, Higenbottam TW, Dinh Xuan AT, et al. Pulmonary hypertension in a lupus clinic: experience with twenty-four patients. J Rheumatol 1990; 17:1292–8.

23. Merkel PA, Chang Y, Pierangeli SS, et al. The prevalence and clinical associations of anticardiolipin antibodies in a large inception cohort of patients with connective tissue diseases. Am J Med 1996; 101(6):576–83.

24. Atsumi T, Khamashta MA, Haworth RS, et al. Arterial disease and thrombosis in the antiphospholipid syndrome: a pathogenic role for endothelin 1. Arthritis Rheum 1998;41(5):800–7.

25. Libman E, Sacks B. A hitherto undescribed form of valvular and mural endocarditis. Arch Intern Med 1924;33:701–37.

26. Galve E, Ordi J, Barquinero J, et al. Valvular heart disease in the primary antiphospholipid syndrome. Ann Intern Med 1992;116:293–8.

27. Khamashta MA, Cervera R, Asherson RA, et al. Association of antibodies against phospholipids with heart valve disease in systemic lupus erythematosus. Lancet 1990;335:1541–4.

28. Leung W-H, Wong K-L, Lau C-P, et al. Association between antiphospholipid antibodies and cardiac abnormalities in patients with systemic lupus erythematosus. Am J Med 1990;89:411–9.

29. Brenner B, Blumenfeld Z, Markiewicz W, et al. Cardiac involvement in patients with primary antiphospholipid syndrome. J Am Coll Cardiol 1991; 18(4):931–6.

30. Delgado JF, Conde E, Sanchez V, et al. Pulmonary vascular remodeling in pulmonary hypertension due to chronic heart failure. Eur J Heart Fail 2005; 7(6):1011–6.

31. Nesher G, Ilany J, Rosenmann D, et al. Valvular dysfunction in antiphospholipid syndrome: prevalence, clinical features, and treatment. Semin Arthritis Rheum 1997;27(1):27–35.

32. McLaughlin VV, Archer SL, Badesch DB, et al. ACCF/AHA 2009 expert consensus document on pulmonary hypertension a report of the American College of Cardiology Foundation Task Force on Expert Consensus Documents and the American Heart Association developed in collaboration with the American College of Chest Physicians; American Thoracic Society, Inc.; and the Pulmonary Hypertension Association. J Am Coll Cardiol 2009; 53(17):1573–619.

33. Asherson RA, Cervera R, Piette JC, et al. Catastrophic antiphospholipid syndrome: clues to the pathogenesis from a series of 80 patients. Medicine (Baltimore) 2001;80(6):355–77.

34. Bucciarelli S, Espinosa G, Cervera R, et al. Mortality in the catastrophic antiphospholipid syndrome: causes of death and prognostic factors in a series of 250 patients. Arthritis Rheum 2006; 54(8):2568–76.

35. Espinosa G, Bucciarelli S, Cervera R, et al. Thrombotic microangiopathic haemolytic anaemia and antiphospholipid antibodies. Ann Rheum Dis 2004; 63(6):730–6.

36. Bayraktar UD, Erkan D, Bucciarelli S, et al. The clinical spectrum of catastrophic antiphospholipid syndrome in the absence and presence of lupus. J Rheumatol 2007;34(2):346–52.

37. A pilot study of Rituximab for the Anticoagulation Resistant Manifestations of Antiphospholipid Syndrome (RITAPS). Available at: http://clinical trials.gov/ct2/show/NCT00537290. Accessed March 22, 2010.

38. Ware LB, Matthay MA. The acute respiratory distress syndrome. N Engl J Med 2000;342(18):1334–49.

39. Bucciarelli S, Espinosa G, Asherson RA, et al. The acute respiratory distress syndrome in catastrophic antiphospholipid syndrome: analysis of a series of 47 patients. Ann Rheum Dis 2006;65(1):81–6.

40. Pugin J, Verghese G, Widmer MC, et al. The alveolar space is the site of intense inflammatory and profibrotic reactions in the early phase of acute respiratory distress syndrome. Crit Care Med 1999;27(2): 304–12.

41. Holter JF, Weiland JE, Pacht ER, et al. Protein permeability in the adult respiratory distress syndrome. Loss of size selectivity of the alveolar epithelium. J Clin Invest 1986;78(6):1513–22.

42. Maneta-Peyret L, Kitsiouli E, Lekka M, et al. Autoantibodies to lipids in bronchoalveolar lavage fluid of patients with acute respiratory distress syndrome. Crit Care Med 2001;29(10):1950–4.

43. Nakos G, Kitsiouli E, Maneta-Peyret L, et al. The characteristics of bronchoalveolar lavage from a patient with antiphospholipid syndrome who developed acute respiratory distress syndrome. Clin Rheumatol 2001;20(2):91–7.

44. Gertner E. Diffuse alveolar hemorrhage in the antiphospholipid syndrome: spectrum of disease and treatment. J Rheumatol 1999;26(4):805–7.

45. Asherson RA, Cervera R, Wells AU. Diffuse alveolar hemorrhage: a nonthrombotic antiphospholipid

lung syndrome? Semin Arthritis Rheum 2005;35(3): 138–42.

46. Deane KD, West SG. Antiphospholipid antibodies as a cause of pulmonary capillaritis and diffuse alveolar hemorrhage: a case series and literature review. Semin Arthritis Rheum 2005; 35(3):154–65.

47. Waterer GW, Latham B, Waring JA, et al. Pulmonary capillaritis associated with the antiphospholipid antibody syndrome and rapid response to plasmapheresis. Respirology 1999;4(4):405–8.

48. Mark EJ, Ramirez JF. Pulmonary capillaritis and hemorrhage in patients with systemic vasculitis. Arch Pathol Lab Med 1985;109(5):413–8.

49. Girardi G, Berman J, Redecha P, et al. Complement C5a receptors and neutrophils mediate fetal injury in the antiphospholipid syndrome. J Clin Invest 2003; 112(11):1644–54.

50. Kelion AD, Cockcroft JR, Ritter JM. Antiphospholipid syndrome in a patient with rapidly progressive fibrosing alveolitis. Postgrad Med J 1995;71(834): 233–5.

51. Savin H, Huberman M, Kott E, et al. Fibrosing alveolitis associated with primary antiphospholipid syndrome. Br J Rheumatol 1994;33(10):977–80.

52. Kochenour NK, Branch DW, Rote NS, et al. A new postpartum syndrome associated with antiphospholipid antibodies. Obstet Gynecol 1987;69:460–8.

53. Kupferminc MJ, Lee MJ, Green D, et al. Severe postpartum pulmonary, cardiac, and renal syndrome associated with antiphospholipid antibodies. Obstet Gynecol 1994;83(5 Pt 2):806–7.

Pulmonary Manifestations of Ankylosing Spondylitis

Naveen Kanathur, MD, Teofilo Lee-Chiong, MD*

KEYWORDS
- Ankylosing spondylitis • Apical fibrobullous disease
- Chest wall restriction • Spontaneous pneumothorax

Ankylosing spondylitis is a chronic multisystem inflammatory disorder with articular and extra-articular features. It mainly affects the joints of the axial skeleton.[1–7] Inflammation and arthritic destruction of the costovertebral, apophyseal, and sacroiliac joints result in pain and progressive stiffening of the spine, chest, and pelvis.[2] In addition, ocular, pulmonary, cardiovascular, renal, and neurologic complications have been described. Ankylosing spondylitis can affect the tracheobronchial tree and the pulmonary parenchyma and is associated with several unique pulmonary manifestations, such as chest wall restriction and upper lobe fibrocystic disease.

DEMOGRAPHIC FEATURES

Ankylosing spondylitis is estimated to affect 0.1% of the general population.[8] However, there is significant variability in prevalence, ranging from approximately 2 per 1000 individuals among black South Africans to 63 per 1000 individuals among Canadian Bella Bella Indians.[9] A strong familial pattern has been described with an estimated 10% increased likelihood of the disease identified among first-degree relatives of an affected individual.[3]

The disorder affects men more commonly than women. The male/female ratio has been estimated to range from 10:1[5] to 16:1.[10] Symptoms are also generally milder among women.[5]

PATHOPHYSIOLOGY

Ankylosing spondylitis has been described in persons with amyloidosis, psoriasis, regional enteritis, systemic sclerosis, ulcerative colitis, and urogenital infections. These associations suggest that an inflammatory or immunologic process is responsible for its pathogenesis.[2] It has been proposed that cross reactivity between microbial elements and specific histocompatibility antigens may trigger an altered immune reaction. *Klebsiella*-related antigens have been identified in persons with ankylosing spondylitis.[11]

Most patients possess the HLA-B27 antigen.[2–5] Nearly 90% to 95% of Caucasian patients with ankylosing spondylitis are positive for the HLA-B27 antigen; in contrast, the antigen is present in only 6% to 10% of healthy individuals.[3] Furthermore, the presence of this antigen may increase the risk of ankylosing spondylitis, with about 2% to 20% of affected persons developing the disorder.[5]

CLINICAL FEATURES

Inflammation of the sacroiliac joints is an early manifestation, and patients may present with back pain or morning stiffness. Other joints of the axial skeleton and extremities may eventually be affected also. About 30% of the patients have peripheral joint involvement.[3] Pain on inspiration secondary to limited chest wall expansion and straightening of the lumbar spine can occur.[2]

Department of Medicine, National Jewish Health, 1400 Jackson Street, Denver, CO 80206, USA
* Corresponding author.
E-mail address: lee-chiongt@njhealth.org

Clin Chest Med 31 (2010) 547–554
doi:10.1016/j.ccm.2010.05.002

chestmed.theclinics.com

Ankylosing spondylitis can affect the ocular, cardiovascular, renal, and neurologic systems (**Box 1**). Nongranulomatous anterior uveitis is encountered in approximately 25% of the patients and seems to be more common in those with peripheral joint disease.[3,5,12] Inflammation of the thoracic aorta can result in dilatation of the aortic root. Extension of the inflammatory process to, and below, the aortic valve can lead to aortitis, aortic insufficiency, and various conduction abnormalities.[5] Aortitis and dilatation of the aortic root have been noted in up to 20% to 30% of the affected individuals.[5] Other extraskeletal complications of ankylosing spondylitis include cardiomyopathy, pericarditis and arteritis,[2,5] amyloidosis,[13,14] urethritis, mucosal ulcerations,[10] cauda equina syndrome,[13] and neuropathy secondary to spinal fracture and trauma-related cord injury.[2]

RESPIRATORY MANIFESTATIONS

The presence of pleuropulmonary disease in patients with ankylosing spondylitis was first described by Dunham and Kautz[15] in 1941 and by Hamilton[16] in 1949. Pulmonary involvement in ankylosing spondylitis consists most frequently of abnormalities of the thoracic cage and lung parenchyma.[5,6] In one study, pleuropulmonary involvement was observed in 28 (1.3%) of 2080 patients with ankylosing spondylitis,[17] including 25 cases of apical fibrobullous changes, 2 of pleural effusions, and 1 of apical fibrosis and pleural effusion. Less commonly, significant cricoarytenoid joint disease can manifest with hoarseness, throat soreness, or, if severe, upper airway obstruction and acute respiratory failure.[18,19] A case of squamous cell carcinoma in a patient with pulmonary fibrosis and ankylosing spondylitis has been reported.[20] Lastly, there is an increase in risk of pneumothorax in ankylosing spondylitis.[17]

Chest Wall Restriction

A restrictive ventilatory impairment can develop in patients with ankylosing spondylitis because of either fusion of the costovertebral joints and ankylosis of the thoracic spine[3,5,6] or anterior chest wall involvement. Fournie and colleagues[21] identified enthesitis of the manubriosternal symphysis and sternoclavicular joints in half of 50 patients with ankylosing spondylitis.

Apical Fibrobullous Disease

Ankylosing spondylitis is a common cause of pulmonary apical fibrocystic disease[22]; conversely, upper lobe fibrobullous disease is commonly associated with ankylosing spondylitis, with a prevalence ranging from 1.3% to 30%.[3,4] In one review, this was the most common pulmonary manifestation in ankylosing spondylitis.[17] Apical fibrobullous disease is seen predominantly in men, with a male/female ratio of 50:1.[1] Wolson and Rohwedder[7] found 2 patients with unexplained upper lung zone fibrosis in their study of 52 patients with ankylosing spondylitis. In another study, 14 cases of ankylosing spondylitis with upper lobe changes during a 10-year period were observed.[23] Lastly, Repo and colleagues[24]

Box 1
Extra-articular manifestations of ankylosing spondylitis

Ocular

   Nongranulomatous anterior uveitis

Pulmonary

   Bronchiolitis obliterans

   Bronchocentric granulomatosis

   Bronchogenic carcinoma

   Chest wall restriction

   Cricoarytenoid arthritis

   Pneumothorax

   Upper lobe fibrocystic changes

Cardiovascular

   Aortic valve abnormalities

   Aortitis

   Arteritis

   Cardiomyopathy

   Conduction abnormalities

   Pericarditis

Genitourinary

   Urethritis

   Chronic prostatism

Neurologic

   Neuropathy

   Spinal stenosis

   Cauda equina syndrome

Others

   Amyloidosis

   Mucosal ulcerations

observed that 3 (25%) of their 12 patients with progressive pulmonary apical changes had ankylosing spondylitis.

Early involvement may be unilateral or asymmetrical, but most cases eventually consist of bilateral apical fibrobullous lesions, many of which are progressive with coalescence of the nodules, formation of cysts and cavities, fibrosis, and bronchiectasis. Apical fibrosis, unless extensive or secondarily infected by bacteria or fungi, is typically clinically silent.[3,6] In more advanced disease, cough, sputum production, or dyspnea may develop. Hemoptysis is more likely in those with bronchiectasis or intracavitary mycetoma and can be massive.[5]

Apical fibrobullous disease generally presents in adulthood, with an average interval of 15 years or more between the onset of arthritic manifestations and emergence of pulmonary lesions. This, however, varies greatly, and pulmonary involvement has been described to occur from 6 to 35 years from presentation,[2,4] before any skeletal symptoms,[25] or in asymptomatic persons with early-stage ankylosing spondylitis.[26]

The mechanism responsible for the apical fibrobullous pulmonary changes is unknown. Proposed causes include reduced ventilation in the upper lobes because of chest wall rigidity,[27] altered mechanical stresses in the lung apices,[5,17] repeated pulmonary infections,[16] prior thoracic irradiation,[28] recurrent aspiration pneumonitis secondary to esophageal muscle dysfunction,[29] and airway inflammation.[30]

Apical hypoventilation does not seem to be chiefly responsible for most upper lobe diseases. Although Stewart and colleagues[27] had reported an overall diminution in lung volume using xenon 133 and a reduction in the proportion of inhaled xenon that reached the lung apices in 9 patients with apparently healthy lungs, Parkin and colleagues[31] failed to demonstrate changes in apical ventilation in 27 individuals with ankylosing spondylitis. In addition, impaired cough mechanisms from altered respiratory mechanics and thoracic rigidity as well as repeated aspiration have been proposed to produce fibrotic changes as a result of recurrent infections.[16] However, several investigators have observed that the lungs of patients with ankylosing spondylitis were essentially healthy and that their lungs were infrequently infected.[32,33] The nondependent lung apices are also less likely to be involved during aspiration when compared with the basal and posterior regions of the lung. Finally, thoracic irradiation of the spine and chest wall has been done in the past to treat ankylosing spondylitis and may have produced scarring of the lung parenchyma;

nonetheless, apical changes are also present in those who have not undergone radiation therapy.[28] Patients with ankylosing spondylitis who underwent therapeutic radiotherapy may have an increased risk of developing pulmonary infections and bronchogenic carcinoma.[34] In one retrospective study, thoracic irradiation was associated with 2.5 to 2.9 times greater respiratory complications, including pulmonary tuberculosis and pneumonia.[34]

Pulmonary Superinfection

Mycobacterial or fungal superinfection of the upper lobe cysts and cavities occurs commonly and has been reported in up to one-third of the patients.[4] Rosenow and colleagues[17] reported 7 cases of superinfection in 26 patients with upper lobe fibrobullous disease. *Aspergillus fumigatus* is the most common pathogen isolated, followed by various species of mycobacteria, including *Mycobacterium kansasii*, *Mycobacterium avium*, *Mycobacterium fortuitum*, and *Mycobacterium scrofulaceum*.[1,17,35] Other microorganisms that have been recovered include *Allescheria boydii*, *Aspergillus niger*, *Aspergillus terreus*, *Candida*, *Geotrichosum candida*, and *Metshnikowia pulcherrima*.[3–5,36,37]

Spontaneous Pneumothorax

Apical fibrobullous disease may increase the likelihood of spontaneous pneumothorax. The estimated incidence of spontaneous pneumothorax in patients with ankylosing spondylitis was 0.29%, which was higher than that in the general population.[38] Bilateral pneumothoraces have also been reported in patients with long-standing histories of ankylosing spondylitis.[39] In one large series of 2080 patients with ankylosing spondylitis, 2 patients were incidentally noted to have spontaneous pneumothorax.[17] In another retrospective observational cohort study of 1028 patients with ankylosing spondylitis, 22 patients had typical apical fibrotic changes as observed from chest radiographs and 3 were found to have pneumothorax. None of the 3 patients had chronic obstructive pulmonary disease or chronic lung infections, but they were current smokers. All were slender and had a low body mass index (mean of 18.5 ± 1.6 kg/m^2). Two patients had recurrent pneumothorax and underwent video-assisted thoracoscopic surgery during the second event.[38]

Obstructive Sleep Apnea

Fatigue is a common symptom in patients with ankylosing spondylitis. Erb and colleagues[40] investigated the prevalence of sleep apnea syndrome in an observational study involving 17 patients with ankylosing spondylitis. Two patients (12%) were diagnosed with sleep apnea syndrome and, compared with those without this diagnosis, had higher mean sleepiness scores, higher fatigue component scores on the Bath Ankylosing Spondylitis Disease Activity Index, larger neck circumference, and greater body mass index.

In another study, 7 (22.6%) of 31 patients with ankylosing spondylitis were diagnosed with obstructive sleep apnea by overnight polysomnography. The prevalence of obstructive sleep apnea was 3 times higher in patients with a disease duration of 5 years or more compared with those with a disease duration of less than 5 years. Patients with obstructive sleep apnea were significantly older (43.4 ± 5.7 years vs 33.2 ± 10.6 years) than persons without sleep-disordered breathing, but no other statistically significant difference was noted in other measured parameters, such as mean body mass index, neck circumference, Epworth Sleepiness Scale score, occiput-wall distance, and mean Schober test measures, between the 2 groups.[41]

Several mechanisms might contribute to the development of obstructive sleep apnea in these patients, including restrictive pulmonary disease, obstruction of the oropharyngeal airway because of temporomandibular joint involvement, and compression of the medullary respiratory centers by cervical spinal disease.[40] Given the higher prevalence of obstructive sleep apnea in persons with advanced ankylosing spondylitis, sleep apnea should be considered and polysomnography performed, if indicated, in persons with fatigue, especially in older (35 years of age or more) patients and in those with a disease duration of greater than 5 years.[41]

CLINICAL COURSE

Onset of symptoms is usually insidious and generally starts between 19 and 40 years of age.[2] The disorder is characterized by progressive loss of functional capacity, with most of the impairment occurring in the first decade of the disease.[42] Gran and Skomsvoll[42] conducted a long-term study of 100 patients with this disorder, more than half of whom remained employed in full-time work after a mean disease duration of 16 years. The presence of "bamboo spine," acute anterior uveitis, and nonrheumatic diseases correlated with cessation of work, as did female gender.[42]

Most deaths are caused by respiratory, renal, and cardiac complications. In one report, the causes of death in 79 patients with ankylosing spondylitis were cardiovascular disease (35%), pulmonary tuberculosis (2.5%), respiratory disease (3.8%), uremia from renal amyloidosis (18%), and ankylosing spondylitis itself (29%).[43]

Prognosis of patients with fibrobullous apical lesions is mainly determined by the presence, extent, and severity of superinfection. Smoking negatively affects several measures of disease severity, including the Schober test measures, total spinal movement, occiput-wall distance, functional index, stiffness, and spine radiographic scores, and is associated with worse long-term clinical, functional, and radiographic outcomes.[44]

EVALUATION

Many inflammatory and connective tissue diseases share features in common with ankylosing spondylitis, and laboratory tests may be required to help distinguish them. Patients with ankylosing spondylitis may demonstrate B-lymphocyte reactivity, circulating immune complexes, elevated levels of immunoglobulins, and increased serum levels of alkaline phosphatase and creatine phosphokinase.[45] Bronchoalveolar lavage may be normal and may show no evidence of alveolitis or may reveal increased levels of B lymphocytes and reduced levels of neutrophil granulocytes.[46,47] Sputum cultures for mycobacteria and fungi should be considered whenever pulmonary superinfection is suspected.

Pulmonary Function and Exercise Testing

Pulmonary function test results are nonspecific and generally parallel the severity of parenchymal involvement. Abnormalities in lung function in patients with isolated apical bullous disease are typically mild and are related principally to mobility of the thoracic cage and duration of the disease.[3] Airflow rates are generally within normal limits, vital capacity and total lung capacity are only decreased mildly to moderately, and functional residual capacity and residual volume are either normal or increased.[3] In one study involving 32 patients with ankylosing spondylitis, mean vital capacity was about 88% of the predicted normal values.[48] Reduction in vital capacity, if present, is primarily because of diminished thoracic cage compliance. Lung diffusing capacity is commonly unaffected.[49,50] There may be reductions in maximal expiratory and inspiratory pressures,[51] increased closing volume/vital capacity ratio, reduced volume airway conductance, and decreased maximal elastic recoil pressures.[48]

Severity of pulmonary function abnormalities is related to several factors, including degree of acute inflammation as measured by the erythrocyte sedimentation rate, duration of disease, mobility of the thoracic cage, diaphragmatic contribution to ventilation, extent of thoracic fixation at greater lung volumes, and maintenance of chest wall symmetry and vertical axis of rib excursion.[3,5,6,48]

Exercise tolerance (maximum oxygen capacity, Vo_2max) correlates directly with changes in vital capacity[52] and is typically preserved if vital capacity is only slightly reduced by no greater than 75% of predicted normal values.[53]

Radiographic Features

Radiographic studies commonly demonstrate the presence of bilateral sacroiliitis, formation of syndesmophytes, ossification of the paravertebral ligaments, and loss of lumbar lordosis.[13]

Chest radiographic findings may mirror the severity of clinical involvement; nonetheless, apical nodular or linear infiltrates, upper lobe fibrosis, and pleural thickening may be present in patients without pulmonary complaints.[3,4] Although abnormalities observed from radiographs may initially be unilateral or asymmetric, many patients eventually develop bilateral disease.[4] With unilateral presentation, the right apex is involved more commonly than the left upper lobe.[2] Infiltrates in the lower half of the lung fields are less frequently encountered.[4]

Pulmonary parenchymal disease is typically progressive. Nodules often coalesce into larger opacities,[7] and cyst formation, cavitation, and fibrosis are seen in advanced cases.[4] Severe fibrosis can result in upper lobe bronchiectasis and upward retraction of the hila.[3,5] Chakera and colleagues[54] reviewed the chest radiographs of persons with ankylosing spondylitis and identified the presence of upper lobe fibrosis in 6 (14%) and focal parenchymal changes (upper zone soft nodular opacities or focal linear shadows in the middle and lower zones) in 13 (31%) of 42 patients. Many of these radiographic changes resemble those found in tuberculous lung involvement, and patients with ankylosing spondylitis may be erroneously believed to have tuberculosis. However, Campbell and MacDonald[30] were unable to find any evidence of tuberculosis in their patients with ankylosing spondylitis. In another study, Appelrouth and Gottlieb[13] detected pulmonary changes evident radiographically in 5 of 39 patients with ankylosing spondylitis; these included apical fibrosis (n = 3), cavitary lesions (n = 2), emphysema, basal atelectasis, and carcinoma.

Computed tomography of the chest, particularly high-resolution techniques, is highly sensitive in defining the extent of airway and pulmonary parenchymal changes and in detecting intracavitary pulmonary mycetomas. It is also useful in identifying pleural thickening, volume loss, cavitation, and bronchiectasis.[4,55] Casserly and colleagues[56] studied 26 patients with ankylosing spondylitis using high-resolution computed tomography and noted pulmonary abnormalities in 19 (73%) patients. Findings include interstitial lung disease (n = 4 patients), bronchiectasis (n = 6), emphysema (n = 4), apical fibrosis (n = 2), mycetoma (n = 1), nonspecific interstitial lung disease (n = 12), saber-sheath trachea (n = 2), and mediastinal adenopathy (n = 3). In contrast, plain radiography revealed abnormalities in only 4 patients. The investigators described 3 patient subgroups based on the findings on high-resolution computed tomography. Four patients were believed to have an interstitial lung disease pattern, and these individuals had respiratory symptoms but normal clinical examination results and no evidence of interstitial disease on plain chest radiographs. Fibrosing alveolitis, characterized by subpleural band opacities, thickened interlobular septae, parenchymal bands, and honeycombing, was noted in 3 patients. Ground glass opacification and pulmonary micronodules were additionally noted in a fourth patient. "Nonspecific interstitial changes" were described in 11 patients; these were defined as changes that were of mild severity and that did not qualify as interstitial lung disease. Bronchiectasis was seen in 6 patients, 2 of whom had apical fibrosis.

Similar findings were noted by Turetschek and colleagues,[57] who reported that 15 (71%) of 21 patients had abnormalities on high-resolution computed tomography, and by Souza and colleagues[58] who found evidence of small airway disease with areas of mosaic perfusion, centrilobular nodules, and bronchiolectasis on inspiratory images and air trapping on expiratory images in 10 of 17 patients evaluated by high-resolution computed tomography. Centrilobular emphysema was seen in 6 patients, 2 of whom were lifelong nonsmokers.[57,58]

Pathologic Features

In articular disease related to ankylosing spondylitis, inflammation is characteristically confined to the tissues adjacent to bones, ligaments, and joint capsules.[5] With disease progression, fibrosis, ligamentous calcification, ossification, and syndesmophyte formation develop and produce additional joint destruction.[5]

Histopathologic features of pulmonary disease associated with ankylosing spondylitis can include bronchial dilatation, bronchiectasis, cavitation, collagen degeneration, fibrosis, patchy pneumonia, scarring, and thin-walled bullae formation.[2,4,6,7] Bronchocentric granulomatosis, bronchiolitis obliterans, and organizing pneumonia have been observed in patients with ankylosing spondylitis.[59,60] Infiltration with round cells, fibroblasts, lymphocytes, and plasma cells may be seen as may the presence of hemosiderin-ladened macrophages and foamy histiocytes within irregular spaces.[2,13] Vasculitis and granulomatous disease are typically absent.[5]

THERAPY OF ANKYLOSING SPONDYLITIS

No treatment has been shown to alter the clinical course of apical fibrobullous disease.[1–3,49] Therapy with antiinflammatory agents, such as phenylbutazone or diflunisal, for arthritic symptoms does not improve pulmonary function or halt the progression of the disease. Management of respiratory complications of ankylosing spondylitis is mainly related to treating pulmonary superinfections using antifungal or antibacterial agents, which are either administered systemically or instilled within existing cavities. Nevertheless, medical management of cavitary lesions secondarily infected with *Aspergillus* is often unsuccessful.[3] Surgical excision of fibrocystic disease is rarely indicated except for major hemoptysis because of an aspergilloma. Thoracotomy and lobectomy can be complicated by bronchopleural fistula and chronic empyema in about 50% of the cases.[3]

The risk of spontaneous pneumothorax is greater in patients with ankylosing spondylitis and apical fibrocystic disease, and prophylactic measures to prevent recurrences should be considered after the first episode of pneumothorax.[38]

Anti–tumor necrosis factor α (TNF-α) therapy has been shown to be effective clinically and radiographically in treating ankylosing spondylitis and is considered as a treatment option in patients unresponsive to therapy using nonsteroidal antiinflammatory agents.[61] Although several agents, such as infliximab,[61] etanercept,[62] and adalimumab,[63] are being used to treat this disorder, their effects on pulmonary manifestations are unclear.

Rare, but serious, side effects can occur with the use of anti–TNF-α agents. Increased risk of infection with mycobacterial and fungal pathogens along with common upper respiratory microorganisms has been noted with this therapy.[64] Extrapulmonary tuberculous infection and disseminated disease are more common than mycobacterial infection in the general population. The risk of reactivation tuberculosis seems to be higher with infliximab than with other TNF-α agents.[65] Therefore, screening for latent mycobacterial infection should be performed routinely before starting anti–TNF-α therapy.[66] Finally, development of autoantibodies, such as antinuclear antibodies and anti–double-stranded DNA antibodies, has been reported with anti–TNF-α therapy.[65] Lupus-like syndrome associated with serositis in the form of pleural effusions and sarcoidosis with bilateral hilar adenopathy and nodular lung infiltrates have been described in patients on anti–TNF-α therapy for ankylosing spondylitis.[67,68]

SUMMARY

Several pulmonary disorders have been described in patients with ankylosing spondylitis, and these can be associated with significant morbidity and mortality. Management is mainly aimed at treating pulmonary superinfections. New antiinflammatory agents for arthritic symptoms seem to have no significant effect on the natural course of pulmonary disorders in these patients.

REFERENCES

1. Bulwark DW, Weissman DN, Doll NJ. Pulmonary manifestations of rheumatic diseases. Clin Rev Allergy 1985;3:249–67.
2. Gupta SM, Johnston WH. Apical pulmonary disease in ankylosing spondylitis. N Z Med J 1978;88:186–8.
3. Hunninghake GW, Fauci AS. Pulmonary involvement in the collagen vascular diseases. Am Rev Respir Dis 1979;119:471–503.
4. Rumancik WM, Firooznia H, Davis MS, et al. Fibrobullous disease of the upper lobes: an extraskeletal manifestation of ankylosing spondylitis. J Comput Tomogr 1984;8:225–9.
5. Tanoue LT. Pulmonary involvement in collagen vascular disease: a review of the pulmonary manifestations of the Marfan syndrome, ankylosing spondylitis, Sjogren's syndrome and relapsing polychondritis. J Thorac Imaging 1992;7:62–77.
6. Wiedemann HP, Matthay RA. Pulmonary manifestations of the collagen vascular diseases. Clin Chest Med 1989;10:677–722.
7. Wolson AH, Rohwedder JJ. Upper lobe fibrosis in ankylosing spondylitis. Am J Roentgenol Radium Ther Nucl Med 1975;124:466–71.
8. Calin A, Fries JF. Striking prevalence of ankylosing spondylitis in "healthy" W27 positive males and females. N Engl J Med 1975;293:835–9.
9. Hurwitz SS, Conlan AA, Krige LP. Fibrocavitating pulmonary lesions in ankylosing spondylitis. S Afr Med J 1982;61:168–70.

10. Prakash S, Mehra NK, Bhargava S, et al. Ankylosing spondylitis in North India: a clinical and immunogenetic study. Ann Rheum Dis 1984;43:381–5.

11. Beaulieu AD, Rousseau F, Israel-Assayag E, et al. Klebsiella related antigens in ankylosing spondylitis. J Rheumatol 1983;10:102–5.

12. Blumberg B, Ragan C. The natural history of rheumatoid spondylitis. Medicine 1956;35:1–31.

13. Appelrouth D, Gottlieb NL. Pulmonary manifestations of ankylosing spondylitis. J Rheumatol 1975; 2:446–53.

14. Blavia R, Toda MR, Vidal F, et al. Pulmonary diffuse amyloidosis and ankylosing spondylitis. Chest 1992;102:1608–10.

15. Dunham CL, Kautz FG. Spondylarthritis ankylopoietica. A review and report of twenty cases. Am J Med Sci 1941;201:232–50.

16. Hamilton KA. Pulmonary disease manifestations of ankylosing spondylarthritis. Ann Intern Med 1949; 31:216–27.

17. Rosenow E, Strimlan CV, Muhm JR, et al. Pleuropulmonary manifestations of ankylosing spondylitis. Mayo Clin Proc 1977;52:641–9.

18. Libby DM, Schley WS, Smith JP. Cricoarytenoid arthritis in ankylosing spondylitis. A cause of acute respiratory failure and cor pulmonale. Chest 1981; 80:641–3.

19. Sinclair JR, Mason RA. Ankylosing spondylitis. The case for awake intubation. Anaesthesia 1984;39:3–11.

20. Shankar PS. Ankylosing spondylitis with fibrosis and carcinoma of the lung. CA Cancer J Clin 1982;32: 177–9.

21. Fournie B, Boutes A, Dromer C, et al. Prospective study of anterior chest wall involvement in ankylosing spondylitis and psoriatic arthritis. Rev Rhum Engl Ed 1997;64:22–5.

22. Kentala E, Repo UK, Lehtipuu AL, et al. HLA-antigens and pulmonary upper lobe fibrocystic changes with and without ankylosing spondylitis. Scand J Respir Dis 1978;59:8–12.

23. Hillerdal G. Ankylosing spondylitis lung disease—an underdiagnosed entity? Eur J Respir Dis 1983;64: 437–41.

24. Repo UK, Kentala E, Koistinen J, et al. Pulmonary apical fibrocystic disease. Eur J Respir Dis 1981; 62:46–55.

25. Crompton GK, Cameron SJ, Langlands AO, et al. Pulmonary fibrosis, mimicking tuberculosis, presenting before joint symptoms in a female with ankylosing spondylitis. Tubercle 1973;54:317–20.

26. Ferdoutis M, Bouros D, Meletis G, et al. Diffuse interstitial lung disease as an early manifestation of ankylosing spondylitis. Respiration 1995;62:286–9.

27. Stewart RM, Ridyard JB, Pearson JD. Regional lung function in ankylosing spondylitis. Thorax 1976;31: 433–7.

28. Jessamine AG. Upper lobe fibrosis in ankylosing spondylitis. Can Med Assoc J 1968;98:25–9.

29. Scobie BA. Disturbed oesophageal manometric responses in patients with ankylosing spondylitis and pulmonary aspergilloma. Australas Ann Med 1970;19:131–4.

30. Campbell AH, MacDonald CB. Upper lobe fibrosis associated with ankylosing spondylitis. Br J Dis Chest 1965;59:90–101.

31. Parkin A, Phil D, Robinson PJ, et al. Regional lung ventilation in ankylosing spondylitis. Br J Radiol 1982;55:833–6.

32. Zorab PA. The lungs in ankylosing spondylitis. Q J Med 1962;31:267–80.

33. Hart FD, Emerson PA, Gregg I. Thorax in ankylosing spondylitis. Ann Rheum Dis 1963;22:11–8.

34. Court-Brown WM, Doll R. Mortality from cancer and other causes after radiotherapy for ankylosing spondylitis. Br Med J 1965;2:1327–32.

35. Zizzo G, Castriota-Scanderbeg A, Zarrelli N, et al. Pulmonary aspergillosis complicating ankylosing spondylitis. Radiol Med 1996;91:817–8.

36. Levy H, Hurwitz MD, Strimling M, et al. Ankylosing spondylitis lung disease and Mycobacterium scrofulaceum. Br J Dis Chest 1988;82:84–7.

37. Libshitz HI, Atkinson GW. Pulmonary cystic disease in ankylosing spondylitis: two cases with unusual superinfection. J Can Assoc Radiol 1978;29:266–8.

38. Lee CC, Lee SH, Chang IJ, et al. Spontaneous pneumothorax associated with ankylosing spondylitis. Rheumatology 2005;44:1538–41.

39. Wang CT, Tsen JC, Lin HJ, et al. Bilateral spontaneous pneumothorax in a patient with ankylosing spondylitis. Eur J Emerg Med 2007;14(2):123–4.

40. Erb N, Karokis D, Delamere JP, et al. Obstructive sleep apnea as a cause of fatigue in ankylosing spondylitis. Ann Rheum Dis 2003;62:183–4.

41. Solak O, Fidan F, Dundar U, et al. The prevalence of obstructive sleep apnea syndrome in ankylosing spondylitis patients. Rheumatology 2009; 48:433–5.

42. Gran JT, Skomsvoll JF. The outcome of ankylosing spondylitis: a study of 100 patients. Br J Rheumatol 1997;36:766–71.

43. Lehtinen K. Cause of death in 79 patients with ankylosing spondylitis. Scand J Rheumatol 1980; 9:145–7.

44. Averns HL, Oxtoby J, Taylor HG, et al. Smoking and outcome in ankylosing spondylitis. Scand J Rheumatol 1996;25:138–42.

45. Eghtedari AA, Davis P, Bacon PA. Immunological reactivity in ankylosing spondylitis: circulating immunoblasts, autoantibodies, and immunoglobulins. Ann Rheum Dis 1976;35:155–7.

46. Scherak O, Kolarz G, Popp W, et al. Lung involvement in rheumatoid factor-negative arthritis. Scand J Rheumatol 1993;22:225–8.

47. Wendling D, Dalphin JC, Toson B, et al. Bronchoalveolar lavage in ankylosing spondylitis. Ann Rheum Dis 1990;49:325–6.

48. Feltelius N, Hedenstrom H, Hillerdal G, et al. Pulmonary involvement in ankylosing spondylitis. Ann Rheum Dis 1986;45:736–40.

49. Franssen MJAM, van Herwaarden CLA, van de Putte LBA, et al. Lung function in patients with ankylosing spondylitis. A study of the influence of disease activity and treatment with nonsteroidal anti-inflammatory drugs. J Rheumatol 1986;13:936–40.

50. Van Noord JA, Cauberghs M, Van de Woestijne KP, et al. Total respiratory resistance and reactance in ankylosing spondylitis and kyphoscoliosis. Eur Respir J 1991;4:945–51.

51. Vanderschueren D, Decramer M, van den Daele P, et al. Pulmonary function and maximal transrespiratory pressures in ankylosing spondylitis. Ann Rheum Dis 1989;48:632–5.

52. Fisher LR, Cawley MID, Holgate ST. Relation between chest expansion, pulmonary function, and exercise tolerance in patients with ankylosing spondylitis. Ann Rheum Dis 1990;49:921–5.

53. Elliott CG, Hill TR, Adams TE, et al. Exercise performance of subjects with ankylosing spondylitis and limited chest expansion. Bull Eur Physiopathol Respir 1985;21:363–8.

54. Chakera TMH, Howarth FH, Kendall MJ, et al. The chest radiograph in ankylosing spondylitis. Clin Radiol 1975;26:455–60.

55. Fenlon HM, Casserly I, Sant SM, et al. Plain radiographs and thoracic high-resolution CT in patients with ankylosing spondylitis. AJR Am J Roentgenol 1997;168:1067–72.

56. Casserly IP, Fenlon HM, Breatnach E, et al. Lung findings on high-resolution computed tomography in idiopathic ankylosing spondylitis—correlation with clinical findings, pulmonary function testing and plain radiography. Br J Rheumatol 1997;36:677–82.

57. Turetschek K, Ebner W, Fleischman D, et al. Early pulmonary involvement in ankylosing spondylitis: assessment with thin-section CT. Clin Radiol 2000;55:632–6.

58. Souza AS Jr, Muller NL, Marchiori E, et al. Pulmonary abnormalities in ankylosing spondylitis. J Thorac Imaging 2004;19:259–63.

59. Rhagae PK, Tarrasa BC. Bronchocentric granulomatosis and ankylosing spondylitis. Thorax 1984;39:317–8.

60. Turner JF, Ensnarer RJ. Bronchiolitis obliterans and organizing pneumonia associated with ankylosing spondylitis. Arthritis Rheum 1994;37:1557–9.

61. Braun J, Brandt J, Listing J, et al. Treatment of active ankylosing spondylitis with infliximab: a randomized controlled multicentre trial. Lancet 2002;359:1187–93.

62. Davis JC Jr, Van Der Heijde D, et al. Recombinant human tumor necrosis factor receptor (etanercept) for treating ankylosing spondylitis: a randomized, controlled trial. Arthritis Rheum 2003;48:3230–6.

63. Van Der Heijde D, Schiff MH, Seiper J, et al. Adalimumab effectiveness for the treatment of ankylosing spondylitis is maintained for up to 2 years: long term results from the ATLAS trial. Ann Rheum Dis 2009;68:922–9.

64. Richly DJ, Dipper JT. Infections associated with tumor necrosis factor-α antagonists. Pharmacotherapy 2005;25(9):1181–92.

65. Desai SB, First DE. Problems encountered during anti-tumor necrosis factor therapy. Best Pract Res Clin Rheumatol 2006;20(4):757–90.

66. Carmona L, Gomez-Rein JJ, Rodríguez-Valverde V, et al. Effectiveness of recommendations to prevent reactivation of latent tuberculosis infection in patients treated with tumor necrosis factor antagonists. Arthritis Rheum 2005;52(6):1766–72.

67. Bodur H, Eser F, Konca S, et al. Infliximab-induced lupus-like syndrome in a patient with ankylosing spondylitis. Rheumatol Int 2009;29(4):451–4.

68. Gonzalez-Lopez MA, Blanco R, González-Vela MC, et al. Development of sarcoidosis during etanercept therapy. Arthritis Rheum 2005;55(5):817–20.

Osteoporosis and Bone Health in Patients with Lung Disease

Marcy B. Bolster, MD

KEYWORDS
- Osteoporosis • Bone health
- Lung disease • Glucocorticoids

Osteoporosis is a condition of low bone mass that places a patient at increased risk of fracture. It is clear that a loss of bone mass occurs in women when they become postmenopausal; however, there are many medical conditions and medications that also increase the likelihood of declining bone mass and increasing fracture risk. Recognition of risk factors for osteoporosis is imperative to improve the detection of this systemic disease, and to thus, improve the management of bone health for patients.

EPIDEMIOLOGY

It is estimated that currently there are 10 million Americans older than 50 with osteoporosis. There are an additional 34 million Americans with low bone mass, or osteopenia.[1] The impact on our society from osteoporosis is huge. The impact however does not relate solely to the low bone mass status of this population, but rather to the relationship that low bone mass has to fracture. In 2005, it is estimated that 2 million osteoporosis-related fractures occurred and the associated health care cost of this approximated $17 billion.[2] The most common sites for an osteoporosis-related fracture are the spine, hip, and forearm. The likelihood of a postmenopausal woman experiencing a fracture each year exceeds the likelihood of her developing one of the following commonly occurring diseases: breast cancer, stroke, and cardiovascular disease.[3] It is

recognized that hip and vertebral insufficiency fractures are associated with an increased 5-year mortality rate of approximately 20%.[4] This mortality rate is associated with comorbidities other than the actual fracture, including lung disease, pneumonia, deep venous thrombosis, and other sequelae associated with the increased debilitated state that occurs after a fracture.

Peak bone mass occurs by the age of 30 years. Approximately 90% of bone growth occurs in adolescence. Adequate calcium and vitamin D intake are essential during the time of bone development to achieve maximal bone density. Also important in bone development is weight-bearing exercise. It is known that in postmenopausal women weight-bearing exercise is important to help maintain bone health; however, it is also important in achieving maximal bone density during adolescence and young adulthood.[5]

Osteoporosis occurs most commonly in women, particularly postmenopausal women, with 80% of patients with osteoporosis being female. Other risk factors for the development of osteoporosis include Caucasian or Asian ethnicity, small body stature (low body mass index), tobacco use, alcohol consumption of 3 or more drinks daily, and a positive family history of osteoporosis. There are certain underlying diseases that are also associated with the development of osteoporosis, including a prolonged hyperthyroid state, hyperparathyroidism, hypogonadism, celiac sprue, and inflammatory diseases such as rheumatoid arthritis

Division of Rheumatology and Immunology, Medical University of South Carolina, 96 Jonathan Lucas Street, Suite 912, Charleston, SC 29425, USA
E-mail address: bolsterm@musc.edu

Clin Chest Med 31 (2010) 555–563
doi:10.1016/j.ccm.2010.04.006

(RA) and systemic lupus erythematosus (SLE). Additionally, several medications are associated with accelerated bone loss, and therefore with osteoporosis, including glucocorticoids, aromatase inhibitors, medroxyprogesterone, and anti-epileptic agents. Importantly, vitamin D insufficiency is also associated with the development of osteoporosis and is independently associated with an increased risk for fracture.[6,7]

EVALUATION

The DXA scan (dual x-ray absorptiometry) is the gold standard for the detection of osteoporosis. The conventional DXA scan measures bone density at 2 different sites to increase the likelihood of detecting bone loss: the lumbar spine and bilateral hips. The DXA scan provides information about the bone density (g/cm^2) at the total lumbar spine (L1–L4), the femoral neck, and the total hip. The T-score is the most clinically useful number provided on the DXA scan. The T-score is defined as the standard deviation of the patient's bone mass from peak bone mass in young patients of the same gender. The Z-score represents the standard deviation of the patient's bone mass from persons of the same gender and the same age. Normal bone density is defined by the World Health Organization (WHO) as a T-score more positive than –1.0. A T-score between –1.0 and –2.5 represents osteopenia, and a T-score less than or equal to –2.5 denotes osteoporosis. If there is evidence by DXA scan of osteoporosis at any of the tested sites, then treatment is warranted and the available pharmacologic options should be considered (**Fig. 1**). A Z-score more negative than –2.0 indicates that the patient's bone density is very low compared with persons of his or her own age; thus, a secondary cause for bone loss should be considered (**Box 1**). Importantly, the Z-score should be used for interpreting bone mass in premenopausal women and men younger than 50. Thus, a Z-score more negative than –2.0 indicates low bone mass for age in either of these populations, and consideration for causes of this bone loss should be given. DXA scans are not only useful for the diagnosis of osteopenia and osteoporosis, but also have a role in following a patient for ongoing bone loss and for evaluating a patient's response to therapy.

The FRAX Tool

It is known that a T-score of –2.5 or lower is associated with an increased risk of sustaining a fracture. However, 50% of fractures occur in patients with osteopenia, ie, with a T-score between –1.0 and –2.5.[8] It is thus important to determine which patients may have risk factors that increase the probability of sustaining a fracture. The WHO has developed a tool for fracture risk assessment termed the FRAX (http://www.sheffield.ac.uk/FRAX/reference.htm) that can be applied to patients aged 40 to 90 years who have osteopenia. The FRAX tool is only applicable to those patients with osteopenia who are not receiving osteoporosis medications. The FRAX tool calculates the 10-year probability that the patient will sustain an osteoporosis-related fracture, either at the hip or what is termed a major osteoporotic fracture (hip, spine, humerus, or forearm), and there is a probability threshold beyond which treatment is recommended. The treatment threshold is determined for each country based on the cost:benefit analysis, and for those countries that do not have a calculated threshold, the closest ethnicity should be applied. For the United States, treatment for osteoporosis is recommended for patients who have a 10-year probability of either a major osteoporotic fracture greater than 20% or of a hip fracture

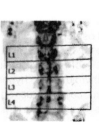

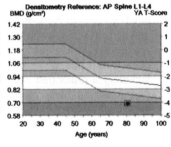

Densitometry Reference: AP Spine L1-L4

Region	BMD (g/cm²)	Young-Adult (%)	Young-Adult T-Score	Age-Matched (%)	Age-Matched Z-Score
L1	0.697	62	-3.6	83	-1.2
L2	0.724	60	-4.0	79	-1.6
L3	0.686	57	-4.3	75	-1.9
L4	0.650	54	-4.6	71	-2.2
L1-L4	0.687	58	-4.1	77	-1.7

Image not for diagnosis

Matched for Age, Weight (females 25-100 kg), Ethnic
NHANES (ages 20-30) / USA (ages 20-40) AP Spine Reference Population (v110)
Statistically 68% of repeat scans fall within 1SD (± 0.010 g/cm² for AP Spine L1-L4)

Fig. 1. DXA scan of the lumbar spine in the 81-year-old woman with osteoporosis pictured in **Fig. 2**. The bone mineral density of L1–L4 is 0.687 g/cm^2 corresponding to a T-score of –4.1 and a Z-score of –1.7. The T-score is consistent with osteoporosis and the Z-score being greater than–2.0 provides information that the bone mineral density is not suggestive of a secondary cause of bone loss.

Box 1
Evaluation for secondary causes of bone loss
Complete metabolic profile (CMP), Phosphorous, Magnesium
Complete blood count
Testosterone (men with osteoporosis)
24-hour urine calcium (and creatinine)
24-hour urine cortisol (and creatinine)
25-hydroxyvitamin D
If low, consider evaluation for celiac sprue
Anti-tissue transglutaminase
Anti-endomysial antibody
Thyroid stimulating hormone (TSH)
Parathyroid hormone (PTH) (and must ensure a normal Vitamin D level)
Erythrocyte sedimentation rate (ESR)
Serum and urine protein electrophoresis (SPEP, UPEP) (if anemia or renal insufficiency)

Box 2
Pharmacotherapy for osteoporosis
Calcium 1200–1500 mg daily in divided doses
Vitamin D3 800–1000 international units daily
Antiresorptive agents
Estrogen
RANK ligand inhibitor
Denosumab
Selective estrogen receptor modulators
Biphosphonates
Alendronate
Risedronate
Ibandronate
Zoledronic acid
Calcitonin
Anabolic agent
Teriparatide

greater than 3%. The tool takes into account body mass index (BMI), gender, age, tobacco use, patient history of an insufficiency fracture, parental history of a hip fracture, glucocorticoid use, patient history of rheumatoid arthritis, 3 or more alcohol-containing beverages daily, and secondary causes of osteoporosis. The calculation is based on the femoral neck bone mineral density. There are several limitations to the FRAX tool including that it does not incorporate the bone density of the lumbar spine, ie, if the T-score of the lumbar spine is –2.1 and that of the femoral neck is –1.1, the calculation incorporates only the information from the higher bone density site for that patient, the femoral neck. Additionally, it does not include such information of family history such as a patient's mother who suffered vertebral insufficiency fractures. Despite its limitations, the FRAX tool provides guidance for the clinician to enhance the ability to treat those patients with low bone mass who may not meet the definition for osteoporosis, but who have a high risk of fracture.

TREATMENT

There are many options available for the treatment of patients with low bone mass or osteoporosis (**Box 2**). The mainstay of therapy for patients to build healthy bone and to maintain good bone health includes calcium and vitamin D supplementation. Patients who have passed the time of peak bone mass, estimated to be about age 30 years, and those of any age on glucocorticoid therapy should receive calcium and vitamin D supplementation. The appropriate dose of calcium supplementation is 1200 to 1500 mg daily in divided doses. Vitamin D supplementation should equal 800 to 1000 international units daily, or a dosage to maintain a serum 25(OH) vitamin D level of 30 ng/mL or higher.

In addition to calcium and vitamin D supplementation, all patients should be encouraged to engage in weight-bearing exercise 3 times weekly if possible. Importantly, fall risk should be minimized to reduce the risk of fracture, and this is also an important feature when considering exercise programs. Reducing the fall risk for a patient may include modification of the home environment to ensure adequate lighting at night, removal of throw rugs, and attention to clutter reduction. Physical therapy offering an osteoporosis program can also provide patients with valuable information on exercises to enhance strength, balance, and mobility, as well as to teach the patient important methods and postures to avoid putting the bones, for example the spine, at risk for fracture.

Pharmacologic therapy includes a choice between several antiresorptive agents and one anabolic agent. Hormone replacement therapy (estrogen) can be considered in a subgroup of patients. It is known that estrogen has a positive effect on maintaining bone mass and has been demonstrated to reduce the risk of hip fracture; however, the coincident cardiovascular and cerebrovascular risks must be weighed against the potential bone benefits.[9]

Selective estrogen receptor modulator agents (SERMs), such as raloxifene, have a positive effect both on bone density and fracture risk reduction; however, the fracture risk reduction is greatest, and statistically significant, at the lumbar spine[10,11] Additionally, raloxifene has been shown to reduce the risk of a woman developing invasive breast cancer.[11]

Pharmacologic therapy also includes the bisphosphonates, potent inhibitors of bone resorption, which are the first line treatment for osteoporosis. Bisphosphonates have been shown to increase the bone mineral density at the hip and lumbar spine, and additionally, to reduce the risk of fracture at both sites.[12] The bisphosphonates currently available include oral agents that may be administered weekly or monthly (alendronate, risedronate, and ibandronate) and the intravenous formulations that are administered quarterly or annually (ibandronate and zoledronic acid, respectively) (see **Box 2**). The bisphosphonates are generally well tolerated. The most common adverse effects of the oral agents include esophageal or gastric irritation manifest as abdominal discomfort, gastroesophageal reflux, or chest pain. The intravenous formulations, ibandronate and zoledronic acid, are indicated for patients who have demonstrated gastrointestinal intolerance to oral bisphosphonates, or who have demonstrated noncompliance with taking the oral medication. Patients may experience bone or muscle pain as a "flulike" illness on the oral agents; however, this is more common following intravenous administration, and perhaps more commonly occurs following zoledronic acid administration. It is evident that premedication with acetaminophen greatly reduces the likelihood of arthralgia, myalgia, and fever following zoledronic acid administration.

Concerns have arisen in the past about the possible causal relationship between bisphosphonates and osteonecrosis of the jaw (ONJ). A large review of cases of ONJ in patients taking bisphosphonates revealed that the vast majority (85%) of patients taking bisphosphonates who experienced ONJ were taking the medication as part of their malignancy treatment (hypercalcemia of malignancy or metastatic disease), and 94% of these patients were receiving intravenous pamidronate or zoledronic acid at higher doses than would be administered to a patient being treated for osteoporosis.[13] Additionally, the risk for ONJ was increased in patients who underwent oral instrumentation or invasive dental procedures. Subsequent studies in patients in clinical trials of zoledronic acid treatment for osteoporosis[14,15] revealed only 1 patient in the treatment group

and 1 patient in the placebo group who developed ONJ; thus, in the management of osteoporosis, it does not appear that zoledronic acid is associated with the development of ONJ. Guidelines have been suggested to have the patient complete invasive oral procedures before initiation of bisphosphonate therapy, particularly intravenous therapy. Because of the very small risk of ONJ developing in patients receiving treatment for osteoporosis, the American Dental Association does not suggest temporary or permanent discontinuation of the bisphosphonate around the time of planned dental work; however, recommends educating patients about the small potential risk and about the importance of routine dental care.[16]

More recent concerns about bisphosphonate use have surfaced with the question of an association between subtrochanteric femur fractures and the prolonged use of alendronate. There have been reports of patients who have taken alendronate for more than 5 years who have sustained an atypical fracture of the femur and thus a link to this medication use has been suggested and/or questioned.[17–19] There is concern that these patients may have had oversuppression of bone turnover owing to prolonged antiresorptive therapy. Others have published that, in fact, subtrochanteric fractures are a rare occurrence in patients with osteoporosis and even in patients with osteoporosis who have received treatment with alendronate.[20,21] The known risk of vertebral and nonvertebral fractures in patients with osteoporosis is significant, and it is not believed that the potential occurrence of these rare fractures should supersede the decision for treatment with bisphosphonates. There may in fact be additional risk factors that predispose certain patients with osteoporosis to experience the atypical femur fractures.[20] It has been suggested that these "atypical fractures" occur in patients with osteoporosis and do not actually occur at a higher rate in patients taking bisphosphonates.[20,21] At the time of this writing the topic remains controversial and further investigation is under way.

The newest anti-resorptive agent is denosumab which is a monoclonal antibody against the receptor activator of nuclear factor-?B ligand (RANKL) which prevents the binding of RANK to RANKL. The RANK/RANKL pathway is important for osteoclast differentiation and function, thus by inhibiting this binding, denosumab inhibits both the differentiation and activity of the osteoclast. Denosumab has been shown in postmenopausal women with osteoporosis to significantly increase bone mineral density and reduce the incidence of new vertebral fractures, hip fractures and non-vertebral fractures.[22] It has been FDA approved for the treatment of postmenopausal osteoporosis in patients who have a high risk of fracture, including those patients with a history of fracture or those with multiple risk factors for fracture, as well as patients who may have failed or are not able to tolerate other medications available for treating osteoporosis. Denosumab is administered twice yearly as a subcutaneous injection by a health care provider. Its side-effects relate to the occurrence of infections which occurred more frequently in the pivotal trial[22] in the denosumab group as compared to the placebo group.

Teriparatide is the only available anabolic agent for the treatment of osteoporosis and it is indicated for treating osteoporosis in men or women at a high risk for fracture. It has been shown to have a particular benefit in patients who have already sustained a greater number or severity of vertebral insufficiency fractures.[23,24] Its efficacy has been demonstrated in patients who have sustained 2 or more prior vertebral compression fractures, and in these patients, teriparatide treatment resulted in a reduction of new vertebral fracture occurrence by 84%. It also reduced the incidence of multiple new vertebral insufficiency fractures by 94%, and in those patients who sustained further vertebral fractures, these were reported to be of a lesser severity.[23] Thus, teriparatide provides an excellent choice for treatment of patients who have had vertebral insufficiency fractures and is also an excellent option for patients who are intolerant of or are not responding to bisphosphonate therapy. Additionally, teriparatide is the agent of choice if a patient sustains a fracture despite bisphosphonate therapy upon confirming compliance with the bisphosphonate, evaluating the patient for secondary causes of bone loss, and determining no contraindications to the use of teriparatide.

HOW ARE WE DOING?

Equally important to the knowledge of medications available for treating osteoporosis is the evaluation of "how we are doing" in providing successful treatment. Osteoporosis is a common disease that is underdiagnosed and undertreated. It is a silent disease and it is thus important to screen for osteoporosis to institute treatment and reduce fracture incidence. However, in addition to the underrecognition of the disease, the treatment of osteoporosis in those patients who have already fractured is, historically, surprisingly low. It has been shown that a low percentage of patients who have had a hip fracture undergo DXA scan evaluation, and, similarly, a low percentage receive pharmacologic treatment. A study in Copenhagen used a national registry and evaluated prescriptions filled by patients who had suffered osteoporosis-related fractures, comparing compliance rates in 1997 to 2004.[25] This study found a low rate of medication prescriptions for both hip and spine fractures. The initiation rate of osteoporosis medication following a hip fracture in women improved from 3.4% to 9.2% between 1997 and 2004. Similarly, there was an improvement in prescriptions for men who had sustained a hip fracture from 0.7% in 1997 to 4.1% in 2004. The Copenhagen study also demonstrated improved treatment initiation of osteoporosis medications after vertebral insufficiency fractures from 1997 to 2004; however, the rate of treatment initiation in men was inferior to women and less than 40% of women were receiving treatment at the 2004 time point. There was a notable improvement in the practice of prescribing, although the prescribing rate remained disappointingly low. Another study, performed in the United States, demonstrated an improvement in prescribing rates within 6 months following hip fracture from 7% to 31% between 1995 and 2002, and this prescribing rate was stable at the conclusion of the study in 2004.[26] Although improved, it is evident that less than one-third of patients were receiving osteoporosis treatment within 6 months of a hip fracture. Thus, in addition to implementing a focus on early detection of osteoporosis, it is also important to ensure pharmacologic treatment for those patients at the highest risk of fracture, including, of course, those patients who have already sustained a fracture.

Glucocorticoid-Induced Osteoporosis

Glucocorticoids are used to treat many inflammatory diseases and pulmonologists comprise one of the specialties most likely to institute glucocorticoid treatment in their patients. Glucocorticoid therapy is a well-documented risk factor for bone loss and occurs because of alterations in bone metabolism including both an increase in bone resorption and a decline in bone formation.[27] The bone loss in a patient taking glucocorticoids occurs early and rapidly. In addition to the rapid loss of bone density that occurs, there is a rapid increase in the risk of fractures with the increase beginning in the first 3 months of glucocorticoid therapy.[28] The greatest early loss of bone occurs in trabecular bone, thus vertebral bone is at a particularly high risk of fracture. It is definitively known that postmenopausal women are at a high risk for bone loss; however, it is clear that men and premenopausal women are also at risk for glucocorticoid-induced osteoporosis. Thus, prophylactic measures should be considered for any patient undergoing treatment with glucocorticoids.

All patients receiving glucocorticoid therapy should receive calcium (1200–1500 mg daily in divided doses) and vitamin D3 supplementation (800–1000 international units daily, or to maintain a serum 25(OH) vitamin D level of 30 ng/mL or higher). A DXA scan is also warranted in a patient taking glucocorticoid therapy to establish a baseline bone mineral density, and follow-up DXA scans to detect ongoing bone loss should be considered at 1- to 2-year intervals. The American College of Rheumatology has delineated guidelines to be used in postmenopausal women and in men taking glucocorticoid therapy such that bisphosphonate treatment should be considered in any patient initiating prednisone (or the prednisone equivalent) of 5 mg or more planned for 3 months or longer.[27] In patients who have been on long-term glucocorticoid therapy, a bisphosphonate should be considered if the patient's T-score on DXA scan is more negative than –1.5.[29] Careful consideration should be given to bisphosphonate therapy use in women of childbearing potential because of the unknown effects of bisphosphonates on the unborn fetus.

More recently, the utility of teriparatide has been investigated for the treatment of glucocorticoid-induced osteoporosis. A study of teriparatide compared with alendronate revealed a significant increase in the bone mineral density of the lumbar spine and of the hip and a significant reduction in vertebral compression fracture occurrence in those patientson glucocorticoids treated with teriparatide.[30,31]

Lung Disease and Bone Loss

Any discussion of lung disease and bone health poses a 2-sided approach. Patients with lung disease are at a high risk for developing osteoporosis, which relates to many factors including but not limited to glucocorticoid therapy. Also, importantly, patients who sustain osteoporosis-related fractures, such as vertebral fragility fractures, are at risk for pulmonary complaints and the development of restrictive lung disease. Additionally, a patient with underlying lung disease who sustains a hip fracture has perioperative pulmonary risks associated with surgical repair of the fracture.

Patients with lung disease, including chronic obstructive pulmonary disease (COPD), asthma, sarcoidosis, or other diseases treated with glucocorticoid therapy, are at a high risk for bone loss, osteoporosis, and fractures. Additionally, patients who undergo organ transplantation, including lung or heart/lung, are treated with chronic glucocorticoid therapy and warrant consideration of their bone health.

The prevalence of osteoporosis in patients with COPD ranges from 9% to 69% in different studies with a mean prevalence of approximately 35%, and this represents a higher occurrence as compared with patients with asthma or healthy control subjects.[32] Risk factors for the development of osteoporosis in patients with COPD include low body mass index (BMI), increased severity of lung disease, tobacco use, and glucocorticoid use.[32,33] Patients with severe underlying lung disease have an increased risk of osteoporosis and of fracture, the etiologies of which are likely multifactorial, and would also include increased immobility. Thus, in patients with COPD it seems that the body habitus, immobility, tobacco use, severity of lung disease, and glucocorticoid therapy are contributing factors to ongoing bone loss and increased risk for osteoporosis-related fractures. In patients with severe COPD (GOLD Stage 3 or 4), contrary to what occurs in the general population, the high incidence of osteoporosis has in fact been shown to be independent of gender or ethnicity. In a multivariate analysis, osteoporosis in this population related solely to % forced vital capacity (FVC) percent predicted. Also unusual was that the incidence of fractures did not differ between men and women, whereas it is known in the general population that fractures in women exceed those in men.[34] Li and colleagues[34] evaluated patients with severe COPD and found that vertebral fractures were the most common fracture site. They also found in this population of 179 patients with severe COPD that low bone mass (osteopenia or osteoporosis) was present in 97% of the patients, yet less than 15% of the patients were receiving either calcium plus vitamin D supplementation or bisphosphonate therapy. It is clear that patients with COPD, particularly those with severe COPD, have many underlying risk factors for osteoporosis and consideration for evaluation and treatment should be broadened to include men as well as women, and patients of all ethnicities. Specific studies to evaluate treatment of osteoporosis in patients with COPD are lacking.[32]

Osteoporosis can be linked not only to tobacco use, low BMI, and glucocorticoids, all known to be significant risk factors for bone loss, but it can also be linked to severity of lung disease as described previously in studies in COPD[32,34] and additionally in patients with pulmonary artery hypertension (PAH)[35] and pretransplantation evaluations of patients with varied underlying lung diseases.[36]

There is good evidence that systemic glucocorticoid therapy is associated with osteoporosis; however, the role that inhaled corticosteroids play in bone loss and fracture risk is more controversial. Certainly, many patients who receive treatment with inhaled corticosteroids have also been exposed to oral prednisone; thus, it is difficult to evaluate the unique role of the inhaled steroids in the measures of bone loss. Scanlon and colleagues[37] found in a group of smokers with COPD treated with inhaled triamcinolone acetonide that there was a significant loss of bone density at the lumbar spine and at the femoral neck at 3 years of follow-up; however, the prevalence of osteoporosis or of fracture did not differ from the control group at this time point. Other studies in patients with asthma have assessed the impact of inhaled corticosteroids on bone density and have found that there may be several important contributing factors, one of which may be menopausal status. Fujita and colleagues[38] found that early postmenopausal women with asthma treated with inhaled corticosteroids had a significant loss of bone density as compared with age- and menopausal status–matched controls and that this decline also differed from premenopausal women with asthma treated similarly. There may be a dose relationship between inhaled corticosteroids and loss of bone mineral density; thus, it is recommended that the lowest possible dose of inhaled steroids be administered, without the use of oral glucocorticoids, to minimize any potential risk of bone loss or of fracture.[39]

Patients with osteoporosis and vertebral insufficiency fractures experience pulmonary effects. The accentuation of the thoracic kyphosis (**Fig. 2**) owing to vertebral insufficiency fractures causes patients to more easily develop dyspnea. These patients also are known to have reduced lung function, specifically a restrictive pattern on pulmonary function tests (PFTs).[40,41] It has been estimated that for every thoracic vertebral compression fracture that a loss of approximately 9% in percent predicted of FVC occurs,[40] thus emphasizing the impairment in lung function that may occur in a patient with little reserve who has COPD and suffers from one or more vertebral insufficiency fracture(s).

Coordination of Care

The first step in the early identification of osteopenia and osteoporosis, and thus in the prevention of fractures and debility, is the consideration of a patient's risk factors for bone loss. A discussion of bone health are appropriate in a patient of any age, and particularly in a patient older than 30 years who has attained peak bone mass. It is important to consider medications used to treat patients and to evaluate if these are contributing to the risk of bone loss and thus to the risk of fracture. Every patient receiving glucocorticoids should receive calcium and vitamin D3 supplementation, unless contraindicated, and consideration for bisphosphonate therapy should also be given. The situation becomes more challenging if the patient receiving osteoporosis therapy suffers a fracture despite therapy. This patient warrants further evaluation to determine if there is a secondary cause for bone loss, such as vitamin D insufficiency, hyperparathyroidism, hypogonadism, or other etiology, or if the patient has had an inadequate response to therapy. In this situation, consideration should be given to referral of the patient to a specialist in osteoporosis. Additionally, treatment with teriparatide has limitations including specific contraindications associated with the Food and Drug Administration's black box warning on the medication (related to the risk of osteosarcoma) and the limitation to the time recommended for its administration (2 years). Patients who warrant treatment with teriparatide also should be considered for referral to an osteoporosis specialist.

There are many challenges to the treatment of osteoporosis. Key to overcoming these challenges

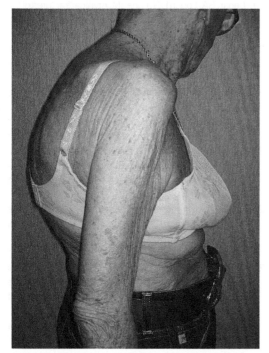

Fig. 2. An 81-year-old woman with osteoporosis and vertebral compression fractures demonstrating an accentuated thoracic kyphosis and reduced distance anteriorly between the lower ribcage and upper pelvis.

includes educating patients about bone health, early identification of patients at risk for osteoporosis, using bone density testing (DXA scan) to detect osteopenia or osteoporosis before a fracture occurs, instituting pharmacologic therapy appropriately, and making modifications to therapy if a patient fractures while taking osteoporosis medications, and appropriate referral to a specialist to achieve enhanced interdisciplinary care. Osteoporosis is a disease that affects many patients, crossing many medical specialties, and thus its evaluation and treatment should also be addressed by any and all of the physicians caring for a patient to optimize the chance of fracture reduction, and in hand, modifying morbidity and mortality.

REFERENCES

1. Services, UDoHaH. Bone health and osteoporosis: a report of the surgeon general. Rockville (MD): Office of the Surgeon General; 2004.
2. Burge R, Dawson-Hughes B, Solomon DH, et al. Incidence and economic burden of osteoporosis-related fractures in the United States. J Bone Miner Res 2007;22:2005–25.
3. Cauley JA, Wampler NS, Barnhart JM, et al. Incidence of fractures compared to cardiovascular disease and breast cancer: the Women's Health Initiative Observational Study. Osteoporos Int 2008; 19(12):1717–23.
4. Cooper C, Atkinson EJ, Jacobsen SJ, et al. Population-based study of survival after osteoporotic fractures. Am J Epidemiol 1993;137:1001–5.
5. Pettersson U, Nordström P, Alfredson H, et al. Effect of high impact activity on bone mass and size in adolescent females: a comparative study between two different types of sports. Calcif Tissue Int 2000;67(3):207–14.
6. Dawson-Hughes B, Heaney RP, Holick MF, et al. Estimates of optimal vitamin D status. Osteoporos Int 2005;16(7):713–6.
7. Bischoff-Ferrari HA, et al. Fracture prevention with vitamin D supplementation: a meta-analysis of randomized controlled trials. JAMA 2005;293(18): 2257–64.
8. Wainwright SA, Marshall LM, Ensrud KE, et al. Hip fracture in women without osteoporosis. J Clin Endocrinol Metab 2005;90:2787–93.
9. Beral V, Reeves G, Banks E. Current evidence about the effect of hormone replacement therapy on the incidence of major conditions in postmenopausal women. BJOG 2005;112(6):692–5.
10. Maricic M, Adachi JD, Sarkar S, et al. Early effects of raloxifene on clinical vertebral fractures at 12 months in postmenopausal women with osteoporosis. Arch Intern Med 2002;162:1140–3.
11. Goldstein SR, Duvernoy CS, Calaf J, et al. Raloxifene use in clinical practice: efficacy and safety. Menopause 2009;16(2):413–21.
12. NIH Consensus Development Panel on Osteoporosis Prevention, Diagosis, and Therapy. JAMA 2001;285:785–95.
13. Woo SB, Hellstein JW, Kalmar JR. Narrative [corrected] review: bisphosphonates and osteonecrosis of the jaws. Ann Intern Med 2006;144(10):753–61.
14. Black DM, Delmas PD, Eastell R, et al. Once-yearly zoledronic acid for treatment of postmenopausal osteoporosis. N Engl J Med 2007;356(18):1809–22.
15. Lyles KW, Colón-Emeric CS, Magaziner JS, et al. Zoledronic acid in reducing clinical fracture and mortality after hip fracture. N Engl J Med 2007;357nihpa40967.
16. Edwards BJ, Hellstein JW, Jacobsen PL, et al. Updated recommendations for managing the care of patients receiving oral bisphosphonate therapy: an advisory statement from the American Dental Association Council on Scientific Affairs. J Am Dent Assoc 2008;139(12):1674–7.
17. Lenart BA, Neviaser AS, Lyman S, et al. Association of low-energy femoral fractures with prolonged bisphosphonate use: a case control study. Osteoporos Int 2009;20(8):1353–62.
18. Neviaser AS, Lane JM, Lenart BA, et al. Low-energy femoral shaft fractures associated with alendronate use. J Orthop Trauma 2008;22(5):346–50.
19. Lenart BA, Lorich DG, Lane JM. Atypical fractures of the femoral diaphysis in postmenopausal women taking alendronate. N Engl J Med 2008;358(12):1304–6.
20. Black DM, Kelly MP, Genant HK, et al. Bisphosphonates and fractures of the subtrochanteric or diaphyseal femur. N Engl J Med 2010;362:1761.
21. Abrahamsen B, Eiken P, Eastell R. Subtrochanteric and diaphyseal femur fractures in patients treated with alendronate: a register-based national cohort study. J Bone Miner Res 2009;24(6):1095–102.
22. Cummings SR, San Martin R, McClung MR, et al. Denosumab for prevention of fractures in postmenopausal women with osteoporosis. N Engl J Med 2009;361:756–65.
23. Prevrhal S, Krege JH, Chen P, et al. Teriparatide vertebral fracture risk reduction determined by quantitative and qualitative radiographic assessment. Curr Med Res Opin 2009;25(4):921–8.
24. Neer RM, Amaud CD, Zanchetta JR, et al. Effect of parathyroid hormone (1–34) on fractures and bone mineral density in postmenopausal women with osteoporosis. N Engl J Med 2001;344(19):1434–41.
25. Roerholt C, Eiken P, Abrahamsen B. Initiation of antiosteoporotic therapy in patients with recent fractures: a nationwide analysis of prescription rates and persistence. Osteoporos Int 2009;20(2):299–307.
26. Cadarette SM, Katz JN, Brookhart MA, et al. Trends in drug prescribing for osteoporosis after hip fracture, 1995–2004. J Rheumatol 2008;35(2):319–26.

27. Osteoporosis, American College of Rheumatology Ad Hoc Committee on Glucocorticoid-Induced Osteoporosis, recommendations for the prevention and treatment of glucocorticoid-induced osteoporosis: 2001 update. Arthritis Rheum 2001;44: 1496–503.

28. Buckley L. In: Maricic M, Gluck OS, editors. Bone disease in rheumatology. Philadelphia: Lippincott Williams & Wilkins; 2005. p. 99–103.

29. Saag KG. Glucocorticoid-induced osteoporosis. Endocrinol Metab Clin North Am 2003;32(1): 135–57, vii.

30. Saag KG, Shane E, Boonen S, et al. Teriparatide or alendronate in glucocorticoid-induced osteoporosis. N Engl J Med 2007;357(20):2028–39.

31. Saag KG, Zanchetta JR, Devogelaer JP, et al. Effects of teriparatide versus alendronate for treating glucocorticoid-induced osteoporosis: thirty-six-month results of a randomized, double-blind, controlled trial. Arthritis Rheum 2009;60(11):3346–55.

32. Graat-Verboom L, Wouters EF, Smeenk FW, et al. Current status of research on osteoporosis in COPD: a systematic review. Eur Respir J 2009; 34(1):209–18.

33. de Vries F, van Staa TP, Bracke MS, et al. Severity of obstructive airway disease and risk of osteoporotic fracture. Eur Respir J 2005;25(5):879–84.

34. Li L, Brennan KJ, Gaughan JP, et al. African Americans and men with severe COPD have a high prevalence of osteoporosis. COPD 2008;5(5):291–7.

35. Tschopp O, Schmid C, Speich R, et al. Pretransplantation bone disease in patients with primary pulmonary hypertension. Chest 2006;129(4):1002–8.

36. Tschopp O, Boehler A, Speich R, et al. Osteoporosis before lung transplantation: association with low body mass index, but not with underlying disease. Am J Transplant 2002;2(2):167–72.

37. Scanlon PD, Connett JE, Wise RA, et al. Loss of bone density with inhaled triamcinolone in Lung Health Study II. Am J Respir Crit Care Med 2004; 170(12):1302–9.

38. Fujita K, Kasayama S, Hashimoto J, et al. Inhaled corticosteroids reduce bone mineral density in early postmenopausal but not premenopausal asthmatic women. J Bone Miner Res 2001;16(4):782–7.

39. Weldon D. The effects of corticosteroids on bone growth and bone density. Ann Allergy Asthma Immunol 2009;103(1):3–11 [quiz: 11–3, 50].

40. Leech JA, Dulberg C, Kellie S, et al. Relationship of lung function to severity of osteoporosis in women. Am Rev Respir Dis 1990;141(1):68–71.

41. Schlaich C, Minne HW, Bruckner T, et al. Reduced pulmonary function in patients with spinal osteoporotic fractures. Osteoporos Int 1998;8(3):261–7.

Toxicity and Monitoring of Immunosuppressive Therapy Used in Systemic Autoimmune Diseases

Keith C. Meyer, MD, MS, FCCP[a],*,
Catherine Decker, PharmD, AE-C[b],
Robert Baughman, MD, FCCP[c]

KEYWORDS

- Immunosuppressive drugs • Adverse drug reactions
- Connective tissue disease • Autoimmunity

In addition to the extrapulmonary disease manifestations and nonpulmonary organ system dysfunction patterns that characterize specific forms of connective tissue disease (CTD), systemic autoimmune disorders frequently involve the lung and can lead to pulmonary fibrosis and/or pulmonary hypertension or vasculitic hemorrhage. Corticosteroids continue to be a mainstay of therapy, especially for acute flares of lung disease. However, other agents may be more effective in achieving remission and stability of the disease and allow corticosteroid dosages to be reduced to low levels, particularly in chronic phases of the disease (**Table 1**).

Corticosteroids and nonsteroidal antiinflammatory drugs (NSAIDs), once primary therapies for many of the systemic autoimmune diseases such as rheumatoid arthritis (RA), were eventually supplanted in the 1980s and 1990s by antimetabolite/cytotoxic agents. These disease-modifying antirheumatic drugs can be steroid-sparing and induce/maintain remission. In the 1990s and beyond, biologic agents have come into widespread use[1] and have revolutionized the treatment of many forms of systemic autoimmune disease. However, all of these agents, nonbiologic and biologic, can cause serious adverse reactions that can be life threatening. Knowledge of their potential toxicities and interactions with other drugs combined with the adoption of a systematic approach to monitoring therapy can minimize the likelihood that a life-threatening reaction occurs.

This article provides an overview of the potential major toxicities (**Table 2**) and drug-drug interactions of the various drugs used to treat systemic autoimmune disorders and recommends an approach to monitoring for adverse reactions to these agents. The article focuses predominantly on antimetabolite/cytotoxic (nonbiologic) and

[a] Section of Allergy, Pulmonary and Critical Care Medicine, Department of Medicine, University of Wisconsin School of Medicine and Public Health, 600 Highland Avenue, Madison, WI 53792, USA
[b] Department of Pharmacy, University of Wisconsin Hospital and Clinics, University of Wisconsin School of Pharmacy, Adult Pulmonary Clinic, 600 Highland Avenue, Madison, WI 53792, USA
[c] Interstitial Lung Disease and Sarcoidosis Clinic, Department of Medicine, University of Cincinnati Medical Center, Eden Avenue & Albert Sabin Way, Cincinnati, OH 45267, USA
* Corresponding author.
E-mail address: kcm@medicine.wisc.edu

Clin Chest Med 31 (2010) 565–588
doi:10.1016/j.ccm.2010.05.006
0272-5231/10/$ – see front matter © 2010 Elsevier Inc. All rights reserved.

Table 1
Summary of mechanism of action, routes of administration, and metabolism

Drug Class	Specific Drug	Mechanism of Action	Route of Administration			Metabolism and Elimination
			IV	Oral	Other	
Corticosteroid	Prednisone or methylprednisolone	• Glucocorticoid analog; suppresses inflammatory mediator production and immune effector cells • Promotes T-lymphocyte apoptosis	+	+		• Prednisone converted to active form of drug (prenisolone) • Excreted in the urine
Anti-TNF Agents	Adalimumab	• Monoclonal antibody that binds TNF-α • Blocks interaction of TNF-α with p55 and p75 cell surface receptors			SC	• Systemic clearance ~ 12 ml/h • Terminal half-life ~ 2 weeks. • No kinetic info for renal/hepatic disorder
	Etanercept	• Soluble form of p75 TNF receptor; inhibits binding of TNF-α and TNF-β to cell surface receptors • Modulates adhesion molecules expression			SC	• Speculated to be metabolized through the RES system
	Infliximab	• Monoclonal antibody that binds TNF-α • Blocks interaction of TNF-α with p55 and p75 cell surface receptors	+			• Elimination by unspecified proteases (?) • Systemic clearance ~11ml/h • Linear pharmacokinetics are suspected
Antimetabolite/ Cytotoxic Agents	AZA	• Antagonizes purine metabolism and may inhibit synthesis of DNA, RNA and proteins; interferes with cellular metabolism and mitosis	+	+		• Metabolism by systemic and hepatic routes • Elimination via systemic, hepatic, and renal pathways
	Cyclophosphamide	• Nitrogen mustardlike alkylating agent • Cross-links DNA and RNA strands, thus inhibiting cell functions and protein synthesis	+	+		• Metabolized extensively by liver • Renal (5%–25% unchanged in urine) and systemic elimination
	Leflunomide	• Inhibits dihydroorotate dehydrogenase • May inhibit T-cell pyrimidine biosynthesis		+		• Metabolized by liver and gut wall • Undergoes enterohepatic recirculation • Eliminated renally and via total body clearance
	MTX	• Reversible inhibition of dihydrofolate reductase	+	+	SC IM	• Metabolized via liver, intracellular metabolism, and gut. • Excreted via kidneys, bile and feces
	MPA derivatives	• Blockade of de novo guanosine nucleotide synthesis impairs NA synthesis and inhibits T- and B-lymphocyte proliferative responses	+	+		• Extensive liver metabolism • Eliminated via the kidney
Other	Chloroquines	• Antimalarial agents • Immunosuppressant mechanism unclear		+		• Metabolized by liver • Eliminated primarily via kidney
	Imatinib mesylate	• Protein-tyrosine kinase inhibitor		+		• Metabolized by liver P-450 enzymes (CYP3A4, CYP1A2, CYP2D6, CYP2C9, and CYP2C19) • Eliminated via feces (68%) and kidney (13%)
	Rituximab	• Promotes B-cell lysis by binding to CD-20 antigen on B lymphocytes	+			• Excretion pathway is uncertain • May undergo phagocytosis and catabolism via RES

Abbreviations: IM, intramuscular; NA, nucleic acid; RES, reticuloendothelial system; SC, subcutaneous; TNF, tumor necrosis factor.

Table 2
Adverse drug reactions (ADR) associated with immunosuppressant agent administration

Drug Class	Specific Drug	Injection Site/Infusion Reactions	Infection	Bone-marrow Suppression	Neurologic Effects	GI Effects	Hepatic Effects	Renal/Genitourinary Effects	Cardio-vascular Effects	Dyslipidemia	Malignancy	Pulmonary Toxicity	Ocular Toxicity	Skin Reactions/Rash
Corticosteroids	Prednisone Methylprednisolone		+	+	±	+		?	±	±	?		+	+
Anti-TNF agents	Adalimumab	+	+	±	+	±	±	+	+	+	?	±	?	+
	Etanercept	+	+	±	+	+	±		?	+	?	±	?	+
	Infliximab	±	+	±	±	±	±	?	+		?	±	±	+
Antimetabolite/ cytotoxic agents	AZA	?	+	+	?	++	++	?	?		+	+	?	±
	Cyclophosphamide	?	+	++		+	±	++	+		+	+	±	+
	Leflunomide	NA	+	+	+	+	+		++				?	+
	MTX	?	+	+	+	++	++	+	+		?	+	+	+
	MPA derivatives		+	+	+	+	+	++	++	++	?	+	+	+
Other agents	Chloroquine/ hydroxychloroquine		+	?	+	+	+		+				+	+
	Imatinib mesylate	NA	+	+	+	+	+	+	+			+	++	+
	Rituximab	+	+	±	+	++	±	±	+			+	?	+

Abbreviations: Bblank, no medication-associated ADR reported; NA, not applicable; ±, ADR suspected to be associated with medication use, yet is infrequent; +, ADR associated with medication use exists ; ++, ADR associated with medication use exists and is noted in greater frequency than +; ?, unknown association of ADR with medication use.

biologic (immunomodulatory/antibody-based) agents.

SPECIFIC AGENTS
Corticosteroids

Systemic corticosteroids are valuable in treating acute disease but may have serious side effects.[2] A myriad of complications (**Box 1**) may and often do occur when high doses and/or prolonged therapy with corticosteroids are prescribed. Some of these complications can be controlled and even prevented, such as fluid retention and weight gain. Steroid-sparing agents may allow control of disease processes and thereby minimize systemic corticosteroid administration and associated adverse effects. Patients should be educated about potential side effects and informed of strategies that may limit some of the adverse effects of corticosteroids. In addition, patients should be monitored for the onset of systemic hypertension, excessive weight gain/fluid retention, gastrointestinal (GI) symptoms, increased blood glucose, osteoporosis, hip pain, and dyslipidemia (**Table 3**). A diet and regular aerobic exercise that diminishes risk for heart disease should be followed along with periodic monitoring of a peripheral blood lipid profile. A bone mineral density scan should be obtained at baseline and at subsequent periodic intervals,

---

Box 1
Complications of corticosteroid therapy

Osteopenia/osteoporosis

Systemic hypertension

Weight gain

Glucose intolerance/diabetes

Dyslipidemia

Accelerated atherosclerosis

Myopathy

Infection

Avascular necrosis of bone

Cataracts

Glaucoma

Atrophy of skin

Adverse psychological effects

Disrupted sleep

Growth retardation

Cushingoid changes

Dyspepsia

---

and vitamin D levels should be obtained (and testosterone levels in men). Vitamin D and supplemental calcium should be given if indicated.

BIOLOGIC AGENTS
Antitumor Necrosis Factor Agents

Biologic agents directed against tumor necrosis factor α (TNF-α) have proved successful in treating various manifestations of RA. These include the TNF receptor antagonist etanercept[3] as well as the chimeric, humanized monoclonal anti-TNF antibody infliximab[4] and the humanized monoclonal antibodies adalimumab[5] and golimumab.[6] Etanercept is a soluble, fully human recombinant form of the p75 tumor necrosis factor receptor fused with the Fc portion of IgG$_1$. In contrast to the anti-TNF antibodies, etanercept acts by binding to endogenous-soluble and membrane-bound TNF, thereby preventing its interaction with TNF receptors and rendering it biologically inactive.[7] In addition to treatment of RA, anti-TNF antibodies also have regulatory approval for the treatment of psoriasis, ankylosing spondylitis, ulcerative colitis, and Crohn disease.[8]

In the past 10 years, anti-TNF agents have been given to more than a million patients, and several guidelines for monitoring their use have been proposed.[9–11] Potential toxicities linked to the administration of these drugs include infection, infusion or injection reactions, worsened congestive heart failure (CHF), demyelination syndromes, lupus-like reactions, and increased risk of malignancy.[12–16]

Infliximab

An estimated 2-fold risk of infection is the most common adverse event associated with infliximab use.[17,18] Most upper respiratory tract or urinary tract infections have not been serious, but case-controlled studies have suggested an increased incidence of opportunistic infections.[17] Although no prospective, randomized data exist, some reports have suggested that the risk of developing tuberculosis may be greater with infliximab than with other anti-TNF agents,[19–21] and tuberculosis infections are also more likely to be extrapulmonary.[19,21,22]

Existent data are not sufficient to determine if lymphoma or nonlymphomatous malignancies are increased.[17] Hepatosplenic T-cell lymphomas have been reported in rare postmarketing reports, particularly in adolescent[23] and young adult patients with Crohn disease,[24] and have exclusively occurred in patients concomitantly treated with azathioprine (AZA) or 6-mercaptopurine.

Table 3
Summary of monitoring precautions

Drug Class	Specific Drug	Recommended Precautions and Monitoring
Corticosteroids	Methylprednisolone Prednisone	• Assess diabetes risk, blood glucose, BMD at baseline • Periodically monitor: blood glucose, blood pressure, body weight, BMD, weight, muscle strength (proximal), mental status
Anti-TNF agents	Adalimumab Etanercept Infliximab	• Assess tuberculosis risk; tuberculin skin test and chest radiograph before therapy • Avoid use during active infection (eg, viral hepatitis) • Hepatitis serology before therapy if increased risk of infection; monitor for viral hepatitis reactivation in patients with history of viral hepatitis or chronic carrier state
Antimetabolite/ cytotoxic agents	AZA Cyclophosphamide Leflunomide MTX MPA derivatives	• Dose reduction (eg, 25%–35%) if coadministered with allopurinol • Monitor CBC with platelets and hepatic function • CBC with platelets and differential cell count at baseline • Monitor CBC, renal function, and urinalysis at least twice monthly • Increase fluid intake on the day of therapy (eg, 2 L per 24 h) • If hematuria occurs, evaluate for cause • Screen for use of alcohol and viral hepatitis before onset of therapy • Perform periodic assessment of CBC and liver function • Screen for use of alcohol and viral hepatitis before onset of therapy • Provide folic acid supplementation • Perform periodic assessment of CBC (eg, monthly) and liver function (eg, every 1–2 months) • Monitor CBC periodically • Monitor for gastrointestinal toxicity and neurotoxicity • Avoid concomitant use of AZA
Other agents	Chloroquine/ hydroxychloroquine Imatinib mesylate Rituximab	• Monitor for ocular toxicity every 6–12 months • Periodic therapy during prolonged therapy • CBC weekly for first month of therapy; biweekly for second month, then periodically • Liver function at baseline and at subsequent monthly intervals • Monitor for infusion reactions (eg, cardiac rhythm disturbance) • Monitor CBC and liver function

Caution has been recommended in treating patients with a previous history of malignancy.[25]

A large, placebo-controlled trial of infliximab (5–10 mg/kg) in New York Heart Classification III or IV heart failure (ATTACH trial) showed no benefit, and the risk of all-cause death or hospitalization for heart failure was increased in patients treated with infliximab (10 mg/kg).[26] In addition, numerous postmarketing reports have described worsening heart failure during therapy.[17] Recent reports suggest that infliximab therapy can alter plasma lipids with increases in total cholesterol and high-density lipoprotein,[27,28] but the potential effect of infliximab therapy on atherogenesis is not clear.

Central nervous system events, including demyelination disorders, have been reported sporadically with TNF inhibitors.[16,17,29] Rare cases of systemic lupus erythematosus-like syndromes have been reported with anti-TNF therapy and generally resolved within 6 weeks to 14 months of discontinuation.[25] In addition, hematological side effects such as leukopenia, neutropenia, thrombocytopenia, and pancytopenia have been occasionally reported.[17] Severe hepatic reactions have also been reported, and infliximab has been associated with reactivation of hepatitis B virus infection.[24,30]

Adalimumab

As with infliximab, adalimumab administration has been associated with increased infection risk, especially tuberculosis,[31] and serious infections have been associated with the use of adalimumab.[32,33] However, the rate of serious infection was not statistically different from that encountered in the comparator groups in 2 different trials.[34,35] Adalimumab has been associated with a cluster of cases of Legionella pneumophila pneumonia,[36] and Pneumocystis jiroveci pneumonia occurred in a patient receiving adalimumab.[37]

Autoimmune disease seems to be induced by anti-TNF agents.[13] In a detailed analysis of a large cohort of cases, 15 of 92 cases of a lupuslike reaction were treated with adalimumab[13] and vasculitis was in reported in 113 patients, 5 of whom were treated with adalimumab. Nervous system events, including demyelination disorders, have been sporadically reported in patients treated with adalimumab.[17,38]

Etanercept

Serious injection site reactions can occur, and injection site-associated necrotizing fasciitis has been reported.[39] Reactivation of latent tuberculosis has been associated with TNF inhibitors,[40] but it is not clear whether etanercept therapy increases the risk more than the already increased risk of reactivation tuberculosis for patients with RA.[41] In the available case series, infection with tuberculosis was extrapulmonary in half the cases, suggesting that etanercept does have a role in inhibiting control of this organism.[41] However, the soluble TNF fusion receptors, which include etanercept, seem to be associated with less risk of reactivation TB than the monoclonal TNF antagonists, infliximab and adalimumab.[41] It is not clear whether etanercept has adverse effects if given to patients with CHF, but there have been case reports of de novo cardiac failure or worsening of preexisting cardiac dysfunction in patients treated with etanercept.[42] Sarcoidosislike reactions have been reported, and seem to occur more frequently with etanercept than with other anti-TNF agents.[43]

Non-Hodgkin lymphomas have been reported in patients treated with etanercept, including several in whom the lymphoma regressed following cessation of the drug.[44,45] However, the baseline incidence of lymphoma is increased in individuals with the chronic inflammatory diseases that are treated with etanercept. In addition, a large study on patients with RA did not show a statistically significant increased incidence of lymphoma in individuals who received etanercept.[46] Demyelination syndromes have not been clearly linked to etanercept.

Monitoring therapy with anti-TNF agents

Early observations of the association of anti-TNF therapy and tuberculosis infection noted that patients receiving infliximab had a higher risk than those receiving etanercept. Most cases appeared to be reactivated latent tuberculosis rather than new infection.[20,47] These observations led to an intense effort to screen for latent tuberculosis, and this screening effort has been successful in reducing the rate of active tuberculosis in patients receiving anti-TNF therapy. In one registry of 5198 patients treated with a TNF antagonist, 15 cases of active tuberculosis were noted. The calculated rate of active tuberculosis was 172 per 100,000 patient-years.[48] Recommendations for monitoring were fully followed in about half of the patients in this study, and the risk for developing active tuberculosis was 7 times higher for those who did not undergo the proposed monitoring. The most common reason for failing to comply with the recommendations was the failure to perform a tuberculin skin test.[48] Although these results support the value of a tuberculin skin test to detect latent tuberculosis, patients receiving immunosuppressive drugs may become anergic. Antigen-specific testing for M tuberculosis via an interferon-γ immunogold enzyme-linked immunosorbent assay test has been developed, and these tests were more specific and sensitive than routine tuberculin skin testing in immunocompromised patients.[49]

Routine blood chemistries should be obtained before the onset of therapy, and a careful history should be taken, with a focus on risk factors for tuberculosis. A chest roentgenograph and skin testing with purified protein derivative should be obtained in all patients, and immunogold testing should be considered for immunocompromised patients. If the testing is positive, alternative therapies should be considered. If anti-TNF agents are administered to positive patients, treatment of latent TB should commence before initiation of therapy. We also recommend screening for chronic hepatitis B infection before initiating therapy, and any neurologic symptoms should raise concern about a possible demyelination syndrome. The administration of live viruses should be avoided.

Other Biologic Agents

Rituximab

Rituximab is a humanized murine antibody to the membrane-bound cell surface CD-20 glycoprotein on B lymphocytes. Rituximab is administered intravenously and has regulatory approval for the treatment of CD-20-positive non-Hodgkin lymphomas and refractory RA, and it has also been used to treat antineutrophil cytoplasmic antibody (ANCA)-associated vasculitis. Antibody responses to recall antigens are dramatically lower in patients treated with rituximab.[50]

Fatal infusion reactions have been reported but primarily occur with the initial infusion.[51,52] Serum sickness has been reported with rituximab treatment in a variety of autoimmune diseases.[53–56] In addition, progressive multifocal leukoencephalopathy, a rare, demyelinating disease of the central nervous system that results from reactivation of latent Jakob-Creutzfeldt virus, has been linked to rituximab therapy in patients with malignancy as well as patients with RA.[57,58] Interstitial pneumonitis has been reported in several patients with non-Hodgkin lymphoma.[59–61] Recovery of lung function has been reported with ceasing rituximab treatment and administering corticosteroids,[59] but fatal cases have been reported.[60,61] Frequent monitoring of vital signs during infusions may be prudent, and clinicians should be vigilant for signs of new infection, reactivation of latent infections, and bowel perforation.[62]

ANTIMETABOLITE/CYTOTOXIC AGENTS

AZA

AZA is a purine analog that is cleaved in vivo to its active antimetabolite, 6-mercaptopurine. Its mechanisms of action remain unclear, but it suppresses delayed hypersensitivity responses and cell-mediated cytotoxicity via its effects on purine metabolism, which likely inhibit DNA and RNA synthesis, and, consequently, protein synthesis.[63] Recent investigations suggest that AZA and its metabolites induce T-cell apoptosis by binding to the guanidine triphosphatase, Rac1.[64] AZA and mercaptopurine are degraded in erythrocytes and the liver via oxidation or methylation. Mercaptopurine undergoes thiol methylation intracellularly via thiopurine methyltransferase (TPMT), which converts it to thiopurine analogs. Deficiency of this enzyme occurs in approximately 1 in 300 individuals and may lead to severe myelosuppression.[65] Intermediate concentrations of TPMT have been linked to severe side effects related to AZA, and measuring TPMT activity

before initiating AZA therapy has been suggested to reduce the likelihood of serious side effects.[66]

Common adverse reactions associated with AZA include leucopenia,[67] pancreatitis,[68] and hepatitis.[69] Thrombocytopenia, anemia, megaloblastic anemia, aplastic anemia, eosinophilia, myelodysplastic syndrome, and fatal acute myeloid leukemia have also been reported.[67,70–72] The incidence of hepatitis or pancreatitis for patients receiving AZA for Crohn disease has been reported to range from 4% to 17% for both side effects independently,[73–75] and AZA treatments were discontinued in approximately 10% to 20% of patients because of side effects.[67,75] Other adverse reactions that have been linked to AZA include skin rash, alopecia, nausea, vomiting, hypersensitivity reactions, muscle weakness, and interstitial pneumonitis/fibrosis. In addition, risk for lymphoma, skin cancer, and infection may be increased.

Concomitant administration of allopurinol can greatly increase the effect of AZA and the risk of associated toxicities.[76] The use of angiotensin-converting enzyme inhibitors with AZA has been associated with myelosuppression,[77] and patients receiving AZA may be at increased risk of infection from administration of live virus vaccines. Inhibitors of TPMT (eg, mesalamine) can considerably increase the risk of myelosuppression and should be avoided. Similarly, coadministration of other inhibitors of purine metabolism (eg, mycophenolate) is not recommended, and concomitant administration of other potentially hepatotoxic agents, such as methotrexate (MTX), should also be avoided. Monitoring of complete blood counts (CBCs) has been recommended every 2 weeks for the first 4 weeks and then monthly thereafter.[78] Similarly, liver function testing has been recommended every 2 weeks for the first 4 weeks and then monthly.[78]

Cyclophosphamide

Cyclophosphamide (CYC), a synthetic alkylating agent, is chemically related to the nitrogen mustards and was originally developed for treatment of malignant tumors. It has antineoplastic and immunosuppressive properties and has received regulatory approval for the treatment of various hematologic and nonhematologic malignancies. It has a dose-dependent, bimodal effect on the immune system. High doses have been shown to induce an antiinflammatory immune deviation (ie, suppression of TH1 and enhancement of TH2 lymphocyte activity), affect CD4CD25(high) regulatory T cells, and establish a state of marked immunosuppression.[79] It has been used to treat various CTD-associated lung diseases such as scleroderma[80,81] and other forms of interstitial lung disease (ILD).[82,83] It has also been used as a standard treatment of ANCA-associated vasculitis.[84]

CYC is metabolized in the kidney and liver. The liver converts CYC to the active metabolites aldophosphamide and phosphoramide mustard, which cause cell death by binding DNA and thereby inhibiting DNA replication. CYC and its metabolites are excreted via the kidney. CYC can be administered via either continuous daily dosage (oral) or intermittent intravenous (IV) pulse therapy. For several conditions, which include ANCA-associated vasculitis[84,85] and scleroderma-associated lung disease,[80,81] the pulse therapy seems to be as effective as and less toxic than daily oral regimens. One of the disadvantages of IV pulse therapy is the associated cost and need for support staff to administer IV CYC. One of the advantages of pulse therapy is that individual doses of the drug can be adjusted based on the patient's individual white blood cell (WBC) count. In one study, dosage adjustments were made in almost one-third of visits.[83] Regardless of the method of administration (IV vs oral), the same guidelines for monitoring apply.

Hemorrhagic cystitis and fibrosis of the urinary bladder can occur, and hematuria frequently occurs. Although hemorrhagic cystitis is an infrequent complication, it can be severe and life threatening. Bladder toxicity likely occurs from the CYC parent compound and several CYC metabolites including acrolein. Measures that are recommended to limit hemorrhagic cystitis include ingesting more than 3 L of water or other fluids daily. Sodium 2-sulfanylethanesulfonate (MESNA) binds acrolein and some other CYC metabolites in the urinary bladder and can attenuate toxicity.[81] A large, prospective study of patients with Wegener granulomatosis reported that hematuria occurred in a time- and dose-dependent manner.[86] Of 145 patients studied, 73 (50%) developed nonglomerular hematuria, 7 of whom had bladder cancer. Hematuria occurred a median of 37 months after initiating CYC. Overall, 15% of the patients developed hematuria within the first year of treatment. In the placebo-controlled trial of oral CYC versus placebo for scleroderma-associated lung disease, 9 of the CYC-treated patients developed hematuria versus 3 of the placebo group.[80]

Bladder cancer is increased in individuals who have received CYC, and cigarette smoking further increases risk. Bladder cancer is also increased in frequency in CYC-treated patients who have had hemorrhagic cystitis.[86] Bladder cancer seems to be dose and duration dependent, with at least a 2-fold increased risk occurring with each 10 g of cumulative drug exposure,[87] and further increases occur over time after a total dose of 20 g.[86] Cancers have been known to occur many years following CYC cessation. Bladder cancer screening with urinalysis seems to be sufficient to detect cancer as long as subjects with hematuria receive additional evaluation.[86]

CYC may cause major bone-marrow suppression, including leukopenia, anemia, and/or thrombocytopenia. Leukopenia is a dose-related complication of the drug and can occur even with lower drug doses.[88] In a randomized trial comparing oral CYC versus placebo for scleroderma-associated pulmonary fibrosis, 19 of 79 (24%) of CYC-treated patients developed leukopenia and 7 (9%) had neutropenia during the year of CYC therapy, whereas none of the patients given placebo had any form of leukopenia.[80] Anemia was more common with CYC, but the difference from placebo was not significant. These rates are higher than those reported for intermittent IV CYC.[81,83,84,89,90]

Lymphomas, leukemias, skin cancers, and probably other solid-organ malignancies are likely increased in frequency in individuals receiving CYC.[91] In a retrospective study of long-term follow-up of patients with Wegener granulomatosis treated with CYC, increased cancer incidence was seen for squamous cell skin cancer (odds ratio [OR] = 7.3; 95% confidence interval [CI] 4.4–12), leukemias (OR = 5.7; 95% CI 2.3–12) and for malignant lymphomas (OR = 4.2; 95% CI 4.2–8.3).[92] Many such studies are complicated by some increase in cancer incidence with the baseline disease state. In a Swedish registry study of scleroderma, no increase in malignancy was seen in 246 patients comparing CYC users with those treated with other medications and followed for up to 13 years.[93] In a prospective 15-year evaluation of 726 lung patients with lung cancer treated with busulfan, CYC, or placebo, no additional malignancies were seen in the CYC arm above the placebo rate.[94]

CHF, hemopericardium, and hemorrhagic myocarditis have been seen after high doses of CYC. These side effects usually resolve after stopping therapy. Alopecia is common and hair may return with a different texture or color. Skin rashes may be seen and rare cases of toxic epidermal necrolysis have been seen. The frequency of bacterial, fungal, viral, and protozoan infections are increased on CYC. There is no consensus that prophylaxis for any of these infections is necessary in patients receiving CYC, although some case series have used prophylaxis for pneumocystis jerocomia.

Lung fibrosis has been a consistent finding in animal studies of CYC use.[95,96] However, the frequency of this complication in humans has been difficult to define in part because of the presence of confounding variables such as concomitant use of other cytotoxic drugs, opportunistic infections, diffuse pulmonary malignancy, radiation pneumonitis, and oxygen toxicity. Therefore, the literature is limited to case reports and small case series[97] that suggest drug withdrawal with or without corticosteroids usually resolves early manifestations of this side effect. A large prospective study in which 192 patients received CYC failed to find any case of lung fibrosis in 5 years using chest radiography.[98]

A CBC with platelets should be monitored frequently (at least every 2 weeks at initiation of therapy) and is the most reproducible method available for CYC dose adjustment. WBC count should be kept greater than 2000 cells/mm^3 and higher WBC counts (eg, >4000 cells/mm^3) decrease the incidence of infectious complications. A urinalysis to evaluate for microscopic hematuria should be obtained monthly beginning before initiation of therapy. Although hemorrhagic cystitis is an infrequent complication, it can be severe and life threatening and carries an increased risk of bladder cancer. Because these side effects are dose and time dependent, intermittent monitoring of urinalysis at least every 3 months is recommended. This complication is decreased by fluid intake that should consist of a 3-L minimum daily. If hemorrhagic cystitis has occurred or a greater than 10 g cumulative dose of CYC has occurred, urinalysis should be obtained yearly and microscopic hematuria evaluated with more comprehensive testing. Because CYC therapy, particularly if sustained over long periods, increases risk of developing urothelial tumors, urine cytology could be performed on a yearly basis to facilitate early detection of bladder cancer.

MTX

MTX is approved in the United States for treatment of RA, psoriasis, and several malignancies. It has also been used to treat pulmonary sarcoidosis,[99,100] and for induction and maintenance therapy for Wegener granulomatosis[101,102] and for ILD associated with polymyositis-dermatomyositis.[103]

MTX is converted to polyglutamates in the liver, and polyglutamate-mediated inhibition of extracellular adenosine metabolism is believed to account for its immunosuppressive effects.[104,105] The plasma half-life of MTX is only 8 to 15 hours, but its immunosuppressive actions can be measured in peripheral blood cells ex vivo for up to 1 week. Adenosine receptor antagonists (eg, caffeine and theophylline) have been shown to inhibit the antiinflammatory effect of MTX in animal models.[106]

Major toxicities attributed to MTX include liver damage, pneumonitis, and cytopenias. Nausea, diarrhea, fatigue, rash, headaches, cognitive impairment, and alopecia are also common side effects. Because most large, randomized clinical trials have monitored subjects for a maximum of 1 to 2 years, the cumulative toxicity profile may underestimate the potential for adverse reactions to occur with prolonged MTX treatment. Side effects have led to drug discontinuation in approximately 30% of subjects in clinical trials for RA and psoriasis. Adverse reactions during MTX therapy for RA included increase in transaminase levels (21%), nausea (18%), and diarrhea (12%),[107] and advanced age and/or impaired renal function have been identified as risk factors for toxicity.[108,109] In a British registry study of 673 individuals prescribed MTX for long-term treatment of rheumatologic diseases, side effects attributed to MTX led to discontinuation in 36.3%.[110] The most common reasons for discontinuing therapy were GI symptoms (10.8%), abnormal liver function tests (5.5%), peripheral blood cytopenias (5.5%), pulmonary symptoms (3%), and cutaneous abnormalities (2.1%). Life-threatening adverse events occurred in 1.7% of this patient cohort.

Pulmonary toxicity is a well-documented potential side effect of MTX treatment,[111-113] and pulmonary toxicity does not seem to be preventable with folic acid supplementation. Potential patterns of pulmonary toxicity include pneumonitis, bronchitis with airways hyperreactivity, pulmonary fibrosis, bronchiolitis obliterans with organizing pneumonia, and diffuse alveolar damage. The most commonly reported manifestation is hypersensitivity pneumonitis, which has a reported incidence of 1% to 5%.[114] Routine high-resolution computed tomography and/or serial pulmonary function tests have not been shown to be useful in monitoring patients for toxicity.[115]

Hepatic toxicity has also been reported with prolonged MTX treatment. MTX was stopped in one prospective study of patients with RA as a result of hepatotoxicty in 5% of patients.[110] Severe hepatic toxicity is uncommon but may occur. Severe liver failure and cirrhosis was detected in 24 patients in this large cohort of patients with RA; the cumulative incidence was 1 per 1000 patients.[110] Roenigk and colleagues[116] have developed a histologic classification (grade 0–IV) to assess MTX toxicity, and a meta-analysis of

636 total patients with RA or psoriasis from 15 published studies concluded that 28% of patients progressed at least one grade while on therapy.[117] Five percent of the patients had advanced liver disease (grade IIIB or IV), and the major risk factors for developing liver damage included a large cumulative dose of MTX, heavy alcohol use, and underlying psoriasis. Patients had a 6.7% chance of progressive liver damage for each cumulative gram of MTX. These data led to the recommendation that liver biopsy should be considered after each 1 to 1.5 g of cumulative MTX.[116] However, monitoring liver function tests on a regular basis for patients with RA has been found to be sufficient to screen for potential MTX-associated liver toxicity,[118] which may be because of a lower incidence rate of severe liver toxicity in patients with RA versus patients with psoriatic arthritis.[119]

Duration of exposure to MTX likely accounts for a substantial proportion of its toxicity. Therefore, once-weekly regimens are favored, and lead to fewer side effects. Delayed clearance of the medication (because of renal insufficiency, the presence of third-space effusions, or GI obstruction) leads to prolonged circulating MTX levels and increases the risk of toxicity.[120–122] Risk for many of the bothersome side effects can be minimized by using folic acid. Typical doses are 1 to 2 mg/d, although daily doses up to 5 mg have been described. Because MTX is a dihydrofolate reductase inhibitor, folic acid supplementation may bypass the MTX-induced blockade of nucleic acid synthesis. A well-designed randomized trial of folic acid supplementation versus placebo in RA patients showed that MTX at 5 mg or 27.5 mg/wk with folate supplementation had no effect on drug efficacy in patients with RA, but it significantly reduced toxicity scores for both doses.[123] A second, larger study (n = 434) in patients with RA reported similar results; MTX-related toxicity led to discontinuation in 38% of placebo-treated subjects versus 17% of those taking 1 to 2 mg of folic acid daily and had no effect on efficacy.[124]

Patients on MTX should undergo routine CBCs and renal function,[125,126] and the dose of MTX should be adjusted if leukopenia is detected. In one study, 26% of patients had one or more hematologic abnormality. More than 95% of these cases had symptoms consistent with viral infection, and the observed abnormality resolved within a month of withholding MTX and did not recur with rechallenge.[127] Liver function, especially the transaminases, should also be monitored, with routine liver function testing usually performed every 4 to 12 weeks while the patient is taking the drug.[118,126,128] Liver biopsies to monitor for irreversible hepatotoxicity (eg, after every 1–2 cumulative grams) have been recommended by some,[116] but liver biopsies are no longer recommended by the American College of Rheumatology (ACR).[118] The current ACR recommendation is to monitor transaminases. If transaminase levels show a sustained increase, biopsy is then recommended.[118] Monitoring exclusively with peripheral blood transaminase levels only may miss an occasional patient with advanced liver disease.[129] Patients should be asked about nausea, diarrhea, and stomatitis. If present, these side effects usually respond to dose reduction and the addition or increase in dosage of 1 mg folic acid.[123]

Leflunomide

Several large clinical trials led to regulatory approval of leflunomide for treatment of RA,[130–133] and clinical trials have been reported for psoriasis and psoriatic arthritis, Sjögren syndrome, systemic lupus erythematosis, ankylosing spondylitis, and Wegener granulomatosis.[130,132,134–138] Its use has also been described for antisynthetase syndrome, relapsing polychondritis, adult-onset Still disease, and scleroderma.[139–142] It antagonizes T- and B-lymphocyte activation and proliferation by inhibiting de novo pyrimidine synthesis.[143] Leflunomide is metabolized in the liver and bowel wall to an active metabolite that is primarily eliminated via the biliary tract, although some renal excretion also occurs.[144] It undergoes extensive enterohepatic recirculation, with an elimination half-life of approximately 2 weeks.

The most common side effects reported in controlled trials include nausea, diarrhea, alopecia, hypertension, increased liver enzymes, and rash. These side effects seem to be dose related, and often resolve with dose reduction. Postmarketing experience has shown rare instances of serious infection, cytopenias, angioedema, fulminant hepatitis, interstitial pneumonitis, peripheral neuropathy, and severe dermatologic syndromes (Stevens-Johnson syndrome, erythema multiforme, toxic epidermal necrolysis). However, postmarketing data are severely limited by ascertainment bias, concomitant immunosuppressive use, and the presence of the underlying disease; therefore, attribution of these toxicities to leflunomide remains unclear. Although leflunomide increases renal excretion of uric acid and decreases tubular reabsorption of phosphate,[145] clinically significant hypophosphatemia was not identified in a large clinical trial.[131]

Hepatic toxicity generally occurs within the first 6 months of therapy, and it is more common in patients with preexisting liver dysfunction or when concomitantly treated with MTX.[146] Increases of alanine aminotransferase levels greater than 3 times the upper limits of normal were observed in 2% to 4% of patients in clinical trials for treatment of RA,[130,131,133] and these usually normalized with dose adjustment or discontinuation of the drug. The incidence of hepatocellular necrosis seems to be 100-fold less than for increases in transaminase levels.[147] When used in combination with MTX, increases in liver function tests occur more frequently in the absence of folic acid supplementation.

Peripheral neuropathy has been reported [148,149] and occurred in a range of 3 days to 3 years following initiation of therapy. The neuropathy associated with leflunomide may be caused by perineural vasculitis,[148] and outcome is best if leflunomide is stopped soon after symptom onset. A recent, controlled, prospective clinical trial reported neuropathic symptoms in 54% versus 8% of patients with RA treated with other disease-modifying agents.[150] When severe neuropathy occurs, administration of oral cholestyramine (see later discussion) is recommended in addition to discontinuing the drug.[150] Several cases of interstitial pneumonitis have been reported,[151–153] some of which have been fatal. However, these data are confounded by the frequent association of ILD and RA combined with physician preference to treat patients with CTD-associated ILD with leflunomide versus MTX.[153]

A CBC, liver function panel, phosphate, and creatinine tests are recommended before starting leflunomide therapy and they should be repeated every 4 to 6 weeks for the first 6 months of treatment. If stable, these parameters can be checked every 6 to 12 weeks beyond 6 months. Clinical monitoring for infection and signs of hepatoxicity should continue throughout the course of therapy, and laboratory examinations should be performed every month indefinitely if leflunomide is coadministered with MTX. If serious toxicity develops, elimination of the active metabolite may be necessary. Cholestyramine at 8 g 3 times daily is recommended because of the enterohepatic recirculation of leflunomide. Activated charcoal, although not so palatable as cholestyramine, is an acceptable alternative.

Mycophenolate

Mycophenolic acid (MPA) selectively and potently inhibits T- and B-lymphocyte proliferation by inhibiting the de novo purine pathway,[154] and it has regulatory approval for the prophylaxis of organ rejection in cardiac, liver, and renal transplantation in combination with cyclosporine and corticosteroids. MPA has been used to treat lupus nephritis,[155] RA,[156] Wegener granulomatosis,[157] systemic lupus erythematosus,[158] and pulmonary disease associated with various collagen vascular disorders.[159]

Two forms of mycophenolate are currently available for prescription.[160] Mycophenolate mofetil (MMF), which is administered orally, is the morpholinoethyl ester prodrug of MPA, and it is rapidly hydrolyzed (within 5 minutes) in the GI tract to MPA. Mycophenolate sodium is a delayed-release enteric formulation of MPA. MPA may accumulate in end-state renal failure, requiring hemodialysis or peritoneal dialysis, and dose attenuation may be required. MPA is extensively conjugated to glucuronide, which is predominantly cleared via renal excretion, and MPA pharmacokinetics do not seem to be altered in patients with hepatic dysfunction.[161] Cardiovascular (systemic hypertension, peripheral edema, tachycardia), dermatologic (rash, neoplasm), endocrinologic (hyperglycemia, cushingoid change, hirsutism), metabolic (hypercholesterolemia, hypophosphatemia, hypokalemia, hyperkalemia), GI (nausea, anorexia, vomiting, abdominal pain, diarrhea, constipation), hematologic (anemia, red blood cell aplasia, leukopenia, thrombocytopenia, leukocytosis), infectious (opportunistic infection), musculoskeletal (bone pain, myalgias, cramps), neurologic (headache, tremor, insomnia, dizziness, anxiety), ocular (blurred vision, cataracts, blepharitis, keratitis, glaucoma, macular abnormalities), genitourinary (infection, hematuria, tubular necrosis, urinary frequency, burning on urination, kidney stones, vaginal burning, vaginal bleeding), and respiratory (cough, dyspnea, infection, pneumonitis, fibrosis) abnormalities have all been associated with MPA administration. Mycophenolate usually lacks a significant effect on hematopoiesis and neutrophil populations because other cell types (nonlymphocytic) can use salvage pathways to obtain guanine. However, neutropenia can occur and may respond to simple modification of mycophenolate dosage.[162]

Several drug interactions can occur with mycophenolate.[163] Activated charcoal, aluminum or magnesium salts, cholestyramine, colesevalam, colestipol, or iron can inhibit absorption from the GI tract.[164] Mycophenolate should not be coadministered with AZA because of increased inhibition of purine metabolism, and mycophenolate can increase plasma concentration of acyclovir or ganciclovir, especially when renal impairment is present. Mycophenolate may decrease exposure to hormonal therapies, and live attenuated virus vaccines should not be given concomitantly with MPA. Patients receiving MPA may have an inadequate immunologic response to vaccination.[165]

CBCs have been recommended on a weekly basis for the first month, twice monthly for the second and third months of treatment, and then once a month for the remainder of the first year of treatment. However, when mycophenolate is not given together with other agents that can synergistically depress bone-marrow function, such as calcineurin inhibitors, obtaining CBCs on such a frequent schedule is probably not necessary. Plasma levels of MPA can be used to guide therapy as well as to detect toxicity.[166,167] In addition, MPA serum concentrations may be useful in patients with impaired renal function to prevent toxicity caused by high levels and graft rejection caused by low levels.[168] However, it has not been conclusively shown that monitoring levels minimizes toxicity or risk for rejection.[169,170]

OTHER AGENTS
Chloroquine/Hydroxychloroquine

Chloroquine and hydroxychloroquine are synthetic 4-aminoquinoline antimalarial agents that have antiinflammatory properties.[171] Chloroquine is well absorbed from the GI tract and rapidly absorbed from subcutaneous and intramuscular sites. Chloroquine is sequestered in various tissues (lung, liver, spleen, kidney, melanin-containing tissues, brain, and spinal cord).[171] The rates of absorption and elimination are closely balanced for orally administered drug. Peak chloroquine plasma levels are reached 3 to 5 hours after oral administration. The half-life of chloroquine has been reported to increase with sustained drug administration. Its half-life has been reported to begin at 30 to 60 days and can extend for years, and prolonged half-lives have been reported with sustained and prolonged administration.[171,172]

Prolonged therapy with chloroquine or hydroxychloroquine can cause toxic myopathy, cardiomyopathy, and peripheral neuropathy; these reactions improve if the drug is promptly withdrawn.[173,174] Cardiovascular effects may progress through vasodilation, hypotension, suppressed myocardial function, cardiac arrhythmia, and cardiac arrest. Central nervous system effects may progress through confusion, convulsions, and coma. Oral therapy may cause GI upset, headache, visual disturbances, urticaria, and pruritus. Prolonged treatment may cause headache, blurring of vision, diplopia, confusion, convulsions, lichenoid skin eruptions, bleaching

of the hair, and electrocardiographic abnormalities such as widening of the QRS interval and T-wave changes. These side effects usually reverse with discontinuation of therapy. Chloroquine may also cause discoloration of the nail beds and mucous membranes and may also interfere with selected vaccines.[175–177] When chloroquines are used as chronic therapy for inflammatory disorders, irreversible retinopathy and ototocity may occur with higher oral doses if in excess of 250 mg/d.[178–180]

Because hydroxychloroquine may cause less ocular toxicity than chloroquine,[180] hydroxychloroquine has been preferred to chloroquine for treating inflammatory disorders. In addition to interval evaluations of patients on chronic therapy to screen for adverse drug reactions, routine ocular screening has been recommended for patients receiving antimalarial agents with a frequency of every 6 to 12 months.[181]

Imatinib Mesylate

Imatinib mesylate, a protein-tyrosine kinase inhibitor, inhibits cellular proliferation and induces apoptosis in a variety of abnormal cell lines. It has received regulatory approval for the treatment of chronic myeloid leukemia and GI stromal tumor. In addition to suppressing the specific kinase dysfunction created by the gene mutations for those malignancies, imatinib inhibits receptor tyrosine kinases for platelet-derived growth factor (PDGF) and stem cell factor (SCF), and it inhibits PDGF- and SCF-mediated cellular events. Imatinib has been used in fibrotic lung diseases and pulmonary arterial hypertension.[182–184]

Imatinib has high oral bioavailability (98%), and the parent and active N-desmethyl derivative are cleared predominantly via hepatic CYP3A4 enzymes. Bullous dermatologic reactions (including erythema multiforme and Stevens-Johnson syndrome), significant fluid retention, GI complications, and hematologic abnormalities have been reported.[185–187] Fluid retention (which can manifest as pleural effusions, ascites, pulmonary edema, or peripheral edema) occurs more frequently in patients older than 65 years. Neutropenia, anemia, and thrombocytopenia have been linked to imatinib therapy, and the package insert recommends a CBC weekly for the first month, biweekly for the second month, and periodically thereafter as clinically indicated.

Hepatic impairment, which can be severe, has been reported. Liver function testing (transaminases, bilirubin, and alkaline phosphatase) is recommended at baseline and then monthly and/or as clinically indicated per the package insert. Available data are insufficient to determine if lymphoma or nonlymphomatous malignancies are increased, although some carcinogenesis, mutagenesis, and impairment of fertility studies are suggestive. Drug-induced pneumonitis has been reported,[188,189] but only dyspnea has been reported in randomized clinical trials for treatment of malignancies. Peripheral edema may occur, especially in elderly patients, and can be managed with diuretic therapy.

DRUG-DRUG INTERACTIONS

Numerous drug-drug interactions may occur, especially with use of the nonbiologic agents. These interactions are summarized in **Table 4**. Drug-drug interactions must be considered when new drugs are administered as well as when coadministered drugs are withdrawn or doses are altered, which is particularly important for drugs that are metabolized by the cytochrome P-450CYP3A4 enzyme system. Drug levels of CYP3A4-metabolized agents (eg, imatinib) can be significantly increased by administration of drugs that are also metabolized via this pathway or reduced by coadministration of CYP3A4 inducers. Appropriate dose adjustment and monitoring should be observed if a CYP3A4 drug is administered and inhibitors or inducers of this enzyme are coadministered. Many commonly prescribed agents (eg, imidazole antifungal agents, macrolide antibiotics) can significantly affect blood levels of the CYP3A4-metabolized imatinib mesylate. In addition, most of the agents covered in this article can suppress antibody responses to vaccines. In addition, recipients may be endangered if live virus vaccines are given while the patients are receiving pharmacologic immunosuppression. Potentially significant interactions have been documented for some of these agents with ingested substances such as grapefruit juice, echinacea, and herbal preparations or supplements. Patients should be aware of these potential interactions.

PREGNANCY

All of the nonbiologic immunosuppressive agents may have teratogenic or embryocidal effects on the fetus and have been placed in the US Food and Drug Administration (FDA) categories of C, D, or X; none has been assigned to category A (**Table 5**).[190] CYC is teratogenic during pregnancy (FDA category D), and it should not be given to women with childbearing potential without adequate measures to prevent pregnancy. However, CYC has been administered successfully during the third trimester when considered necessary to control severe disease requiring treatment. Men should not father a child during CYC therapy or for a few months following cessation of CYC administration. Because posttreatment sterility may occur in men or women during treatment with CYC, consideration should be given before treatment to bank sperm or oocytes if future pregnancy is desired. MTX and the anti-TNF agents have been shown to be directly toxic to the fetus,[190] as has mycophenolate. AZA has, however, been given throughout the course of successful pregnancies.[191,192] However, pregnancy should be discouraged and avoided when patients are taking these medications, and these agents should not be prescribed for pregnant women unless the treatment benefit clearly outweighs the risk of teratogenic effects on the developing fetus.

PEDIATRIC DOSING

There are limited data on the use of immunosuppressive drugs for the treatment of inflammatory disorders in children. Antimalarial agents have been used to treat rheumatologic diseases in children for many years, and these drugs are generally felt to be safe despite limited published literature. Toxicities for older children are generally believed to parallel those for adults. However, this may not be the case for certain situations. Pharmacokinetic parameters and mycophenolate levels were found to be similar for adults and children in one study, but mycophenolate levels were disproportionately increased in children when kidney function was impaired and/or albumin levels were depressed.[193] Pharmacokinetic monitoring in children receiving MTX revealed that the maximum dose appeared to be 10 mg/m^2 for children and differed from dosing for adult patients.[194] In addition, newer approaches to treating children with immunosuppressive therapies are evolving in which certain agents, such as corticosteroids, are minimized.[195,196] Monitoring strategies may also be helpful in children to help avoid toxicity from some drugs. Monitoring metabolite levels in patients treated with AZA may help to minimize toxicity and enhance treatment efficacy.[197]

MONITORING AND PREVENTION OF TOXICITY

Specific recommendation for pretherapy evaluation and monitoring of clinical and laboratory parameters during therapy are given in **Table 3** for the various drugs. Reactivation of latent infection (eg, tuberculosis, herpesviruses, endemic fungi) or the onset of new infection (eg,

Table 4
Summary of drug-drug interactions

Specific Drug	Metabolized by CYP3A4*	Imidazole Antifungal Agents	Psychiatric Therapies	Antibacterial Agents	Steroidal Therapies	Antiarrythmic Therapies	Anticonvulsants	Vaccines	Anakinra/MTX/Mycophenolate/AZA	NSAIDs	ACE Inhibitors	Thiazide Diuretics	GI Acid Reducers (Proton Pump Inhibitor; H-2, Elements)	Allopurinol	Coumadin	Hydroxymethylglutaryl Coenzyme A Reductase Inhibitors	Herbal Supplements
Adalimumab								+	+								
Etanercept								+	+								
Infliximab								+	+								
AZA								+	+		+			+	+		+
Cyclophosphamide	+			Chloramphenicol		+		+	+	+		+		+	+		+
Leflunomide				Rifampin Rifapentine				+	+						+		
MTX				Penicillins, Doxycyline		+	+	+	+	+		+	+		+		
Mycophenolate				Norfloxacin				+	+				+				+
Chloroquines			+	Quinolones Trimethoprim sulfa/Sulfa macrolides Pentamidine		+							+				
Imatinib mesylate	+	+		Macrolides Rifampin Rifabutin Rifapentine			+	+							+	+	+
Rituximab								+								+	

CYP3A4-metabolized drugs (competitors; increased levels of other drugs metabolized by CYP3A4): nefazodone, macrolides, imidazoles, metronidazole, cisapride, cimetidine, chloramphenicol, grapefruit juice, calcium channel-blockers, theophylline. CYP3A4 inducers (decreased drug level caused by increased activity of CYP3A4): phenytoin, phenobarbitol, modafinil, carbamazepine, quinopristine, rifampin, sulfasalazine, sulfinpyrazone.

Table 5
Effects on pregnancy and pregnancy classification

Specific Drug	Pregnancy Category FDA (United States)	Australia	Category Definitions (FDA)
Prednisone	None	A	A. Controlled studies in women fail to show a risk to the fetus in the first trimester (and there is no evidence of a risk in later trimesters), and the possibility of fetal harm seems remote
Methyprednisolone			B. Either animal-reproduction studies have not shown a fetal risk but there are no controlled studies in pregnant women or animal-reproduction studies have shown adverse effect (other than a decrease in fertility) that was not confirmed in controlled studies in women in the first trimester (and there is no evidence of a risk in later trimesters)
Adalimumab	B	C	C. Either studies in animals have revealed adverse effects on the fetus (teratogenic or embryocidal or other) and there are no controlled studies in women, or studies in women and animals are not available. Drugs should be given only if the potential benefit justifies the potential risk to the fetus
Etanercept	B	B	D. There is positive evidence of human fetal risk, but the benefits from use in pregnant women may be acceptable despite the risk (eg, if the drug is needed in a life-threatening situation or for a serious disease for which safer drugs cannot be used or are ineffective)
Infliximab	B	None	X. Studies in animals or human beings have demonstrated fetal abnormalities or there is evidence of fetal risk based on human experience or both, and the risk of the use of the drug in pregnant women clearly outweighs any possible benefit. The drug is contraindicated in women who are or may become pregnant
AZA	D	D	
Cyclophosphamide	D	D	
Leflunomide	X	None	
MTX	X	D	
Mycophenolate	D	D	
Chloroquines	C	D	
Imatinib	D	D	
Rituximab	C	C	

aspergillosis, histoplasmosis, other endemic fungi, pneumocystis pneumonia, cytomegalovirus pneumonia, viral hepatitis) during the course of treatment presents significant risks for patients undergoing intensive pharmacologic immunosuppression. Infection may occur because of suppression of immune cell function (eg, T lymphocytes), bone-marrow toxicity with neutropenia, or a combination of depressed cell function and decreased numbers of immune effector cells. Pneumocystis pneumonia may complicate the course of patients with systemic autoimmune disease who are treated with intense immunosuppression.[198–200] If intensive immunosuppressive therapy is prescribed, prophylaxis for *P jiroveci* should be strongly considered.[201,202] Although screening for active or latent tuberculosis is supported only by the literature for anti-TNF therapy, the administration of other potent immunosuppressive regimens could lead to reactivation of latent infection. Ideally, patients should be uniformly and carefully screened for evidence of active or latent tuberculosis before the initiation of any intense immunosuppressive therapies.

Many of the nonbiologic agents can significantly depress bone-marrow function. Granulocytic cell lines are most susceptible, and neutropenia may complicate therapy by predisposing patients to infection. Other hematopoietic cell lineages may also be affected and lead to anemia or thrombocytopenia. Other drugs (eg, trimethoprim sulfa or ganciclovir) given for prophylaxis or treatment of infection may contribute to bone-marrow suppression and potentiate the effect of immunosuppressive drug therapies. Intermittent monitoring of bone-marrow function via CBC with differential cell count is advised for all patients receiving drugs that are associated with potential bone-marrow suppression.

GI toxicity including severe hepatotoxicity can occur as a consequence of several nonbiologic agents. MPA derivatives can significantly affect intestinal transit times and often cause diarrhea, which can be severe in some instances and not necessarily correlate well with mycophenolate blood levels. Although blood levels of mycophenolate are not routinely obtained to monitor this agent, a level can be obtained if diarrhea complicates therapy, and a high level would implicate mycophenolate as a potential cause of this complication if other causes such as infection are excluded. Serious hepatic injury can occur with MTX, AZA, or leflunomide, and hepatic function should be intermittently monitored (eg, once monthly) with appropriate testing while patients are receiving agents that can potentially cause serious hepatotoxicity.

Patient education is an important aspect of monitoring for infection and other adverse drug reactions. Patients need to be informed of the increased risk of infection and report in a timely fashion symptoms such as fever, new onset or change in cough, or shortness of breath. Because many of the noncorticosteroid drugs discussed earlier may be pneumotoxic,[97,114,151,152,203–206] increasing dyspnea or other respiratory symptoms should be reported promptly. In addition, patients need to be aware that taking new medications may lead to significant drug-drug interactions, and they should question the possibility of drug interactions whenever a change in their medications is made while they are on therapy with the noncorticosteroid agents discussed earlier.

SUMMARY

Immunosuppressive drug therapy for systemic autoimmune disorders considerably increases the risk of infection and various other complications that range from bone-marrow suppression and hepatic dysfunction to pulmonary toxicity. Provider knowledge of potential adverse reactions to these drugs combined with the use of strategies for pretherapy screening before drug administration plus appropriate interval clinical evaluation and laboratory testing while on therapy are key to avoiding severe complications of immunosuppressive drug therapy. In addition, patient education is important, and prophylactic measures to prevent complications (eg, administration of folic acid, trimethoprime-sulfa prophylaxis, appropriate screening and treatment of osteopenia/osteoporosis) can benefit the patient.

REFERENCES

1. Kourbeti IS, Boumpas D. Biological therapies of autoimmune diseases. Curr Drug Targets Inflamm Allergy 2005;4:41–6.
2. McDonough AK, Curtis JR, Saag KG. The epidemiology of glucocorticoid-associated adverse events. Curr Opin Rheumatol 2008;20:131–7.
3. Lovell DJ, Giannini EH, Reiff A, et al. Etanercept in children with polyarticular juvenile rheumatoid arthritis. Pediatric Rheumatology Collaborative Study Group. N Engl J Med 2000;342:763–9.
4. Kavanaugh A, Clair EW, McCune WJ, et al. Chimeric anti-tumor necrosis factor-alpha monoclonal antibody treatment of patients with rheumatoid arthritis receiving methotrexate therapy. J Rheumatol 2000;27:841–50.
5. Furst DE, Schiff MH, Fleischmann RM, et al. Adalimumab, a fully human anti tumor necrosis factor-alpha monoclonal antibody, and concomitant

standard antirheumatic therapy for the treatment of rheumatoid arthritis: results of STAR (Safety Trial of Adalimumab in Rheumatoid Arthritis). J Rheumatol 2003;30:2563–71.

6. Keystone EC, Genovese MC, Klareskog L, et al. Golimumab, a human antibody to tumour necrosis factor {alpha} given by monthly subcutaneous injections, in active rheumatoid arthritis despite methotrexate therapy: the GO-FORWARD Study. Ann Rheum Dis 2009;68:789–96.

7. Goldenberg MM. Etanercept, a novel drug for the treatment of patients with severe, active rheumatoid arthritis. Clin Ther 1999;21:75–87.

8. Weaver A. Efficacy and safety of the anti-TNF biologic agents. Mod Rheumatol 2004;14:101–12.

9. Pham T, Claudepierre P, Deprez X, et al. Anti-TNF alpha therapy and safety monitoring. Clinical tool guide elaborated by the Club Rhumatismes et Inflammations (CRI), section of the French Society of Rheumatology (Société Française de Rhumatologie, SFR). Joint Bone Spine 2005;72(Suppl 1): S1–58.

10. Saag KG, Teng GG, Patkar NM, et al. American College of Rheumatology 2008 recommendations for the use of nonbiologic and biologic disease-modifying antirheumatic drugs in rheumatoid arthritis. Arthritis Rheum 2008;59:762–84.

11. Smith CH, Anstey AV, Barker JN, et al. British Association of Dermatologists' guidelines for biologic interventions for psoriasis 2009. Br J Dermatol 2009;161:987–1019.

12. Favalli EG, Desiati F, Atzeni F, et al. Serious infections during anti-TNFalpha treatment in rheumatoid arthritis patients. Autoimmun Rev 2009;8:266–73.

13. Ramos-Casals M, Brito-Zeron P, Soto MJ, et al. Autoimmune diseases induced by TNF-targeted therapies. Best Pract Res Clin Rheumatol 2008; 22:847–61.

14. Danila MI, Patkar NM, Curtis JR, et al. Biologics and heart failure in rheumatoid arthritis: are we any wiser? Curr Opin Rheumatol 2008;20:327–33.

15. Bongartz T, Sutton AJ, Sweeting MJ, et al. Anti-TNF antibody therapy in rheumatoid arthritis and the risk of serious infections and malignancies: systematic review and meta-analysis of rare harmful effects in randomized controlled trials. JAMA 2006;295:2275–85.

16. Fromont A, De Seze J, Fleury MC, et al. Inflammatory demyelinating events following treatment with anti-tumor necrosis factor. Cytokine 2009; 45:55–7.

17. Reddy J, Loftus E Jr. Safety of infliximab and other biologic agents in the inflammatory bowel diseases. Gastroenterol Clin North Am 2006;35:837–55.

18. Strangfeld A, Listing J. Bacterial and opportunistic infections during anti-TNF therapy. Best Pract Res Clin Rheumatol 2006;20:1181–95.

19. Winthrop K, Siegel J, Jereb J, et al. Tuberculosis associated with therapy against tumor necrosis factor α. Arthritis Rheum 2005;52(10):2978–84.

20. Keane J, Gershon S, Wise R, et al. Tuberculosis associated with infliximab, a tumor necrosis factor-a-neutralizing agent. N Engl J Med 2001; 345:1098–104.

21. Gomez-Reino J, Carmona L, Valverde V, et al. on behalf of the DASER Group. Treatment of rheumatoid arthritis with tumor necrosis factor inhibitors may predispose to significant increase in tuberculosis risk. A multicenter active-surveillance report. Arthritis Rheum 2003;48(8):2122–7.

22. Gardam M, Keystone E, Menzies R, et al. Anti-tumour necrosis factor agents and tuberculosis risk: mechanisms of action and clinical management. Lancet Infect Dis 2003;3:148–53.

23. Badesch DB, Raskob GE, Elliott CG, et al. Pulmonary arterial hypertension: baseline characteristics from the REVEAL Registry. Chest 2009; 137:376–87.

24. Available at: www.remicade.com/remicade/assets/ HCP_PPI.pdf. Accessed December 5, 2009.

25. Ledingham J, Deighton C, British Society for Rheumatology Standards GaAWGS. Update on the British Society for Rheumatology guidelines for prescribing TNFa blockers in adults with rheumatoid arthritis (update of previous guidelines of April 2001). Rheumatology 2005;44:157–63.

26. Chung E, Packer M, Lo K, et al. Randomized, double-blind, placebo-controlled, pilot trial of infliximab, a chimeric monoclonal antibody to tumor necrosis factor-alpha, in patients with moderate-to-severe heart failure: results of the anti-TNF Therapy Against Congestive Heart Failure (ATTACH) trial. Circulation 2003;107: 2133–40.

27. Peters M, Vis M, van Halm V, et al. Changes in lipid profile during infliximab and corticosteroid treatment in rheumatoid arthritis. Ann Rheum Dis 2007;66:958–61.

28. Allanore Y, Kahan A, Sellam J, et al. Effects of repeated infliximab therapy on serum lipid profile in patients with refractory rheumatoid arthritis. Clin Chim Acta 2006;365:143–8.

29. Mohan N, Edwards E, Cupps T, et al. Demyelination occurring during anti-tumor necrosis factor alpha therapy for inflammatory arthritides. Arthritis Rheum 2001;44:2862–9.

30. Carroll MB, Bond MI. Use of tumor necrosis factor-alpha inhibitors in patients with chronic hepatitis B infection. Semin Arthritis Rheum 2008;38(3):208–17.

31. Dixon WG, Hyrich KL, Watson KD, et al. Drug-specific risk of tuberculosis in patients with rheumatoid arthritis treated with anti-TNF therapy: results from the British Society for Rheumatology

Biologics Register (BSRBR). Ann Rheum Dis 2009; 69:522–8.

32. Baughman RP, Lower EE. Novel therapies for sarcoidosis. Semin Respir Crit Care Med 2007;28: 128–33.

33. Sandborn WJ, Hanauer SB, Rutgeerts P, et al. Adalimumab for maintenance treatment of Crohn's disease: results of the CLASSIC II trial. Gut 2007; 56:1232–9.

34. Breedveld FC, Weisman MH, Kavanaugh AF, et al. The PREMIER study: a multicenter, randomized, double-blind clinical trial of combination therapy with adalimumab plus methotrexate versus methotrexate alone or adalimumab alone in patients with early, aggressive rheumatoid arthritis who had not had previous methotrexate treatment. Arthritis Rheum 2006;54:26–37.

35. Sandborn WJ, Rutgeerts P, Enns R, et al. Adalimumab induction therapy for Crohn disease previously treated with infliximab: a randomized trial. Ann Intern Med 2007;146:829–38.

36. Tubach F, Ravaud P, Salmon-Ceron D, et al. Emergence of Legionella pneumophila pneumonia in patients receiving tumor necrosis factor-alpha antagonists. Clin Infect Dis 2006; 43:e95–100.

37. Kalyoncu U, Karaday O, Akdogan A, et al. Pneumocystic carinii pneumonia in a rheumatoid arthritis patient treated with adalimumab. Scand J Infect Dis 2007;39:475–8.

38. Stubgen JP. Tumor necrosis factor-alpha antagonists and neuropathy. Muscle Nerve 2008;37: 281–92.

39. Baghai M, Osmon DR, Wolk DM, et al. Fatal sepsis in a patient with rheumatoid arthritis treated with entanercept. Mayo Clin Proc 2001;76:653–6.

40. Furst DE, Breedveld FC, Kalden JR, et al. Updated consensus statement on biological agents, specifically tumour necrosis factor-alpha (TNF-alpha) blocking agents and interleukin-1 receptor antagonist (IL-1ra), for the treatment of rheumatic diseases. Ann Rheum Dis 2005; 64(Suppl 4):v2–14.

41. Mohan AK, Broder MS, Wong JY, et al. Granulomatous infectious diseases associated with tumor necrosis factor antagonists. Clin Infect Dis 2004; 38:1261–5.

42. Kwon HJ, Cote TR, Cuffe MS, et al. Case reports of heart failure after therapy with a tumor necrosis factor antagonist. Ann Intern Med 2003;138:807–11.

43. Daien CI, Monnier A, Claudepierre P, et al. Sarcoid-like granulomatosis in patients treated with tumor necrosis factor blockers: 10 cases. Rheumatology (Oxford) 2009;48(8):883–6.

44. Brown SL, Greene MH, Gershon SK, et al. Tumor necrosis factor antagonist therapy and lymphoma development: twenty-six cases reported to the Food and Drug Administration. Arthritis Rheum 2002;46:3151–8.

45. Utz JP, Limper AH, Kalra S, et al. Etanercept for the treatment of stage II and III progressive pulmonary sarcoidosis. Chest 2003;124:177–85.

46. Wolfe F, Michaud K. Lymphoma in rheumatoid arthritis: the effect of methotrexate and anti-tumor necrosis factor therapy in 18,572 patients. Arthritis Rheum 2004;50:1740–51.

47. Wallis RS, Broder MS, Wong JY, et al. Granulomatous infectious diseases associated with tumor necrosis factor antagonists. Clin Infect Dis 2004; 38:1261–5.

48. Gomez-Reino JJ, Carmona L, Angel DM. Risk of tuberculosis in patients treated with tumor necrosis factor antagonists due to incomplete prevention of reactivation of latent infection. Arthritis Rheum 2007;57:756–61.

49. Matulis G, Juni P, Villiger PM, et al. Detection of latent tuberculosis in immunosuppressed patients with autoimmune diseases performance of a mycobacterium tuberculosis antigen specific IFN-gamma assay. Ann Rheum Dis 2008;67:84–90.

50. van der Kolk LE, Baars JW, Prins MH, et al. Rituximab treatment results in impaired secondary humoral immune responsiveness. Blood 2002; 100:2257–9.

51. Dillman RO. Infusion reactions associated with the therapeutic use of monoclonal antibodies in the treatment of malignancy. Cancer Metastasis Rev 1999;18:465–71.

52. Schwartzberg LS, Stepanski EJ, Fortner BV, et al. Retrospective chart review of severe infusion reactions with rituximab, cetuximab, and bevacizumab in community oncology practices: assessment of clinical consequences. Support Care Cancer 2008;16:393–8.

53. Bennett CM, Rogers ZR, Kinnamon DD, et al. Prospective phase 1/2 study of rituximab in childhood and adolescent chronic immune thrombocytopenic purpura. Blood 2006;107:2639–42.

54. Herishanu Y. Rituximab-induced serum sickness. Am J Hematol 2002;70:329.

55. Wang J, Wiley JM, Luddy R, et al. Chronic immune thrombocytopenic purpura in children: assessment of rituximab treatment. J Pediatr 2005;146:217–21.

56. Hellerstedt B, Ahmed A. Delayed-type hypersensitivity reaction or serum sickness after rituximab treatment. Ann Oncol 2003;14:1792.

57. Carson KR, Evens AM, Richey EA, et al. Progressive multifocal leukoencephalopathy after rituximab therapy in HIV-negative patients: a report of 57 cases from the Research on Adverse Drug Events and Reports project. Blood 2009;113(20): 4834–40.

58. Fleischmann RM. Progressive multifocal leukoencephalopathy following rituximab treatment in

a patient with rheumatoid arthritis. Arthritis Rheum 2009;60(11):3225–8.

59. Burton C, Kaczmarski R, Jan-Mohamed R, et al. Interstitial pneumonitis related to rituximab therapy. N Engl J Med 2003;348:2690–1.

60. Herishanu Y, Polliack A, Leider-Trejo L, et al. Fatal interstitial pneumonitis related to rituximab-containing regimen. Clin Lymphoma Myeloma 2006;6:407–9.

61. Lee Y, Kyung SY, Choi SJ, et al. Two cases of interstitial pneumonitis caused by rituximab therapy. Korean J Intern Med 2006;21(3):183–6.

62. Fleischmann RM. Safety of biologic therapy in rheumatoid arthritis and other autoimmune diseases: focus on rituximab. Semin Arthritis Rheum 2009;38:265–80.

63. Lennard L. The clinical pharmacology of 6-mercaptopurine. Eur J Clin Pharmacol 1992;43:329–39.

64. Tiede I, Fritz G, Strand S, et al. CD28-dependent Rac1 activation is the molecular target of azathioprine in primary human CD4+ T lymphocytes. J Clin Invest 2003;111:133–45.

65. Carrico CK, Sartorelli AC. Effects of 6-thioquanine on macromolecular events in regenerating rat liver. Cancer Res 1977;37:1868–75.

66. Stolk JN, Boerbooms AM, de Abreu RA, et al. Reduced thiopurine methyltransferase activity and development of side effects of azathioprine treatment in patients with rheumatoid arthritis. Arthritis Rheum 1998;41(10):1858–66.

67. Connell WR, Kamm MA, Ritchie JK, et al. Bone marrow toxicity caused by azathioprine in inflammatory bowel disease: 27 years of experience. Gut 1993;34:1081–5.

68. Sturdevant R, Singleton JW, Daren JL, et al. Azathioprine-related pancreatitis in patients with Crohn's disease. Gastroenterology 1979;77:883–6.

69. Dubinsky MC, Vasiliauskas EA, Singh H, et al. 6-Thioguanine can cause serious liver injury in inflammatory bowel disease patients. Gastroenterology 2003;125:298–303.

70. Kibukamusoke JW. Malaria prophylaxis and immunosuppressant therapy in management of nephrotic syndrome associated with Guartan Malaria. Arch Dis Child 1968;43:598.

71. Jeurissen ME, Boerbooms AM, van de Putte LB. Pancytopenia related to azathioprine in rheumatoid arthritis. Ann Rheum Dis 1988;47:503–5.

72. Swanson M, Cook R. Drugs, chemicals, and blood dyscrasias. Hamilton (IL): Drug Intelligence Publications; 1977.

73. Dubinsky MC, Lamothe S, Yang HY, et al. Pharmacogenomics and metabolite measurement for 6-mercaptopurine therapy in inflammatory bowel disease. Gastroenterology 2000;118:705–13.

74. Cuffari C, Theoret Y, Latour S, et al. 6-Mercaptopurine metabolism in Crohn's disease: correlation with efficacy and toxicity. Gut 1996;39:401–6.

75. Kirschner BS. Safety of azathioprine and 6-mercaptopurine in pediatric patients with inflammatory bowel disease. Gastroenterology 1998;115:813–21.

76. Rundles RW, Wyngaarden JB, Hitchings GH. Effects of a xanthine oxidase inhibitor on thiopurine metabolism, hyperuricemia and gout. Trans Assoc Am Physicians 1963;76:126.

77. Gossman J, Kachel HG, Schoepe W, et al. Anemia in renal transplant recipients caused by concomitant therapy with azathioprine and angiotensin-converting enzyme inhibitors. Transplantation 1993;56:585–9.

78. Gaffney K, Scott DG. Azathioprine and cyclophosphamide in the treatment of rheumatoid arthritis. Br J Rheumatol 1998;37:824–36.

79. Baughman RP, Peddi R, Lower EE. Therapy: general issues. In: Baughman RP, du Bois RM, Lynch JP III, et al, editors. Diffuse lung disease: a practical approach. London: Arnold; 2004. p. 78–105.

80. Tashkin DP, Elashoff R, Clements PJ, et al. Cyclophosphamide versus placebo in scleroderma lung disease. N Engl J Med 2006;354: 2655–66.

81. Hoyles RK, Ellis RW, Wellsbury J, et al. A multicenter, prospective, randomized, double-blind, placebo-controlled trial of corticosteroids and intravenous cyclophosphamide followed by oral azathioprine for the treatment of pulmonary fibrosis in scleroderma. Arthritis Rheum 2006;54: 3962–70.

82. Kondoh Y, Taniguchi H, Yokoi T, et al. Cyclophosphamide and low-dose prednisolone in idiopathic pulmonary fibrosis and fibrosing nonspecific interstitial pneumonia. Eur Respir J 2005;25: 528–33.

83. Baughman RP, Lower EE. Use of intermittent, intravenous cyclophosphamide for idiopathic pulmonary fibrosis. Chest 1992;102:1090–4.

84. Haubitz M, Schellong S, Gobel U, et al. Intravenous pulse administration of cyclophosphamide versus daily oral treatment in patients with antineutrophil cytoplasmic antibody-associated vasculitis and renal involvement: a prospective, randomized study. Arthritis Rheum 1998;41:1835–44.

85. Adu D, Pall A, Luqmani RA, et al. Controlled trial of pulse versus continuous prednisolone and cyclophosphamide in the treatment of systemic vasculitis. QJM 1997;90:401–9.

86. Talar-Williams C, Hijazi YM, Walther MM, et al. Cyclophosphamide-induced cystitis and bladder cancer in patients with Wegener granulomatosis. Ann Intern Med 1996;124:477–84.

87. Radis CD, Kahl LE, Baker GL, et al. Effects of cyclophosphamide on the development of malignancy and on long-term survival of patients with

rheumatoid arthritis. A 20-year followup study. Arthritis Rheum 1995;38:1120–7.

88. Martin-Suarez I, D'Cruz D, Mansoor M, et al. Immunosuppressive treatment in severe connective tissue diseases: effects of low dose intravenous cyclophosphamide. Ann Rheum Dis 1997; 56:481–7.

89. Martin F, Lauwerys B, Lefebvre C, et al. Side-effects of intravenous cyclophosphamide pulse therapy. Lupus 1997;6:254–7.

90. de Groot K, Adu D, Savage CO. The value of pulse cyclophosphamide in ANCA-associated vasculitis: meta-analysis and critical review. Nephrol Dial Transplant 2001;16:2018–27.

91. Dorr FA, Coltman CA Jr. Second cancers following antineoplastic therapy. Curr Probl Cancer 1985;9: 1–43.

92. Knight A, Askling J, Ekbom A. Cancer incidence in a population-based cohort of patients with Wegener's granulomatosis. Int J Cancer 2002;100: 82–5.

93. Hesselstrand R, Scheja A, Akesson A. Mortality and causes of death in a Swedish series of systemic sclerosis patients. Ann Rheum Dis 1998; 57:682–6.

94. Girling DJ, Stott H, Stephens RJ, et al. Fifteen-year follow-up of all patients in a study of post-operative chemotherapy for bronchial carcinoma. Br J Cancer 1985;52:867–73.

95. Siemann DW, Macler L, Penney DP. Cyclophosphamide-induced pulmonary toxicity. Br J Cancer Suppl 1986;7:343–6.

96. Gould VE, Miller J. Sclerosing alveolitis induced by cyclophosphamide. Ultrastructural observations on alveolar injury and repair. Am J Pathol 1975;81: 513–53.

97. Malik SW, Myers JL, DeRemee RA, et al. Lung toxicity associated with cyclophosphamide use. Two distinct patterns. Am J Respir Crit Care Med 1996;154:1851–6.

98. Stott H, Stephens R, Fox W, et al. An investigation of the chest radiographs in a controlled trial of busulphan, cyclophosphamide, and a placebo after resection for carcinoma of the lung. Thorax 1976; 31:265–70.

99. Baughman RP, Winget DB, Lower EE. Methotrexate is steroid sparing in acute sarcoidosis: results of a double blind, randomized trial. Sarcoidosis Vasc Diffuse Lung Dis 2000;17:60–6.

100. Lower EE, Baughman RP. The use of low dose methotrexate in refractory sarcoidosis. Am J Med Sci 1990;299:153–7.

101. de Groot K, Rasmussen N, Bacon PA, et al. Randomized trial of cyclophosphamide versus methotrexate for induction of remission in early systemic antineutrophil cytoplasmic antibody-associated vasculitis. Arthritis Rheum 2005;52:2461–9.

102. de Groot K, Reinhold-Keller E, Tatsis E, et al. Therapy for the maintenance of remission in sixty-five patients with generalized Wegener's granulomatosis. Methotrexate versus trimethoprim/sulfamethoxazole. Arthritis Rheum 1996;39: 2052–61.

103. Douglas WW, Tazelaar HD, Hartman TE, et al. Polymyositis-dermatomyositis-associated interstitial lung disease. Am J Respir Crit Care Med 2001; 164(7):1182–5.

104. Chan ES, Cronstein BN. Molecular action of methotrexate in inflammatory diseases. Arthritis Res 2002;4(4):266–73.

105. Montesinos MC, Desai A, Delano D, et al. Adenosine A2A or A3 receptors are required for inhibition of inflammation by methotrexate and its analog MX-68. Arthritis Rheum 2003;48:240–7.

106. Montesinos MC, Yap JS, Desai A, et al. Reversal of the antiinflammatory effects of methotrexate by the nonselective adenosine receptor antagonists theophylline and caffeine: evidence that the antiinflammatory effects of methotrexate are mediated via multiple adenosine receptors in rat adjuvant arthritis. Arthritis Rheum 2000;43:656–63.

107. Weinblatt ME, Coblyn JS, Fox DA, et al. Efficacy of low-dose methotrexate in rheumatoid arthritis. N Engl J Med 1985;312:818–22.

108. Wijnands MJ, van Riel PL, Gribnau FW, et al. Risk factors of second-line antirheumatic drugs in rheumatoid arthritis. Semin Arthritis Rheum 1990;19: 337–52.

109. McKendry RJ, Dale P. Adverse effects of low dose methotrexate therapy in rheumatoid arthritis. J Rheumatol 1993;20:1850–6.

110. Kinder AJ, Hassell AB, Brand J, et al. The treatment of inflammatory arthritis with methotrexate in clinical practice: treatment duration and incidence of adverse drug reactions. Rheumatology (Oxford) 2005;44:61–6.

111. McKendry RJ, Cyr M. Toxicity of methotrexate compared with azathioprine in the treatment of rheumatoid arthritis: a case-control study of 131 patients. Arch Intern Med 1989;149:685–9.

112. Hargreaves MR, Mowat AG, Benson MK. Acute pneumonitis associated with low dose methotrexate treatment for rheumatoid arthritis: report of five cases and review of published reports. Thorax 1992;47(8):628–33.

113. Salaffi F, Manganelli P, Carotti M, et al. Methotrexate-induced pneumonitis in patients with rheumatoid arthritis and psoriatic arthritis: report of five cases and review of the literature. Clin Rheumatol 1997;16:296–304.

114. Zisman DA, McCune WJ, Tino G, et al. Drug-induced pneumonitis: the role of methotrexate. Sarcoidosis Vasc Diffuse Lung Dis 2001;18: 243–52.

115. Dawson JK, Graham DR, Desmond J, et al. Investigation of the chronic pulmonary effects of low-dose oral methotrexate in patients with rheumatoid arthritis: a prospective study incorporating HRCT scanning and pulmonary function tests. Rheumatology (Oxford) 2002;41:262–7.

116. Roenigk HH, Auerbach R, Mailbach HI, et al. Methotrexate guidelines revised. J Am Acad Dermatol 1982;6:145–55.

117. Whiting-O'Keefe QE, Fye KH, Sack KD. Methotrexate and histologic hepatic abnormalities: a meta-analysis. Am J Med 1991;90:711–6.

118. Kremer JM, Alarcon GS, Lightfoot RW Jr, et al. Methotrexate for rheumatoid arthritis. Suggested guidelines for monitoring liver toxicity. American College of Rheumatology. Arthritis Rheum 1994; 37(3):316–28.

119. Walker AM, Funch D, Dreyer NA, et al. Determinants of serious liver disease among patients receiving low-dose methotrexate for rheumatoid arthritis. Arthritis Rheum 1993;36(3):329–35.

120. Evans WE, Pratt CB. Effect of pleural effusion on high-dose methotrexate kinetics. Clin Pharmacol Ther 1978;23:68–72.

121. Li J, Gwilt P. The effect of malignant effusions on methotrexate disposition. Cancer Chemother Pharmacol 2002;50(5):373–82.

122. Evans WE, Tsiatis A, Crom WR, et al. Pharmacokinetics of sustained serum methotrexate concentrations secondary to gastrointestinal obstruction. J Pharm Sci 1981;70:1194–8.

123. Morgan SL, Baggott JE, Vaughn WH, et al. Supplementation with folic acid during methotrexate therapy for rheumatoid arthritis. Ann Intern Med 1994;121:833–41.

124. van Ede AE, Laan RF, Rood MJ, et al. Effect of folic or folinic acid supplementation on the toxicity and efficacy of methotrexate in rheumatoid arthritis: a forty-eight week, multicenter, randomized, double-blind, placebo-controlled study. Arthritis Rheum 2001;44:1515–24.

125. Pavy S, Constantin A, Pham T, et al. Methotrexate therapy for rheumatoid arthritis: clinical practice guidelines based on published evidence and expert opinion. Joint Bone Spine 2006;73: 388–95.

126. Baughman RP, Lower EE. A clinical approach to the use of methotrexate for sarcoidosis. Thorax 1999;54:742–6.

127. Ortiz-Alvarez O, Morishita K, Avery G, et al. Guidelines for blood test monitoring of methotrexate toxicity in juvenile idiopathic arthritis. J Rheumatol 2004;31:2501–6.

128. Aithal GP, Haugk B, Das S, et al. Monitoring methotrexate-induced hepatic fibrosis in patients with psoriasis: are serial liver biopsies justified? Aliment Pharmacol Ther 2004;19:391–9.

129. Erickson AR, Reddy V, Vogelgesang SA, et al. Usefulness of the American College of Rheumatology recommendations for liver biopsy in methotrexate-treated rheumatoid arthritis patients. Arthritis Rheum 1995;38:1115–9.

130. Smolen JS, Kalden JR, Scott DL, et al. Efficacy and safety of leflunomide compared with placebo and sulphasalazine in active rheumatoid arthritis: a double-blind, randomised, multicentre trial. European Leflunomide Study Group. Lancet 1999;353: 259–66.

131. Emery P, Breedveld FC, Lemmel EM, et al. A comparison of the efficacy and safety of leflunomide and methotrexate for the treatment of rheumatoid arthritis. Rheumatology (Oxford) 2000;39: 655–65.

132. Cohen S, Cannon GW, Schiff M, et al. Two-year, blinded, randomized, controlled trial of treatment of active rheumatoid arthritis with leflunomide compared with methotrexate. Utilization of Leflunomide in the Treatment of Rheumatoid Arthritis Trial Investigator Group. Arthritis Rheum 2001; 44:1984–92.

133. Strand V, Cohen S, Schiff M, et al. Treatment of active rheumatoid arthritis with leflunomide compared with placebo and methotrexate. Leflunomide Rheumatoid Arthritis Investigators Group. Arch Intern Med 1999;159:2542–50.

134. Nash P, Thaci D, Behrens F, et al. Leflunomide improves psoriasis in patients with psoriatic arthritis: an in-depth analysis of data from the TO-PAS study. Dermatology 2006;212:238–49.

135. van Woerkom J, Kruize AA, Geenen R, et al. Safety and efficacy of Leflunomide in primary Sjögren's syndrome: a phase II pilot study. Ann Rheum Dis 2007;66:1026–32.

136. Tam LS, Li EK, Wong CK, et al. Double-blind, randomized, placebo-controlled pilot study of leflunomide in systemic lupus erythematosus. Lupus 2004;13:601–4.

137. van Denderen JC, van der Paardt M, Nurmohamed MT, et al. Double blind, randomised, placebo controlled study of leflunomide in the treatment of active ankylosing spondylitis. Ann Rheum Dis 2005;64:1761–4.

138. Metzler C, Fink C, Lamprecht P, et al. Maintenance of remission with leflunomide in Wegener's granulomatosis. Rheumatology (Oxford) 2004;43:315–20.

139. Lange U, Piegsa M, Muller-Ladner U, et al. Anti-Jo-1 antibody positive polymyositis–successful therapy with leflunomide. Autoimmunity 2006;39:261–4.

140. Handler RP. Leflunomide for relapsing polychondritis: successful longterm treatment. J Rheumatol 2006;33:1916–7.

141. Pirildar T. Treatment of adult-onset Still's disease with leflunomide and chloroquine combination in two patients. Clin Rheumatol 2003;22:157.

142. Sebastiani M, Giuggioli D, Vesprini E, et al. Successful treatment with leflunomide of arthritis in systemic sclerosis patients. Rheumatology (Oxford) 2006;45:1175–6.

143. Cherwinski HM, Cohn RG, Cheung P, et al. The immunosuppressant leflunomide inhibits lymphocyte proliferation by inhibiting pyrimidine biosynthesis. J Pharmacol Exp Ther 1995;275:1043–9.

144. Li EK, Tam LS, Tomlinson B. Leflunomide in the treatment of rheumatoid arthritis. Clin Ther 2004;26:447–59.

145. Perez-Ruiz F, Nolla JM. Influence of Leflunomide on renal handling of urate and phosphate in patients with rheumatoid arthritis. J Clin Rheumatol 2003; 9:215–8.

146. Prakash A, Jarvis B. Leflunomide: a review of its use in active rheumatoid arthritis. Drugs 1999;58:1137–64.

147. Olsen NJ, Stein CM. New drugs for rheumatoid arthritis. N Engl J Med 2004;350:2167–79.

148. Bharadwaj A, Haroon N. Peripheral neuropathy in patients on leflunomide. Rheumatology (Oxford) 2004;43:934.

149. Bonnel RA, Graham DJ. Peripheral neuropathy in patients treated with leflunomide. Clin Pharmacol Ther 2004;75:580–5.

150. Richards BL, Spies J, McGill N, et al. Effect of leflunomide on the peripheral nerves in rheumatoid arthritis. Intern Med J 2007;37(2):101–7.

151. Takeishi M, Akiyama Y, Akiba H, et al. Leflunomide induced acute interstitial pneumonia. J Rheumatol 2005;32:1160–3.

152. Sakai F, Noma S, Kurihara Y, et al. Leflunomide-related lung injury in patients with rheumatoid arthritis: imaging features. Mod Rheumatol 2005;15:173–9.

153. Suissa S, Hudson M, Ernst P. Leflunomide use and the risk of interstitial lung disease in rheumatoid arthritis. Arthritis Rheum 2006;54:1435–9.

154. Allison AC, Eugui EM. The design and development of an immunosuppressive drug, mycophenolate mofetil. Springer Semin Immunopathol 1993; 14:353–80.

155. Contreras G, Pardo V, Leclercq B, et al. Sequential therapies for proliferative lupus nephritis. N Engl J Med 2004;350:971–80.

156. Goldblum R. Therapy of rheumatoid arthritis with mycophenolate mofetil. Clin Exp Rheumatol 1993; 11(Suppl 8):S117–9.

157. Langford CA, Talar-Williams C, Sneller MC. Mycophenolate mofetil for remission maintenance in the treatment of Wegener's granulomatosis. Arthritis Rheum 2004;15:278–83.

158. Samad AS, Lindsley CB. Treatment of pulmonary hemorrhage in childhood systemic lupus erythematosus with mycophenolate mofetil. South Med J 2003;96:705–7.

159. Swigris JJ, Olson AL, Fischer A, et al. Mycophenolate mofetil is safe, well tolerated, and preserves lung function in patients with connective tissue disease-related interstitial lung disease. Chest 2006;130:30–6.

160. Staatz CE, Tett SE. Clinical pharmacokinetics and pharmacodynamics of mycophenolate in solid organ transplant recipients. Clin Pharmacokinet 2007;46:13–58.

161. Parker G, Bullingham R, Kamm B, et al. Pharmacokinetics of oral mycophenolate mofetil in volunteer subjects with varying degrees of hepatic oxidative impairment. J Clin Pharmacol 1996;36:332–44.

162. Nogueras F, Espinosa MD, Mansilla A, et al. Mycophenolate mofetil-induced neutropenia in liver transplantation. Transplant Proc 2005;37(3):1509–11.

163. Warrington JS, Shaw LM. Pharmacogenetic differences and drug-drug interactions in immunosuppressive therapy. Curr Opin Drug Metab Toxicol 2005;1:487–503.

164. Morii M, Ueno K, Ogawa A, et al. Impairment of mycophenolate mofetil absorption by iron ion. Clin Pharmacol Ther 2000;68:613–6.

165. Smith KG, Isbel NM, Catton MG, et al. Suppression of the humoral immune response by mycophenolate mofetil. Nephrol Dial Transplant 1998;13:160–4.

166. Kaczmarek I, Bigdeli AK, Vogeser M, et al. Defining algorithms for efficient therapeutic drug monitoring of mycophenolate mofetil in heart transplant recipients. Ther Drug Monit 2008;30:419–27.

167. Meiser BM, Pfeiffer M, Schmidt D, et al. Combination therapy with tacrolimus and mycophenolate mofetil following cardiac transplantation: importance of mycophenolic acid therapeutic drug monitoring. J Heart Lung Transplant 1999; 18:143–9.

168. van Gelder T, le Meur Y, Shaw LM, et al. Therapeutic drug monitoring of mycophenolate mofetil in transplantation. Ther Drug Monit 2006;28:145–54.

169. Filler G, Ehrich J. Mycophenolate mofetil for rescue therapy in acute renal transplant rejection in children should always be monitored by measurement of trough concentration. Nephrol Dial Transplant 1997;12:374–5.

170. van Gelder T, Silva HT, de Fijter JW, et al. Comparing mycophenolate mofetil regimens for de novo renal transplant recipients: the fixed-dose concentration-controlled trial. Transplantation 2008;86(8):1043–51.

171. Furst DE. Pharmacokinetics of hydroxychloroquine and chloroquine during treatment of rheumatic diseases. Lupus 1996;5(Suppl 1):S11–5.

172. Tett SE. Clinical pharmacokinetics of slow-acting antirheumatic drugs. Clin Pharmacokinet 1993;25:392–407.

173. Estes ML, Ewing-Wilson D, Chou SM, et al. Chloroquine neuromyotoxicity. Clinical and pathologic perspective. Am J Med 1987;82:447–55.

174. Ratiff NB, Estes ML, Myles JL, et al. Diagnosis of chloroquine cardiomyopathy by endomyocardial biopsy. N Engl J Med 1987;316:191–3.

175. Brachman PS Jr, Metchock B, Kozarsky PE. Effects of antimalarial chemoprophylactic agents on the viability of the Ty21a typhoid vaccine strain. Clin Infect Dis 1992;15:1057–8.

176. Horowitz H, Carbonaro CA. Inhibition of the Salmonella typhi oral vaccine strain, Ty21a, by mefloquine and chloroquine. J Infect Dis 1992;166:1462–4.

177. Pappaioanou M, Fishbein DB, Dreesen DW, et al. Antibody response to preexposure human diploid-cell rabies vaccine given concurrently with chloroquine. N Engl J Med 1986;314:280–4.

178. Rennie IG. Clinically important ocular reactions to systemic drug therapy. Drug Saf 1993;9:196–211.

179. Elder M, Rahman AM, McLay J. Early paracentral visual field loss in patients taking hydroxychloroquine. Arch Ophthalmol 2006;124:1729–33.

180. Yam JC, Kwok AK. Ocular toxicity of hydroxychloroquine. Hong Kong Med J 2006;12:294–304.

181. Mazzuca SA, Yung R, Brandt KD, et al. Current practices for monitoring ocular toxicity related to hydroxychloroquine (Plaquenil) therapy. J Rheumatol 1994;21:59–63.

182. Daniels CE, Wilkes MC, Edens M, et al. Imatinib mesylate inhibits the profibrogenic activity of TGF-beta and prevents bleomycin-mediated lung fibrosis. J Clin Invest 2004;114:1308–16.

183. Ghofrani HA, Seeger W, Grimminger F. Imatinib for the treatment of pulmonary arterial hypertension. N Engl J Med 2005;353:1412–3.

184. Patterson KC, Weissmann A, Ahmadi T, et al. Imatinib mesylate in the treatment of refractory idiopathic pulmonary arterial hypertension. Ann Intern Med 2006;145:152–3.

185. van Glabbeke M, Verweij J, Casali PG, et al. Predicting toxicities for patients with advanced gastrointestinal stromal tumours treated with imatinib: a study of the European Organisation for Research and Treatment of Cancer, the Italian Sarcoma Group, and the Australasian Gastro-Intestinal Trials Group (EORTC-ISG-AGITG). Eur J Cancer 2006;42:2277–85.

186. Hensley ML, Ford JM. Imatinib treatment: specific issues related to safety, fertility, and pregnancy. Semin Hematol 2003;40:21–5.

187. Chintalgattu V, Patel SS, Khakoo AY. Cardiovascular effects of tyrosine kinase inhibitors used to gastrointestinal stromal tumors. Hematol Oncol Clin North Am 2009;23:97–107.

188. Yamasawa H, Sugiyama Y, Bando M, et al. Drug-induced pneumonitis associated with imatinib mesylate in a patient with idiopathic pulmonary fibrosis. Respiration 2008;75:350–4.

189. Yokoyama T, Miyazawa K, Kurakawa E, et al. Interstitial pneumonia induced by imatinib mesylate: pathologic study demonstrates alveolar destruction and fibrosis with eosinophilic infiltration. Leukemia 2004;18:645–6.

190. Ostensen M, Lockshin M, Doria A, et al. Update on safety during pregnancy of biological agents and some immunosuppressive anti-rheumatic drugs. Rheumatology (Oxford) 2008;47(Suppl 3):iii28–31.

191. Miniero R, Tardivo I, Curtoni ES, et al. Pregnancy after renal transplantation in Italian patients: focus on fetal outcome. J Nephrol 2002;15(6):626–32.

192. Ostensen M, Ramsey-Goldman R. Treatment of inflammatory rheumatic disorders in pregnancy: what are the safest treatment options? Drug Saf 1998;19(5):389–410.

193. Weber LT, Shipkova M, Lamersdorf T, et al. Pharmacokinetics of mycophenolic acid (MPA) and determinants of MPA free fraction in pediatric and adult renal transplant recipients. German Study group on Mycophenolate Mofetil Therapy in Pediatric Renal Transplant Recipients. J Am Soc Nephrol 1998;9:1511–20.

194. Mori M, Naruto T, Imagawa T, et al. Methotrexate for the treatment of juvenile idiopathic arthritis: process to approval for JIA indication in Japan. Mod Rheumatol 2006;19:1–11.

195. Sarwal M, Pascual J. Immunosuppression minimization in pediatric transplantation. Am J Transplant 2007;7:2227–35.

196. Sarwal MM. Out with the old, in with the new: immunosuppresion minimization in children. Curr Opin Organ Transplant 2008;13:513–21.

197. Dubinsky MC, Reyes E, Ofman J, et al. A cost-effectiveness analysis of alternative disease management strategies in patients with Crohn's disease treated with azathioprine or 6-mercaptopurine. Am J Gastroenterol 2005;100:2239–47.

198. Godeau B, Coutant-Perronne V, Le Thi Huong D, et al. *Pneumocystis carinii* pneumonia in the course of connective tissue disease: report of 34 cases. J Rheumatol 1994;21:246–51.

199. Yale SH, Limper AH. *Pneumocystis carinii* pneumonia in patients without acquired immunodeficiency syndrome: associated illness and prior corticosteroid therapy. Mayo Clin Proc 1996;71:5–13.

200. Sen RP, Walsh TE, Fisher W, et al. Pulmonary complications of combination therapy with cyclophosphamide and prednisone. Chest 1991;99:143–6.

201. Rodriguez M, Fishman JA. Prevention of infection due to *Pneumocystis* spp. in human

immunodeficiency virus-negative immunocompromised patients. Clin Microbiol Rev 2004;17:770–82.

202. Ogawa J, Harigai M, Nagasaka K, et al. Prediction of and prophylaxis against Pneumocystis pneumonia in patients with connective tissue diseases undergoing medium- or high-dose corticosteroid therapy. Mod Rheumatol 2005;15:91–6.

203. Bedrossian CW, Sussman J, Conklin RH, et al. Azathioprine-associated interstitial pneumonitis. Am J Clin Pathol 1984;82:148–54.

204. Gross DC, Sasaki TM, Buick MK, et al. Acute respiratory failure and pulmonary fibrosis secondary to administration of mycophenolate mofetil. Transplantation 1997;64:1607–9.

205. Rosado MF, Donna E, Ahn YS. Challenging problems in advanced malignancy. Case 3. Imatinib mesylate-induced interstitial pneumonitis. J Clin Oncol 2003;21:3171–3.

206. Available at: www.pneumotox.com. Accessed December 5, 2009.

Lung Transplantation in Autoimmune Diseases

James C. Lee, MD, Vivek N. Ahya, MD*

KEYWORDS

- Lung transplantation • Autoimmune diseases
- Lung diseases

In the last 45 years, lung transplantation has evolved from its status as a rare, extreme form of surgical therapy for the treatment of advanced lung diseases to an accepted therapeutic option for select patients. Short- and intermediate-term survival is now commonplace and long-term survival is possible. As of June 30, 2008, the registry for the International Society for Heart and Lung Transplantation (ISHLT) had accrued data from more than 29,000 lung transplants (LTxp) performed across the world.[1] Important indications for lung transplantation include idiopathic pulmonary fibrosis (IPF), chronic obstructive pulmonary disease (COPD), cystic fibrosis, and idiopathic pulmonary arterial hypertension (IPAH). Although pulmonary fibrosis and pulmonary vascular disease are common pulmonary manifestations of collagen vascular diseases, in the international registry, the number of LTxp performed for the indication of systemic autoimmune diseases (AID) accounted for only 0.8% of transplants.[1] The reasons for such a low number are multifactorial and are a main subject of this article. Before discussing issues specific to these patients, important topics relevant to all transplant recipients are briefly reviewed.

GENERAL OVERVIEW OF LUNG TRANSPLANTATION

The first lung transplantation procedure was performed by Dr James Hardy and colleagues[2] at the University of Mississippi in 1963 in a patient with advanced emphysema, lung cancer, and renal insufficiency. Although this patient succumbed to multiorgan system failure after 18 days, this initial case highlighted the future potential of lung transplantation by showing that the procedure was technically feasible and that the immunologic barriers associated with acute rejection were not insurmountable. However, the poor outcome also emphasized the importance of selecting appropriate candidates for transplantation.

The modern era of transplantation began in the early 1980s with the first successful heart-lung and unilateral LTxp procedures.[3,4] Both recipients survived more than 5 years, considerably longer than previous experience. This dramatic improvement in outcomes was related to several factors including the introduction of the potent new immunosuppressive agent cyclosporine, recognition of the deleterious effects of high doses of corticosteroids on bronchial anastomotic healing, and optimization of surgical techniques and intensive care unit care. Since the 1980s, there has been continued but gradual improvement in posttransplant survival.

Outcomes

Outcomes after lung transplantation have improved in the past 20 years, but they remain inferior to what has been achieved after other solid organ transplant procedures. Although lung transplantation offers the possibility of longer survival and improved quality of life (QOL) for select patients with advanced lung diseases, the LTxp recipient remains vulnerable to numerous

Lung Transplantation Program, Division of Pulmonary, Allergy, and Critical Care Medicine, Department of Medicine, University of Pennsylvania School of Medicine, 832 West Gates Building, 3400 Spruce Street, Philadelphia, PA 19104, USA
* Corresponding author.
E-mail address: ahyav@uphs.upenn.edu

Clin Chest Med 31 (2010) 589–603
doi:10.1016/j.ccm.2010.05.003
0272-5231/10/$ – see front matter © 2010 Elsevier Inc. All rights reserved.

complications that threaten both of these objectives. These issues are discussed in greater detail later. In the ISHLT 2009 annual report, patients transplanted in the current era (January 2000–June 2008) had an overall 1-year survival rate of 81.4% and a 5-year survival of 54.2%. A 10-year survival rate of 26.8% was reported for the cohort of patients transplanted in the late 1990s.[1] Outcomes also varied depending on the recipient's underlying diagnosis, and this may in part be because of differences in age, comorbidities, and technical issues with performing the transplant procedure. For example, patients with cystic fibrosis had a 1-year survival rate of 82.6% and a 5-year survival of 57.4%. In contrast, recipients with IPF (1- and 5-year survival rates of 74.1% and 45.9%) and IPAH (1 and 5-year survival rate of 71.1% and 51.7%) had inferior outcomes.[1]

Lung Allocation

The success of lung transplantation has resulted in increased demand for the transplant procedure. As with other types of solid organ transplantation, the demand for organs exceeds donor availability.[5] With a shortage of life-saving donor organs, the goal of any organ allocation system is to try to distribute organs in an equitable manner. In the United States, lungs are allocated based on calculation of a lung allocation score (LAS). In general, patients with greater medical urgency and increased likelihood of deriving a benefit with transplantation are given priority. LAS calculation is based on a complex equation using more than 13 clinical and demographic variables. Patients with a higher score are given priority over candidates with lower scores.[6] For more information on the US lung allocation system, the reader is referred to the following document prepared by the United Network of Organ Sharing: http://www.unos.org/SharedContentDocuments/Lung_Professional.pdf.[1]

Complications

The LTxp recipient is subject to several complications that affect survival and QOL, including primary graft dysfunction (PGD), acute and chronic graft rejection, infection, and side effects related to immunosuppressive medications.

PGD

The most feared early complication after transplantation is the development of PGD. Clinical and histopathologic findings of PGD are similar to those seen in patients with the acute respiratory distress syndrome (ARDS). Although its pathogenesis is not fully understood, PGD is believed to be the result of numerous insults to the allograft that encompasses the entire LTxp procedure, beginning with donor injury and brain death, and extending to organ harvesting, hypothermic storage, and subsequent rewarming and reperfusion during implantation. This injury may be amplified further by intraoperative and recipient-specific factors.[7–9] The incidence of PGD ranges from 10% to 25% and it is associated with a 30-day mortality of approximately 50%.[7] In addition, survivors have increased long-term mortality and risk of developing chronic rejection.[10,11] Treatment options are largely supportive and similar to those used in the management of ARDS. No therapeutic intervention has been shown to be useful for preventing PGD or treating it when it does occur.

Acute rejection

Organ transplantation involves the transfer of donor antigens into the recipient, and exposure of these foreign, nonself antigens to the transplant recipient's immune system triggers a potent immunologic attack directed against the allograft. This alloimmune response, also called acute rejection, is commonly seen after lung transplantation, with some reports documenting a rejection rate of more than 75% in the first posttransplant year.[12,13] The alloimmune response is primarily directed by the cell-mediated arm of the immune system, although there is increasing evidence that innate and humoral immunity are also important.[13,14] The diagnosis of acute rejection requires bronchoscopy and is established by the histologic findings of perivascular and/or peribronchiolar mononuclear cellular infiltrates in transbronchial biopsy specimens.[14] Although acute rejection may be readily treated with high doses of corticosteroids or other potent immunosuppressive agents, it remains an important posttransplant complication because its treatment may increase the risk of serious infection and malignancy, and it is the most consistently reported risk factor for chronic rejection, a condition for which there are few therapeutic options.[15]

Chronic rejection

Chronic allograft rejection remains the main obstacle to long-term survival and a major cause of reduced health-related QOL after lung transplantation.[1,16,17] The classic histopathologic finding of chronic rejection on lung biopsy is bronchiolitis obliterans (BO). Approximately half of all LTxp recipients develop chronic rejection within 5 years and almost 75% by 10 years.[1] Although the clinical course of chronic rejection can be variable, median survival after onset is 3 to 4 years.[18–20] Clinically, patients may be asymptomatic during early stages and later develop progressive dyspnea and cough. Although a pathologic determination of chronic rejection is possible on transbronchial biopsy specimens, the sensitivity for detecting BO is poor. Bronchoscopy, however, remains an important diagnostic tool for ruling out other causes of dyspnea and airflow obstruction (eg, acute rejection, infection, or bronchial anastomotic stricture).[14] Surgical lung biopsy specimens have a higher sensitivity for BO, unfortunately performing serial surveillance surgical lung biopsies is not useful or practical because of high procedural risk. In the absence of safe and reliable tools for detecting BO, the LTxp community has established noninvasive criteria based on measurements of pulmonary function to identify patients likely to have chronic rejection.[16] The presence of airflow obstruction on spirometry, as defined by forced expiratory volume after 1 second (FEV_1) of less than 80% of the posttransplant baseline, in the absence of other causes of airflow obstruction, identifies a patient with bronchiolitis obliterans syndrome (BOS) Higher degrees of airflow obstruction correlate with higher grades of BOS.[16] Although BOS is a physiologic rather than a pathologic assessment, the term BOS is often used interchangeably with the terms BO or chronic rejection.

The pathogenesis of chronic rejection is not well understood. BO has been recognized outside the LTxp population and seems to be the result of different types of lung injury. It has been described after toxic inhalation, toxic ingestion, after respiratory infections, as well as in patients with systemic AID and patients who have undergone allogeneic hematopoietic stem cell transplantation.[21–24] In lung transplantation, the development of BO is believed to be the consequence of multiple potentially injurious processes that damage the small airways, trigger inflammation, impair healing, and promote fibroproliferation. Such processes include alloimmune factors (acute rejection), alloindependent factors (respiratory infections, PGD, gastroesophageal reflux disease [GERD]) and autoimmune factors (host immune response to exposure of previously sequestered bronchiolar self antigens such as type V collagen).[15,25]

Treatment options for chronic rejection are limited. Modifying or increasing immunosuppression has generally not been beneficial, although some reports have suggested that this approach may slow the rate of decline in lung function. Most published studies have significant methodologic flaws. Thus, treatment approaches for chronic rejection vary from center to center and are largely based on limited data and institutional biases. More recently, reports have suggested that treatment with the immunomodulatory macrolide antibiotic azithromycin may improve lung function in up to 40% of patients with chronic rejection. Although benefit has not yet been confirmed by large randomized clinical trials, the excellent safety profile of azithromycin has established it as the initial choice for treatment of chronic rejection at many transplant programs.[26–28] Attempts to prevent chronic rejection from occurring have also been disappointing. A small randomized single-center study suggested that treatment with aerosolized cyclosporine improved survival and reduced incidence of BOS.[29] A large, phase III, randomized, multicenter clinical trial is under way to address the important question of whether or not this agent improves outcomes and reduces the risk of developing chronic rejection.

Discussion of many of the other posttransplant complications is beyond the scope of this article but they are briefly summarized in **Table 1**.

Patient Selection

Perhaps one of the most daunting aspects of managing LTxp candidates is determining their suitability for transplantation. These patients have often exhausted all medical options and face the prospects of deteriorating QOL, impending respiratory failure, and poor short-term survival without transplantation. The limited supply of donor organs and significant number of deaths on transplant waiting lists necessitates rigorous selection of patients for transplantation.[5] At the core of the patient selection process are 2 fundamental principles. The first is specific to the individual patient and is a risk-benefit analysis to ascertain potential benefit with transplantation. This analysis requires an understanding of the natural history of the patient's disorder and recognition of other comorbidities that may compromise posttransplant outcome. The second principle reflects a programmatic risk assessment of whether or not the individual patient's predicted posttransplant outcome is acceptable, an assessment that involves taking into account the other patients on the waiting list and the transplant center's overall outcomes and expertise. Making precise predictions on survival and other outcomes such as QOL remains imprecise at best. Complicating matters further, there is not yet consensus in the transplant community regarding which metrics should be used to best judge outcome.[6] Thus, it is not surprising that there is variability in patient selection criteria among different transplant centers. This variability is particularly important and relevant for patients with AID. If a patient is turned down at one

Table 1
Common complications of lung transplantation

Complication	
PGD	Affects 10%–25% of all LTxp[7]
	Leading cause of early mortality: 30-day mortality of 50%[7]
	Survivors have impaired physical function, increased risk for BOS, increased mortality[10,11,108]
Acute rejection	Up to 75% incidence in first year after LTxp[12,13]
	Increased risk of infection with augmented immunosuppression treatment
	Increased risk for chronic rejection[15]
Chronic rejection	Most important limiting factor for long-term survival and QOL
	50% incidence at 5 years, 75% by 10 years[1]
	Median survival after onset of 3–4 years[18–20]
	No proven treatment
Infections	Allograft and native lungs at risk in immunosuppressed patients[109]
	Donor-derived, community-acquired, nosocomial, and opportunistic pathogens
	Impaired cough reflex and mucociliary clearance from lung denervation and disrupted lymphatic drainage from surgery
	Bronchial anastomosis prone to ischemic injury and resulting bacterial and fungal infections
	Viral infections may contribute to development of BOS[110,111]
Malignancy	3- to 4-fold increased risk of developing cancer[112]
	Nonmelanoma skin cancers most common[112–114]
	Posttransplant lymphoproliferative disorders[112–114]
	Greater incidence of bronchogenic carcinoma: especially native lung of single-lung transplant in former smokers[115]
Medication side effects[5]	Renal insufficiency
	Hypertension
	Diabetes mellitus
	Posterior reversible leukoencephalopathy
	Osteoporosis
	Muscle wasting
	Cataracts
	Leukopenia
	Nausea and vomiting
	Diarrhea
	High risk of medication interactions

transplant center, it may be worth exploring their candidacy at an alternative site.

SPECIFIC ISSUES FOR THE LTxP PATIENT WITH AID

Although advanced cardiopulmonary disease is not uncommon in patients with severe AID, only 181 of the 23,528 LTxp procedures reported to the ISHLT registry between January 1995 and June 2008 were performed for a stated indication of connective tissue disease.[1] The reasons for such paucity are likely related to the protean extrapulmonary manifestations of AID, which often pose strong relative or absolute contraindications to lung transplantation. Active vasculitis, severe neurologic, cardiac, or liver disease, and the requirement for high doses of immunomodulatory therapy to control the AID typically preclude consideration for lung transplantation. On rare occasions, a multiorgan transplant procedure (eg, lung/liver or heart/lung transplantation) may be considered.[30,31] In addition, these patients are at increased risk for developing anti-HLA antibodies, are often debilitated (related to the lung disease, chronic steroid use, poor nutritional status, chronic pain, joint deformities, neuromuscular weakness, and so forth), have preexisting renal insufficiency and severe gastroesophageal disease (gastroparesis, esophageal dysmotility, reflux); conditions that further increase the risk for poor posttransplant outcome.[32] A few of these extrapulmonary comorbidities are examined in greater detail in later sections.

Anti-HLA Antibodies

In evaluating potential candidates for lung transplantation, measurement of preformed HLA antibodies is routinely performed. HLA-class I and class II antibodies have been associated with hyperacute rejection, a life-threatening process triggered by binding of preformed donor-specific anti-HLA antibodies to antigens in the graft vasculature, resulting in activation of the complement and coagulation cascades. Within minutes to hours, severe inflammation and thrombosis occur, and graft failure rapidly ensues.[33] Thus, in transplant candidates who are sensitized (ie, have pretransplant anti-HLA antibodies), donor HLA types specific for these antibodies must be avoided. Even if hyperacute rejection does not develop, there is increasing evidence that these patients are at greater risk for other dangerous immunologic complications such as acute and chronic rejection and may have poorer survival.[34–38] In addition to anti-HLA antibodies, the presence of

non-HLA antibodies is also recognized as being potentially detrimental to graft function.[39]

AID, especially systemic lupus erythematosus (SLE), are characterized by autoantibody production. Although many of these antibodies are directed against non-HLA nuclear, cytoplasmic, and cell membrane molecules, reports from the renal transplant literature suggest that these patients are also at greater risk for developing anti-HLA antibodies.[40–42] In clinical practice, the presence of these antibodies increases the difficulty of identifying appropriate organs for transplantation. Highly sensitized patients may wait years for an acceptable donor. The effect of other autoantibodies on posttransplant outcome, or whether or not patients with AID have a greater propensity for developing de novo HLA or non-HLA antibodies has not been established.

Exercise Capacity

The clinical manifestations of many AID include significant joint and musculoskeletal involvement that directly affect pre- and posttransplant exercise capacity. For example, degenerative arthropathies are a common complication of rheumatoid arthritis and the seronegative spondyloarthropathies. Inflammatory myopathies such as dermatomyositis and polymyositis can impair strength and conditioning. In addition, associated diaphragmatic inflammation may contribute to dyspnea, restrictive pulmonary physiology, and reduced functional status.[43,44] It is critically important to consider diaphragmatic weakness because its presence may exaggerate the severity of parenchymal lung disease on pulmonary function testing, increase the likelihood of prolonged mechanical ventilation after transplantation, and most importantly, it is not corrected with lung transplantation.

Exercise capacity, measured by the 6-minute walk test (6MWT), before transplantation has a direct relationship with functional status after transplantation, although the correlation between pretransplant 6MWT distance and posttransplant survival is less clear.[45,46] In practice, the 6MWT is used to help guide timing for active listing for transplantation. Several studies have shown that reduced 6MWT distance in patients with diffuse parenchymal lung disease is associated with disease severity and increased mortality; however, this has not been established in patients with lung disease associated with systemic sclerosis.[47–51] Although data regarding 6MWT distance and posttransplant outcome are lacking, deconditioning and reduced exercise capacity have been associated with increased morbidity after other thoracic surgical procedures.[52] For this reason, many

LTxp programs consider ambulating less than a certain minimum distance (eg, 182 m [600 feet]) on the 6MWT to be a strong relative or absolute contraindication to transplantation.[53]

During the transplant evaluation process, the rehabilitation potential of the transplant candidate must also be taken into account. Patients with AID and musculoskeletal involvement often require intensive and extended physical therapy and pulmonary rehabilitation to promote recuperation and return to normal functional status. If hampered by debilitating joint and muscle problems, rehabilitation potential may be limited. Another consideration is whether musculoskeletal pain related to AID is adequately controlled and if high doses of chronic narcotic treatment are required. In these situations, management of postoperative pain can be difficult and could potentially affect postoperative weaning from mechanical ventilation and subsequent rehabilitation.[54]

Immunosuppressive Therapy for AID

As reviewed in the article by Meyer and colleagues elsewhere in this issue, the potential side effects of immunosuppressive therapies to treat systemic AID are numerous. Many of these agents such as corticosteroids, azathioprine, mycophenolate mofetil, and calcineurin inhibitors are commonly used as part of a post-LTxp immunosuppressive regimen. Before transplant, adequate control of AID flares with these agents might offer reassurance that the AID could be managed with traditional agents after transplantation. The use of potent immunomodulatory agents such as cyclophosphamide or antitumor necrosis factor agents (eg, infliximab) is of greater concern because the risk of infection and bone marrow toxicity (particularly with cyclophosphamide) when administered in combination with other posttransplant antirejection drugs is substantial.

Pretransplant treatment with high doses of corticosteroids and early posttransplant use of sirolimus have been associated with an increased risk of bronchial anastomotic dehiscence.[55,56] Chronic treatment with nonsteroidal antiinflammatory drugs (NSAIDs) may increase the risk of renal insufficiency. LTxp recipients are at particularly high risk for developing renal insufficiency (25% and 37% at 1 and 5 years, respectively) as a result of chronic administration of high doses of calcineurin inhibitors such as tacrolimus and cyclosporine.[1] Thus, pretransplant renal insufficiency is an important relative contraindication to transplantation, and posttransplant use of NSAIDs is strongly discouraged.[32,57] Several of the immunomodulatory agents used in treatment of AID have been associated with acute lung injury syndromes. Agents such as methotrexate, sirolimus, infliximab, and leflunamide have all been reported to cause pneumonitis and must be used cautiously in the LTxp recipient.[58–62]

Venous Thromboembolism

Venous thromboembolism (VTE) is not uncommon after lung transplantation, with reports indicating that 8% to 22% of patients may develop this complication.[63,64] In addition to pulmonary embolism, thrombus formation at the pulmonary venous anastomotic site is a potentially life-threatening early posttransplant complication that can result in respiratory failure as a result of refractory pulmonary edema and increased risk for embolic stroke.[65] The presence of a hypercoaguable state increases the risk for VTE.[64] Patients with AID, especially SLE, seem to have higher rates of thrombotic complications when compared with the general population. Although there are numerous predisposing risk factors (eg, debility, nephrotic syndrome), the antiphospholipid antibody syndrome (APLS) is perhaps of greatest concern.[66] APLS is characterized by the presence of antiphospholipid antibodies in association with thrombotic disorders of the arterial and/or venous system, thrombocytopenia, and recurrent pregnancy loss. Although reports in the literature specific to the LTxp population are sparse, in kidney transplantation, several studies have suggested that patients with APLS are at higher risk for developing posttransplant pulmonary embolism as well as graft thrombosis and graft loss.[67–69] Initiation of anticoagulation in the perioperative period, however, may significantly reduce the risk of postrenal transplant graft thrombosis/loss.[70] With regards to APLS in lung transplantation, there is a single case report of a transplant recipient with APLS who underwent unilateral transplantation and subsequently developed a pulmonary embolism and diffuse alveolar hemorrhage that on lung biopsy showed findings that indicate a necrotizing capillaritis. Treatment with anticoagulation, immunosuppression, and plasmapheresis was required before clinical improvement was seen.[71]

The need for chronic anticoagulation before transplantation or immediately after surgery may be considered a contraindication to lung transplantation, especially for patients who are anticipated to have a complex and difficult explantation procedure and thus are at high risk for significant bleeding complications causing significant bleeding. The use of cardiopulmonary bypass requires administration of high levels of systemic anticoagulation, which can also increase the risk of intraoperative hemorrhage. Reinitiation of anticoagulation in the postoperative period may be problematic if surgically related bleeding (eg, hemothorax) is an issue. Excessive bleeding may require surgical reexploration and blood transfusions. Transfusions have been associated with the development of PGD and transfusion-related acute lung injury.[72–74] Withholding anticoagulation, however, may increase risk for VTE. Long-term anticoagulation also complicates performance of urgent transbronchial biopsies to assess for graft rejection or infection.

Pulmonary Vascular Disease

As described earlier, pulmonary hypertension is a common manifestation of AID (eg, systemic sclerosis and SLE), and is often the main indication for referral for lung transplantation. The presence of severe pulmonary hypertension, however, is itself a significant risk factor for PGD.[75–78] This risk may in part be because of increased mechanical endothelial shear stress in the graft during reperfusion.[72,79]

Another manifestation of vascular dysfunction in patients with AID pertinent to perioperative management is the Raynaud phenomenon. This condition is characterized by periodic arterial vasospasm and vasoconstriction in the digits in response to cold, stress, or temperature changes. Postoperative hypothermia and use of vasopressor agents may result in irreversible ischemic injury to digits. Use of hand warmers and minimized use of vasopressors should be strongly considered.

Gastrointestinal Disease

Gastrointestinal (GI) complications are frequently seen in patients with AID, especially in systemic sclerosis; studies have reported that 50% to 90% of patients may be affected.[80,81] Although any part of the GI tract may be involved, esophageal and gastric disease is most common. Severe GERD, esophageal dysmotility, and gastroparesis may result in heartburn, dysphagia, nausea, vomiting, recurrent aspiration, and weight loss. However, on occasion, patients may be asymptomatic. These complications are associated with reduced QOL and survival and have significant implications for lung transplantation.[80]

Based on studies suggesting an association between GERD and microaspiration of gastric contents in the pathogenesis of asthma and chronic cough, there has been interest in determining whether or not such a link exists for the development of pulmonary fibrosis in patients with scleroderma.[82–84] Data supporting this link have been conflicting. For example, review of the records of 39 patients with scleroderma who had completed testing of pulmonary function, esophageal motility, and pH monitoring showed no association between the presence of lung disease and the severity of reflux.[85] More recently, however, evaluation of 40 consecutive patients with systemic sclerosis with pH-impedance monitoring showed that patients with systemic sclerosis and interstitial lung disease had more severe reflux (acid and nonacid) than those without interstitial lung disease.[81]

There is increasing recognition that GERD is common in patients with advanced lung diseases referred for lung transplantation, especially in patients with AID. In a series of 23 patients with AID referred to a LTxp center, 18 (83%) had pathologic GERD and 78% with manometry data had aperistalsis or abnormal peristalsis.[83] In a larger study of 78 consecutive patients assessed for lung transplantation (10 of whom had scleroderma and 16 of whom had "miscellaneous diseases"), GERD symptoms were present in 63%, the lower esophageal sphincter was hypotensive in 72%, and 33% had esophageal body dysmotility.[86] Reflux disease can also be exacerbated by the transplant procedure itself. Vagal nerve injury (mechanical or thermal) experienced during the surgical procedure can contribute to gastroparesis and esophageal dysmotility. The vagus nerves course posteroinferiorly through the mediastinum and supply branches to the pulmonary and esophageal plexuses before entering the abdomen. They may be inadvertently injured during the explantation procedure, especially if complex dissection of the posterior mediastinum is required.[87] Posttransplant medications, especially narcotics and perhaps the calcineurin inhibitors, may further delay gastric emptying and increase the propensity for aspiration.[83,87] In a study of 23 patients who underwent 24-hour pH monitoring before and after transplantation, there was a significant increase in GERD following surgery, from 35% to 65% of patients studied. Only 20% of those patients with abnormal studies were symptomatic.[88] In another cohort of 43 posttransplant patients, 91% had abnormal gastric emptying studies.[89] Thus, it is clear that gastroesophageal disease is common after transplantation. An important early posttransplant concern is that this population is at high risk for developing severe aspiration pneumonia that compromises graft function; for this reason, severe gastroesophageal disease is an absolute or strong relative

Table 2
Summary of published series of LTxp performed for systemic sclerosis

Author	Study Population	Length of Follow-up	Outcomes/Findings
Levine et al[116] University of Texas at San Antonio–1994	2 patients with limited SSc Dx: 1 with PF, 1 with PF+pHTN Both with mild esophageal dysfunction	2.5 months and 2 years	1 patient alive at 2.75 years after LTxp with no complications and resolution of arthralgias and improvement in Raynaud phenomenon 1 patient died of *Pseudomonas* sepsis, ARDS, and MOSF at POD 90
Pigula et al[117] University of Pittsburgh–1997	6 patients with SSc All patients with pHTN only All patients were free of extrapulmonary disease	18.9 ± 15.6 months	5 of 6 patients alive 6–60 months after LTxp; 1 died at POD 22 from pneumonia and pancreatitis No differences in infection rate compared with patients with pHTN unrelated to systemic disease; lower rate of rejection in patients with pHTN related to systemic disease No differences in 1- and 2-year survival rates compared with patients undergoing LTxp for isolated pulmonary disease
Rosas et al[118] Johns Hopkins University–2000	9 patients with SSc: 6 limited, 3 diffuse SSc Concomitant renal insufficiency, aspiration, or skin breakdown precluded referral for LTxp	4 years	Compared with IPF population: No differences in survival, annual rate of acute rejection, infection, or kidney function
Kubo et al[119] University of Pittsburgh–2001	12 patients with SSc	5 years	3 deaths within 30 days after LTxp, 6 deaths overall Causes of death included pneumonia,[3] PGD,[1] PE,[1] metastatic cholangiocarcinoma[1] Compared with LTxp patients for IPF or COPD: FEV$_1$ at 1 year, and 1- and 5- year survival after LTxp were not statistically different

Study	Details	Follow-up	Findings
Massad et al[120] University of Illinois at Chicago–2005	Review of pooled data of 47 patients with SSc undergoing LTxp at 23 US centers entered into the United Network of Organ Sharing database from October 1987 to March 2004		7 early deaths (≤30 days) and 17 late deaths (>30 days) Causes of early death: PGD,[2] cardiac event,[2] bacterial infection,[1] CVA,[1] not recorded[1] Leading cause of late death: infection[7] 3 of 27 (11%) patients with SSc undergoing LTxp had BOS within first year, not statistically different from BOS incidence in rest of registry in first year (9%) Compared with rest of registry (10,070 patients): 1-, 2-, and 3-year survival was not statistically different
Schachna et al[121] Johns Hopkins University and University of Pittsburgh–2006	29 patients with SSc: 14 new patients added to previously published series of 15 total patients at these institutions[117,118] Concomitant renal insufficiency, aspiration, or skin breakdown precluded referral for LTxp	2 years	11 patients (38%) died in first 2 years 7 died within first month; causes of death: PGD[4]–confined to SLT for pHTN group, pneumonia[3] Estimated mortality at 6 months was increased in SSc patients compared with IPF and PAH patients, but not statistically significant By 24 months, survival rates converged and among all 3 groups (Ssc, IPF, PAH) were not statistically different
Shitrit et al[122] Tel Aviv University–2009	7 patients in new series added to pooled experience of 47 patients in literature[120] 6 of 7 patients had PF+pHTN, 1 had only PF	Up to 50 months	1 of 7 patients had fatal PGD Compared with institutional experience in LTxp for other indications, 1- and 3- year survival rates were similar, as were infection and rejection rates

Abbreviations: CVA, cerebral vascular accident; Dx, diagnosis; MOSF, multiorgan system failure; PAH, idiopathic pulmonary arterial hypertension; PE, pulmonary embolism; PF, pulmonary fibrosis; pHTN, pulmonary hypertension; POD, postoperative day; SLT, single-lung transplant; Ssc, systemic sclerosis.

contraindication to lung transplantation at many LTxp centers.[43,90]

In the past decade, there has also been increasing evidence implicating GERD as a risk factor for chronic allograft dysfunction. Interest in the link between severe GERD and BOS was stimulated by a report from the LTxp center at Duke University describing a patient with severe reflux disease who developed accelerated decline in lung function after retransplantation. Pulmonary function rapidly improved after Nissen fundoplication.[91] Subsequently, these investigators retrospectively examined esophageal pH studies in 43 patients at a median of 558 days after transplant and showed that there was a negative correlation between total or upright acid reflux and FEV_1 ratio.[92] In 2005, the LTxp group at the University of Toronto showed that bile acid levels in bronchoalveolar lavage fluid (BALF) were significantly increased in patients with BOS compared with those patients without BOS. Freedom from BOS was significantly shortened in patients with increased levels of BALF bile acids.[93]

Medical treatment options for GERD are limited. Although proton pump inhibitors (PPIs) may reduce acid reflux, data suggest that nonacid reflux may also be important in the development of graft dysfunction. In a recent study, 18 LTxp patients treated with PPIs were evaluated with pH-impedance monitoring and testing for pepsin and bile acids in BALF (as markers for gastric and duodenogastroesophageal aspiration) and compared with 45 patients not treated with PPIs. Treatment with PPIs did not reduce total reflux events, esophageal volume exposure, or proximal extent of reflux. Pepsin was detected in the BALF of all patients and bile acids in 50%. More importantly, bile acids were detected in 70% of patients with BOS compared with 31% in stable patients without BOS.[94] Thus, treatment approaches that aim to simply reduce acid production are inadequate for management of severe posttransplant GERD and may not reduce the risk of chronic rejection.[89,95]

Surgical interventions for GERD are attractive therapeutic options because they reduce the risk of acid and nonacid reflux. In a small retrospective analysis of 43 LTxp recipients who underwent fundoplication for abnormal pH studies, of the 26 who met criteria for BOS, 16 had improved pulmonary function after surgery.[96] A follow-up analysis of 16 patients with severe GERD who underwent early fundoplication (within 90 days of transplantation) showed improved rates of BOS and survival when compared with patients with reflux who did not undergo fundoplication.[97] These small retrospective studies have lent support to the

practice of aggressive surgical intervention for GERD in LTxp recipients. However, prospective, randomized studies need to be performed and demonstrate benefit before surgery for treatment of GERD can be recommended with confidence.[98] Several major questions remain unanswered, including the optimal timing of surgery and choice of surgical procedure.[99]

Although it may be advantageous to perform fundoplication before transplantation to offer protection against perioperative aspiration, many patients with advanced lung disease may be unable to tolerate general anesthesia or the surgical procedure. Laparascopic fundoplication, however, has been performed safely in stable patients with IPF awaiting lung transplantation (average preoperative FEV_1 of 55% of predicted and average diffusion lung capacity for carbon monoxide of 35% of predicted).[100] The laparascopic approach is generally favored because in experienced hands it seems to have lower operative complications, reduced pain and hospitalization days, and outcomes equivalent to the open approach.[101,102] It remains to be seen if in the future, newer endoscopic techniques will achieve equivalent outcomes without the need for surgery.[103] The ideal timing of surgical intervention after transplantation has not been clearly established; however, as discussed previously, earlier fundoplication may have a greater effect on preserving pulmonary function.[97] Further support for early intervention comes from a recent report of 21 patients who underwent fundoplication for GERD at later time points (mean 768 days after transplant). No improvement in lung function was reported in this group, although the procedure may have slowed the rate of progression to higher grades of chronic rejection.[104]

The high frequency of esophageal dysmotility in patients with systemic sclerosis and GERD may limit the applicability of surgical fundoplication because of concern that narrowing of the lower esophagus could cause mechanical obstruction, especially for patients with esophageal aperistalsis. Although a loose or partial fundoplication has been advocated for these patients, strong evidence supporting this approach is lacking.[104–106] Gastroparesis may also complicate the choice of surgical procedure for reflux and increases the risk for poorly tolerated side effects such as abdominal pain and bloating associated with gastric distension and inability to belch (ie, gas bloat). For these patients, pyloroplasty is recommended, although it may be associated with other undesirable side effects such as diarrhea/dumping syndrome.

There are limited data specific to surgical intervention for GI disease in LTxp candidates or recipients with AID. Most series have few if any patients with underlying AID diagnoses. The most relevant study addressing gastroesophageal issues in patients with collagen vascular diseases was performed by the transplant program at the University of California in San Francisco. They retrospectively reviewed outcomes of 26 patients with a diagnosis of AID referred for LTxp (14 with scleroderma, 6 with dermatomyositis/polymyositis, and 6 with mixed connective tissue disease). Eleven of these patients ultimately underwent lung transplantation, and at a median follow-up of 26 months, only 1 patient had BOS. Six patients underwent fundoplication (1 before and 5 after transplant), and all were alive at follow-up. Three of the 5 fundoplication procedures were performed during the same hospitalization as the transplant and did not delay discharge.[107] Although the investigators concluded that lung transplantation could be safely performed in this population and that in experienced hands, fundoplication was a safe procedure in carefully selected patients, it is clear that more evidence is needed before LTxp selection criteria can be broadened to routinely include patients with severe gastroesophageal complications associated with AID. Future studies will be limited by their ability to accumulate adequate numbers of patients to allow for meaningful conclusions.

PUBLISHED EXPERIENCE OF LUNG TRANSPLANTATION FOR AID

Given the low numbers of transplants performed for any of the 5 major AID (systemic sclerosis, rheumatoid arthritis, SLE, dermatomyositis/polymyositis, mixed connective tissue disease), published accounts of LTxp for AID are mainly individual case reports or small series. The most reported experience has been lung transplantation for scleroderma. However, given the diversity of clinical complications for each AID, it would be unwise to directly apply the experience of LTxp for scleroderma to other AID. **Table 2** summarizes in chronologic order the published series of patients undergoing lung transplantation for scleroderma as well as the investigators' main findings. Several series add onto experience from previously published reports from their own centers or other institutions, illustrating the difficulty in accumulating a large enough cohort of patients to analyze. In total, these studies suggest that in carefully selected patients with scleroderma (usually without significant extrapulmonary manifestations), LTxp is feasible and is associated with comparable short-term survival rates and

complication rates when compared with other groups of patients undergoing LTxp. Many of these series do not clearly state which criteria were used to deny referral to a transplant center or consideration for active listing after evaluation.

SUMMARY

Although lung transplantation offers the possibility of improved survival and QOL for select patients with advanced lung disease, for many patients with systemic AID, the presence of significant extrapulmonary comorbidities limits the availability of this therapeutic option and increases the risk for complications when transplantation is performed. It is hoped that in the future, as new treatment options for AID and related comorbidites are developed, lung transplantation can be considered for greater numbers of patients or perhaps not be necessary at all.

REFERENCES

1. Christie JD, Edwards LB, Aurora P, et al. The registry of the International Society For Heart And Lung Transplantation: Twenty-sixth Official Adult Lung and Heart-Lung Transplantation Report-2009. J Heart Lung Transplant 2009;28(10):1031–49.
2. Hardy JD, Webb WR, Dalton ML Jr, et al. Lung homotransplantation in man. JAMA 1963;186: 1065–74.
3. Reitz BA, Wallwork JL, Hunt SA, et al. Heart-lung transplantation: successful therapy for patients with pulmonary vascular disease. N Engl J Med 1982;306(10):557–64.
4. Unilateral lung transplantation for pulmonary fibrosis. Toronto Lung Transplant Group. N Engl J Med 1986;314(18):1140–5.
5. Bhorade SM, Stern E. Immunosuppression for lung transplantation. Proc Am Thorac Soc 2009; 6(1):47–53.
6. Egan TM, Murray S, Bustami RT, et al. Development of the new lung allocation system in the United States. Am J Transplant 2006;6(5 Pt 2): 1212–27.
7. Lee JC, Christie JD. Primary graft dysfunction. Proc Am Thorac Soc 2009;6(1):39–46.
8. de Perrot M, Bonser RS, Dark J, et al. Report of the ISHLT Working Group on Primary Lung Graft Dysfunction part III: donor-related risk factors and markers. J Heart Lung Transplant 2005; 24(10):1460–7.
9. Barr ML, Kawut SM, Whelan TP, et al. Report of the ISHLT Working Group on Primary Lung Graft Dysfunction part IV: recipient-related risk factors and markers. J Heart Lung Transplant 2005; 24(10):1468–82.

10. Daud SA, Yusen RD, Meyers BF, et al. Impact of immediate primary lung allograft dysfunction on bronchiolitis obliterans syndrome. Am J Respir Crit Care Med 2007;175(5):507–13.

11. Christie JD, Kotloff RM, Ahya VN, et al. The effect of primary graft dysfunction on survival after lung transplantation. Am J Respir Crit Care Med 2005; 171(11):1312–6.

12. Hopkins PM, Aboyoun CL, Chhajed PN, et al. Prospective analysis of 1,235 transbronchial lung biopsies in lung transplant recipients. J Heart Lung Transplant 2002;21(10):1062–7.

13. Martinu T, Chen DF, Palmer SM. Acute rejection and humoral sensitization in lung transplant recipients. Proc Am Thorac Soc 2009;6(1):54–65.

14. Stewart S, Fishbein MC, Snell GI, et al. Revision of the 1996 working formulation for the standardization of nomenclature in the diagnosis of lung rejection. J Heart Lung Transplant 2007;26(12):1229–42.

15. Belperio JA, Weigt SS, Fishbein MC, et al. Chronic lung allograft rejection: mechanisms and therapy. Proc Am Thorac Soc 2009;6(1):108–21.

16. Estenne M, Maurer JR, Boehler A, et al. Bronchiolitis obliterans syndrome 2001: an update of the diagnostic criteria. J Heart Lung Transplant 2002; 21(3):297–310.

17. Kugler C, Fischer S, Gottlieb J, et al. Health-related quality of life in two hundred-eighty lung transplant recipients. J Heart Lung Transplant 2005;24(12):2262–8.

18. Burton CM, Carlsen J, Mortensen J, et al. Long-term survival after lung transplantation depends on development and severity of bronchiolitis obliterans syndrome. J Heart Lung Transplant 2007; 26(7):681–6.

19. Lama VN, Murray S, Mumford JA, et al. Prognostic value of bronchiolitis obliterans syndrome stage 0-p in single-lung transplant recipients. Am J Respir Crit Care Med 2005;172(3):379–83.

20. Jackson CH, Sharples LD, McNeil K, et al. Acute and chronic onset of bronchiolitis obliterans syndrome (BOS): are they different entities? J Heart Lung Transplant 2002;21(6):658–66.

21. Horvath EP, doPico GA, Barbee RA, et al. Nitrogen dioxide-induced pulmonary disease: five new cases and a review of the literature. J Occup Med 1978;20(2):103–10.

22. Kreiss K, Gomaa A, Kullman G, et al. Clinical bronchiolitis obliterans in workers at a microwave-popcorn plant. N Engl J Med 2002;347(5):330–8.

23. Lai RS, Chiang AA, Wu MT, et al. Outbreak of bronchiolitis obliterans associated with consumption of Sauropus androgynus in Taiwan. Lancet 1996; 348(9020):83–5.

24. Visscher DW, Myers JL. Bronchiolitis: the pathologist's perspective. Proc Am Thorac Soc 2006; 3(1):41–7.

25. Shilling RA, Wilkes DS. Immunobiology of chronic lung allograft dysfunction: new insights from the bench and beyond. Am J Transplant 2009;9(8): 1714–8.

26. Vanaudenaerde BM, Meyts I, Vos R, et al. A dichotomy in bronchiolitis obliterans syndrome after lung transplantation revealed by azithromycin therapy. Eur Respir J 2008;32(4):832–43.

27. Crosbie PA, Woodhead MA. Long-term macrolide therapy in chronic inflammatory airway diseases. Eur Respir J 2009;33(1):171–81.

28. Williams TJ, Verleden GM. Azithromycin: a plea for multicenter randomized studies in lung transplantation. Am J Respir Crit Care Med 2005;172(6): 657–9.

29. Iacono AT, Johnson BA, Grgurich WF, et al. A randomized trial of inhaled cyclosporine in lung-transplant recipients. N Engl J Med 2006; 354(2):141–50.

30. Barshes NR, DiBardino DJ, McKenzie ED, et al. Combined lung and liver transplantation: the United States experience. Transplantation 2005; 80(9):1161–7.

31. Levy RD, Guerraty AJ, Yacoub MH, et al. Prolonged survival after heart-lung transplantation in systemic lupus erythematosus. Chest 1993; 104(6):1903–5.

32. Orens JB, Estenne M, Arcasoy S, et al. International guidelines for the selection of lung transplant candidates: 2006 update–a consensus report from the Pulmonary Scientific Council of the International Society for Heart and Lung Transplantation. J Heart Lung Transplant 2006;25(7):745–55.

33. Choi JK, Kearns J, Palevsky HI, et al. Hyperacute rejection of a pulmonary allograft. Immediate clinical and pathologic findings. Am J Respir Crit Care Med 1999;160(3):1015–8.

34. Gammie JS, Pham SM, Colson YL, et al. Influence of panel-reactive antibody on survival and rejection after lung transplantation. J Heart Lung Transplant 1997;16(4):408–15.

35. Lau CL, Palmer SM, Posther KE, et al. Influence of panel-reactive antibodies on posttransplant outcomes in lung transplant recipients. Ann Thorac Surg 2000;69(5):1520–4.

36. Hadjiliadis D, Chaparro C, Reinsmoen NL, et al. Pre-transplant panel reactive antibody in lung transplant recipients is associated with significantly worse post-transplant survival in a multicenter study. J Heart Lung Transplant 2005;24(Suppl 7): S249–54.

37. Shah AS, Nwakanma L, Simpkins C, et al. Pretransplant panel reactive antibodies in human lung transplantation: an analysis of over 10,000 patients. Ann Thorac Surg 2008;85(6):1919–24.

38. Girnita AL, McCurry KR, Iacono AT, et al. HLA-specific antibodies are associated with high-grade

and persistent-recurrent lung allograft acute rejection. J Heart Lung Transplant 2004;23(10):1135–41.

39. Dragun D. Humoral responses directed against non-human leukocyte antigens in solid-organ transplantation. Transplantation 2008;86(8):1019–25.

40. Showkat A, Lo A, Shokouh-Amiri H, et al. Are auto-immune diseases or glomerulonephritis affecting the development of panel-reactive antibodies in candidates for renal transplantation? Transplant Proc 2005;37(2):645–7.

41. Sherer Y, Gorstein A, Fritzler MJ, et al. Autoantibody explosion in systemic lupus erythematosus: more than 100 different antibodies found in SLE patients. Semin Arthritis Rheum 2004;34(2):501–37.

42. Thervet E, Anglicheau D, Legendre C. Recent issues concerning renal transplantation in systemic lupus erythematosus patients. Nephrol Dial Transplant 2001;16(1):12–4.

43. Prakash UB. Respiratory complications in mixed connective tissue disease. Clin Chest Med 1998;19(4):733–46, ix.

44. Gilchrist JM. Overview of neuromuscular disorders affecting respiratory function. Semin Respir Crit Care Med 2002;23(3):191–200.

45. Gonzalez Castro A, Suberviola Canas B, Quesada Suescun A, et al. [Evaluation of the pre-operative exercise capacity as survival marker in the lung transplant recipients]. Med Intensiva 2008;32(2):65–70 [in Spanish].

46. Sager JS, Kotloff RM, Ahya VN, et al. Association of clinical risk factors with functional status following lung transplantation. Am J Transplant 2006;6(9):2191–201.

47. Kadikar A, Maurer J, Kesten S. The six-minute walk test: a guide to assessment for lung transplantation. J Heart Lung Transplant 1997;16(3):313–9.

48. Kawut SM, O'Shea MK, Bartels MN, et al. Exercise testing determines survival in patients with diffuse parenchymal lung disease evaluated for lung transplantation. Respir Med 2005;99(11):1431–9.

49. Lederer DJ, Arcasoy SM, Wilt JS, et al. Six-minute-walk distance predicts waiting list survival in idiopathic pulmonary fibrosis. Am J Respir Crit Care Med 2006;174(6):659–64.

50. Tuppin MP, Paratz JD, Chang AT, et al. Predictive utility of the 6-minute walk distance on survival in patients awaiting lung transplantation. J Heart Lung Transplant 2008;27(7):729–34.

51. Impens AJ, Wangkaew S, Seibold JR. The 6-minute walk test in scleroderma–how measuring everything measures nothing. Rheumatology (Oxford) 2008;47(Suppl 5):v68–9.

52. Benzo R, Kelley GA, Recchi L, et al. Complications of lung resection and exercise capacity: a meta-analysis. Respir Med 2007;101(8):1790–7.

53. Levine SM. A survey of clinical practice of lung transplantation in North America. Chest 2004;125(4):1224–38.

54. Gordon D, Inturrisi CE, Greensmith JE, et al. Perioperative pain management in the opioid-tolerant individual. J Pain 2008;9(5):383–7.

55. King-Biggs MB, Dunitz JM, Park SJ, et al. Airway anastomotic dehiscence associated with use of sirolimus immediately after lung transplantation. Transplantation 2003;75(9):1437–43.

56. McAnally KJ, Valentine VG, LaPlace SG, et al. Effect of pre-transplantation prednisone on survival after lung transplantation. J Heart Lung Transplant 2006;25(1):67–74.

57. Sheiner PA, Mor E, Chodoff L, et al. Acute renal failure associated with the use of ibuprofen in two liver transplant recipients on FK506. Transplantation 1994;57(7):1132–3.

58. Saravanan V, Kelly C. Drug-related pulmonary problems in patients with rheumatoid arthritis. Rheumatology (Oxford) 2006;45(7):787–9.

59. Sawada T, Inokuma S, Sato T, et al. Leflunomide-induced interstitial lung disease: prevalence and risk factors in Japanese patients with rheumatoid arthritis. Rheumatology (Oxford) 2009;48(9):1069–72.

60. Chikura B, Lane S, Dawson JK. Clinical expression of leflunomide-induced pneumonitis. Rheumatology (Oxford) 2009;48(9):1065–8.

61. Champion L, Stern M, Israel-Biet D, et al. Brief communication: sirolimus-associated pneumonitis: 24 cases in renal transplant recipients. Ann Intern Med 2006;144(7):505–9.

62. Taki H, Kawagishi Y, Shinoda K, et al. Interstitial pneumonitis associated with infliximab therapy without methotrexate treatment. Rheumatol Int 2009;30(2):275–6.

63. Yegen HA, Lederer DJ, Barr RG, et al. Risk factors for venous thromboembolism after lung transplantation. Chest 2007;132(2):547–53.

64. Izbicki G, Bairey O, Shitrit D, et al. Increased thromboembolic events after lung transplantation. Chest 2006;129(2):412–6.

65. Schulman LL, Anandarangam T, Leibowitz DW, et al. Four-year prospective study of pulmonary venous thrombosis after lung transplantation. J Am Soc Echocardiogr 2001;14(8):806–12.

66. Burgos PI, Alarcon GS. Thrombosis in systemic lupus erythematosus: risk and protection. Expert Rev Cardiovasc Ther 2009;7(12):1541–9.

67. Stone JH, Amend WJ, Criswell LA. Antiphospholipid antibody syndrome in renal transplantation: occurrence of clinical events in 96 consecutive patients with systemic lupus erythematosus. Am J Kidney Dis 1999;34(6):1040–7.

68. Wagenknecht DR, Becker DG, LeFor WM, et al. Antiphospholipid antibodies are a risk factor for

early renal allograft failure. Transplantation 1999; 68(2):241–6.

69. Ducloux D, Pellet E, Fournier V, et al. Prevalence and clinical significance of antiphospholipid antibodies in renal transplant recipients. Transplantation 1999;67(1):90–3.

70. Morrissey PE, Ramirez PJ, Gohh RY, et al. Management of thrombophilia in renal transplant patients. Am J Transplant 2002;2(9):872–6.

71. Magro CM, Pope-Harman A, Moh P, et al. Primary anti-phospholipid antibody syndrome caused by isolated anti-phosphatidylethanolamine antibodies presenting as cryptogenic fibrosing alveolitis with recurrent pulmonary hemorrhage after single-lung transplantation. J Heart Lung Transplant 2002; 21(11):1232–6.

72. Covarrubias M, Ware LB, Kawut SM, et al. Plasma intercellular adhesion molecule-1 and von Willebrand factor in primary graft dysfunction after lung transplantation. Am J Transplant 2007;7(11): 2573–8.

73. Lee JCKC, Hadjiliadis D, Aahya VN, et al. Risk factors for early vs late primary graft dysfunction. Am J Respir Crit Care Med 2008;177:A396 [abstract].

74. Webert KE, Blajchman MA. Transfusion-related acute lung injury. Transfus Med Rev 2003;17(4): 252–62.

75. Christie JD, Kotloff RM, Pochettino A, et al. Clinical risk factors for primary graft failure following lung transplantation. Chest 2003;124(4):1232–41.

76. King RC, Binns OA, Rodriguez F, et al. Reperfusion injury significantly impacts clinical outcome after pulmonary transplantation. Ann Thorac Surg 2000;69(6):1681–5.

77. Thabut G, Vinatier I, Stern JB, et al. Primary graft failure following lung transplantation: predictive factors of mortality. Chest 2002; 121(6):1876–82.

78. Lee JC, Kuntz C, Kawut SM, et al. Clinical risk factors for the development of primary graft dysfunction. J Heart Lung Transplant 2008;27(2 Suppl 1):S67–8.

79. Kawut SM, Okun J, Shimbo D, et al. Soluble p-selectin and the risk of primary graft dysfunction after lung transplantation. Chest 2009;136(1):237–44.

80. Forbes A, Marie I. Gastrointestinal complications: the most frequent internal complications of systemic sclerosis. Rheumatology (Oxford) 2009; 48(Suppl 3):iii36–9.

81. Savarino E, Bazzica M, Zentilin P, et al. Gastroesophageal reflux and pulmonary fibrosis in scleroderma: a study using pH-impedance monitoring. Am J Respir Crit Care Med 2009;179(5):408–13.

82. Napierkowski J, Wong RK. Extraesophageal manifestations of GERD. Am J Med Sci 2003;326(5): 285–99.

83. Sweet MP, Patti MG, Hoopes C, et al. Gastro-oesophageal reflux and aspiration in patients with advanced lung disease. Thorax 2009;64(2): 167–73.

84. Parsons JP, Mastronarde JG. Gastroesophageal reflux disease and asthma. Curr Opin Pulm Med 2010;16(1):60–3.

85. Troshinsky MB, Kane GC, Varga J, et al. Pulmonary function and gastroesophageal reflux in systemic sclerosis. Ann Intern Med 1994;121(1):6–10.

86. D'Ovidio F, Singer LG, Hadjiliadis D, et al. Prevalence of gastroesophageal reflux in end-stage lung disease candidates for lung transplant. Ann Thorac Surg 2005;80(4):1254–60.

87. Akindipe OA, Faul JL, Vierra MA, et al. The surgical management of severe gastroparesis in heart/lung transplant recipients. Chest 2000;117(3):907–10.

88. Young LR, Hadjiliadis D, Davis RD, et al. Lung transplantation exacerbates gastroesophageal reflux disease. Chest 2003;124(5):1689–93.

89. D'Ovidio F, Mura M, Ridsdale R, et al. The effect of reflux and bile acid aspiration on the lung allograft and its surfactant and innate immunity molecules SP-A and SP-D. Am J Transplant 2006;6(8):1930–8.

90. Cossio M, Menon Y, Wilson W, et al. Life-threatening complications of systemic sclerosis. Crit Care Clin 2002;18(4):819–39.

91. Palmer SM, Miralles AP, Howell DN, et al. Gastroesophageal reflux as a reversible cause of allograft dysfunction after lung transplantation. Chest 2000; 118(4):1214–7.

92. Hadjiliadis D, Duane Davis R, Steele MP, et al. Gastroesophageal reflux disease in lung transplant recipients. Clin Transplant 2003;17(4):363–8.

93. D'Ovidio F, Mura M, Tsang M, et al. Bile acid aspiration and the development of bronchiolitis obliterans after lung transplantation. J Thorac Cardiovasc Surg 2005;129(5):1144–52.

94. Blondeau K, Mertens V, Vanaudenaerde BA, et al. Gastro-oesophageal reflux and gastric aspiration in lung transplant patients with or without chronic rejection. Eur Respir J 2008;31(4):707–13.

95. D'Ovidio F, Keshavjee S. Gastroesophageal reflux and lung transplantation. Dis Esophagus 2006; 19(5):315–20.

96. Davis RD Jr, Lau CL, Eubanks S, et al. Improved lung allograft function after fundoplication in patients with gastroesophageal reflux disease undergoing lung transplantation. J Thorac Cardiovasc Surg 2003;125(3):533–42.

97. Cantu E 3rd, Appel JZ 3rd, Hartwig MG, et al. J. Maxwell Chamberlain Memorial Paper. Early fundoplication prevents chronic allograft dysfunction in patients with gastroesophageal reflux disease. Ann Thorac Surg 2004;78(4):1142–51 [discussion: 1142–51].

98. Robertson AG, Shenfine J, Ward C, et al. A call for standardization of antireflux surgery in the lung transplantation population. Transplantation 2009; 87(8):1112–4.

99. Robertson AG, Griffin SM, Murphy DM, et al. Targeting allograft injury and inflammation in the management of post-lung transplant bronchiolitis obliterans syndrome. Am J Transplant 2009;9(6): 1272–8.

100. Linden PA, Gilbert RJ, Yeap BY, et al. Laparoscopic fundoplication in patients with end-stage lung disease awaiting transplantation. J Thorac Cardiovasc Surg 2006;131(2):438–46.

101. Dallemagne B, Weerts J, Markiewicz S, et al. Clinical results of laparoscopic fundoplication at ten years after surgery. Surg Endosc 2006;20(1):159–65.

102. Kelly JJ, Watson DI, Chin KF, et al. Laparoscopic Nissen fundoplication: clinical outcomes at 10 years. J Am Coll Surg 2007;205(4):570–5.

103. Eckardt AJ, Pinnow G, Pohl H, et al. Antireflux 'barriers': problems with patient recruitment for a new endoscopic antireflux procedure. Eur J Gastroenterol Hepatol 2009;21(10):1110–8.

104. Burton PR, Button B, Brown W, et al. Medium-term outcome of fundoplication after lung transplantation. Dis Esophagus 2009;22(8):642–8.

105. Gasper WJ, Sweet MP, Hoopes C, et al. Antireflux surgery for patients with end-stage lung disease before and after lung transplantation. Surg Endosc 2008;22(2):495–500.

106. Limpert PA, Naunheim KS. Partial versus complete fundoplication: is there a correct answer? Surg Clin North Am 2005;85(3):399–410.

107. Gasper WJ, Sweet MP, Golden JA, et al. Lung transplantation in patients with connective tissue disorders and esophageal dysmotility. Dis Esophagus 2008;21(7):650–5.

108. Christie JD, Sager JS, Kimmel SE, et al. Impact of primary graft failure on outcomes following lung transplantation. Chest 2005;127(1):161–5.

109. Hafkin J, Blumberg E. Infections in lung transplantation: new insights. Curr Opin Organ Transplant 2009;14(5):483–7.

110. Barton TD, Blumberg EA. Viral pneumonias other than cytomegalovirus in transplant recipients. Clin Chest Med 2005;26(4):707–20, viii.

111. Remund KF, Best M, Egan JJ. Infections relevant to lung transplantation. Proc Am Thorac Soc 2009; 6(1):94–100.

112. Penn I. Post-transplant malignancy: the role of immunosuppression. Drug Saf 2000;23(2):101–13.

113. Loren AW, Tsai DE. Post-transplant lymphoproliferative disorder. Clin Chest Med 2005;26(4): 631–45, vii.

114. Lyu DM, Zamora MR. Medical complications of lung transplantation. Proc Am Thorac Soc 2009; 6(1):101–7.

115. Roithmaier S, Haydon AM, Loi S, et al. Incidence of malignancies in heart and/or lung transplant recipients: a single-institution experience. J Heart Lung Transplant 2007;26(8):845–9.

116. Levine SM, Anzueto A, Peters JI, et al. Single lung transplantation in patients with systemic disease. Chest 1994;105(3):837–41.

117. Pigula FA, Griffith BP, Zenati MA, et al. Lung transplantation for respiratory failure resulting from systemic disease. Ann Thorac Surg 1997;64(6): 1630–4.

118. Rosas V, Conte JV, Yang SC, et al. Lung transplantation and systemic sclerosis. Ann Transplant 2000; 5(3):38–43.

119. Kubo M, Vensak J, Dauber J, et al. Lung transplantation in patients with scleroderma. J Heart Lung Transplant 2001;20(2):174–5.

120. Massad MG, Powell CR, Kpodonu J, et al. Outcomes of lung transplantation in patients with scleroderma. World J Surg 2005;29(11):1510–5.

121. Schachna L, Medsger TA Jr, Dauber JH, et al. Lung transplantation in scleroderma compared with idiopathic pulmonary fibrosis and idiopathic pulmonary arterial hypertension. Arthritis Rheum 2006; 54(12):3954–61.

122. Shitrit D, Amital A, Peled N, et al. Lung transplantation in patients with scleroderma: case series, review of the literature, and criteria for transplantation. Clin Transplant 2009;23(2):178–83.

INDEX

Note: Page numbers of article titles are in **boldface** type.

A

Abatacept, lung disease related to, 465
Acute lupus pneumonitis, SLE and, 481
Acute pulmonary embolism, APS and, 537–538
Acute respiratory distress syndrome (ARDS)
    APS and, 541–542
    SLE and, 482–483
Acute reversible hypoxemia, SLE and, 484
Adalimumab, in systemic autoimmune diseases, 570
Airway disease
    RA and, 460–462
    SLE and, 484
Airway obstruction, RA and, 461
Alveolar hemorrhage, mixed connective tissue
    disease and, 445
Alveolar hemorrhage syndromes, APS and, 542
Alveolitis, fibrosing, APS and, 542
Amyloidosis
    RA and, 469
    Sjögren syndrome and, 495–496
ANCAs. See *Antineutrophil cytoplasmic antibodies*
    (ANCAs).
Ankylosing spondylitis
    clinical course of, 550
    clinical features of, 547–548
    demographic features of, 547
    described, 547
    pathologic features of, 551–552
    pathophysiology of, 547
    prevalence of, 547
    pulmonary manifestations of, **547–554**
        apical fibrobullous disease, 548–549
        chest wall restriction, 548
        evaluation of, 550–552
        obstructive sleep apnea, 549–550
        spontaneous pneumothorax, 549
        superinfection, 549
    treatment of, 552
Antibody(ies)
    anti-HLA, lung transplantation in autoimmune
        diseases and, 593
    antiphospholipid, in SLE, 417
Anti-HLA antibodies, lung transplantation in
    autoimmune diseases and, 593
Anti-inflammatory drugs, lung disease related to, 465
Antimetabolite(s), lung disease related to, 465
Antimetabolite/cytotoxic agents, in systemic
    autoimmune diseases, 571–576

Antineutrophil cytoplasmic antibodies
    (ANCAs)—related vasculitides, autoantibody
    testing for, 420–421
Antiphospholipid antibodies (APAs), in SLE, 417
Antiphospholipid syndrome (APS)
    catastrophic, pulmonary manifestations of, 541
    described, 537
    pulmonary manifestations of, **537–545**
        acute pulmonary embolism, 537–538
        alveolar hemorrhage syndromes, 542
        ARDS, 541–542
        chronic pulmonary thromboembolic disease,
            538–539
        fibrosing alveolitis, 542
        PAH, 539–541
        postpartum syndrome, 543
        pulmonary capillaritis, 542
        pulmonary venous hypertension, 539–541
Antitumor necrosis factor agents, in systemic
    autoimmune diseases, 568–570
APAs. See *Antiphospholipid antibodies (APAs)*.
Apical fibrobullous disease, ankylosing spondylitis
    and, 548–549
APS. See *Antiphospholipid syndrome (APS)*.
ARDS. See *Acute respiratory distress syndrome
    (ARDS)*.
Arteritis
    giant cell, 525
    Takayasu, 525
Arthritis, rheumatoid. See *Rheumatoid arthritis (RA)*.
Aspiration pneumonia
    dyspnea and, 504
    in systemic sclerosis, 444
Autoantibody testing
    for ANCAs-related vasculitides, 420–421
    for autoimmune diseases, **415–422**
    for dermatomyositis, 418
    for Goodpasture syndrome, 421–422
    for mixed connective tissue disease, 419
    for polymyositis, 418
    for RA, 418–419
    for Sjögren syndrome, 419
    for SLE, 415–417
    for systemic sclerosis, 418
Autoimmune diseases
    autoantibody testing for, **415–422**. See also
        specific diseases and *Autoantibody testing*.
    lung transplantation in, **589–603**. See also *Lung
        transplantation, in autoimmune diseases*.

doi:10.1016/S0272-5231(10)00096-1

chestmed.theclinics.com

Moving?

Make sure your subscription moves with you!

To notify us of your new address, find your **Clinics Account Number** (located on your mailing label above your name), and contact customer service at:

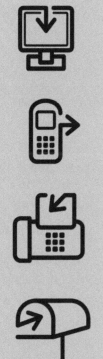

Email: journalscustomerservice-usa@elsevier.com

800-654-2452 (subscribers in the U.S. & Canada)
314-447-8871 (subscribers outside of the U.S. & Canada)

Fax number: 314-447-8029

Elsevier Health Sciences Division
Subscription Customer Service
3251 Riverport Lane
Maryland Heights, MO 63043

Printed and bound by CPI Group (UK) Ltd, Croydon, CR0 4YY

03/10/2024

01040358-0017